S0-BTR-914

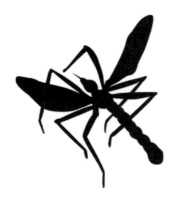

GLOBAL PANDEMICS AND EPIDEMICS AND HOW THEY RELATE TO YOU

First Edition

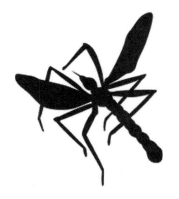

GLOBAL PANDEMICS AND EPIDEMICS AND HOW THEY RELATE TO YOU

First Edition

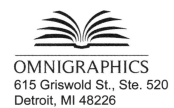

OMNIGRAPHICS
615 Griswold St., Ste. 520
Detroit, MI 48226

Bibliographic Note
Because this page cannot legibly accommodate all the copyright notices, the Bibliographic Note
portion of the Preface constitutes an extension of the copyright notice.

∗ ∗ ∗

OMNIGRAPHICS
Angela L. Williams, *Managing Editor*

∗ ∗ ∗

Copyright © 2020 Omnigraphics
ISBN 978-0-7808-1816-3
E-ISBN 978-0-7808-1817-0

Library of Congress Cataloging-in-Publication Data

Names: Williams, Angela, 1963- editor.

Title: Global pandemics and epidemics and how they relate to you / edited by Angela L. Williams.

Description: First edition. | Detroit, MI: Omnigraphics, [2020] | Series: Health reference series: special edition | Summary: "Offers basic consumer health information about epidemics, pandemics, and notable pseudopandemics over the years and across the world, disease management, including monitoring and planning, and action plan during outbreaks and for future incidents. Along with statistical data, a glossary, and directory of organizations"-- Provided by publisher.

Identifiers: LCCN 2019051760 (print) | LCCN 2019051761 (ebook) | ISBN 9780780818163 (library binding) | ISBN 9780780818170 (ebook)

Subjects: LCSH: Epidemics--United States. | Epidemiology--United States.

Classification: LCC RA650.5.G56 2020 (print) | LCC RA650.5 (ebook) | DDC 614.4/973--dc23

LC record available at https://lccn.loc.gov/2019051760
LC ebook record available at https://lccn.loc.gov/2019051761

Electronic or mechanical reproduction, including photography, recording, or any other information storage and retrieval system for the purpose of resale is strictly prohibited without permission in writing from the publisher.

The information in this publication was compiled from the sources cited and from other sources considered reliable. While every possible effort has been made to ensure reliability, the publisher will not assume liability for damages caused by inaccuracies in the data, and makes no warranty, express or implied, on the accuracy of the information contained herein.

This book is printed on acid-free paper meeting the ANSI Z39.48 Standard. The infinity symbol that appears above indicates that the paper in this book meets that standard.

Printed in the United States

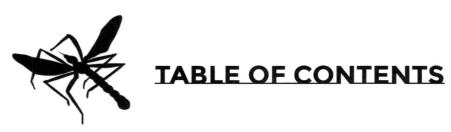

TABLE OF CONTENTS

Part 3: Principles of Disease Management

VII

Part 4: The Next Pandemic: Are We Ready?

Part 5: Additional Help and Information

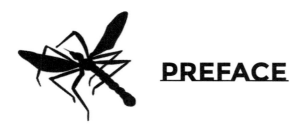 **PREFACE**

About This Book

When an infectious disease spreads rapidly to many people, it is known as an "epidemic." The year 2014 marked the beginning of the West Africa Ebola epidemic, the largest in history when the World Health Organization (WHO) reported Ebola virus disease (EVD) cases in southeastern Guinea. If a disease outbreak occurs globally, it becomes a "pandemic," which often is caused by a new virus that has not been in circulation among people for a long time and that spreads quickly from person to person. People have little to no immunity against it and it causes death in larger numbers.

Global Pandemics and Epidemics and How They Relate to You, First Edition provides information about outbreaks, epidemics, and pandemics and their related threats. It discusses the major epidemics, pandemics, and notable pseudopandemics that have threatened humankind over the years. It provides information about disease management, including various methods of detection, prevention, and treatment of several diseases. Steps taken by humankind to stay protected from any future outbreaks are provided, along with a glossary of related terms and directories of organizations.

How to Use This Book

This book is divided into parts and chapters. Parts focus on broad areas of interest. Chapters are devoted to single topics within a part.

Part 1: Understanding Pandemics and Epidemics presents information about pandemics and epidemics, their history, and their occurrence in the United States and across the world. It also provides information about outbreaks, pandemic threats, and other major issues caused by bioterrorism.

Part 2: Major Pandemics and Epidemics provides information about several of the deadliest outbreaks, including HIV/AIDS, chikungunya, cholera, Ebola, influenza, malaria, meningitis, Nipah virus infection, severe acute respiratory syndrome (SARS)—related to the emerging 2020 coronavirus outbreak in China—smallpox, tuberculosis, yellow fever, and Zika.

Part 3: Principles of Disease Management talks about the steps to be taken to prevent the spread of epidemics. It provides insight into antimicrobial resistance and hospital-based infections. Disease detection, surveillance, and treatment are also discussed in detail.

Part 4: The Next Pandemic: Are We Ready? explains how to get ahead of the next pandemic. It provides information about strategies followed at national and global levels to counter the outbreak of new pandemics and epidemics. It also talks about the 2009 H1N1 pandemic and explains how medical science has made great strides in the fields of disease surveillance, prevention, and treatment since then.

Part 5: Additional Help and Information includes a glossary of terms associated with outbreaks, epidemics, and pandemics, and a directory of organizations.

Bibliographic Note

This volume contains documents and excerpts from publications issued by the following U.S. government agencies: Centers for Disease Control and Prevention (CDC); Fogarty International Center (FIC); National Institute of Neurological Disorders and Stroke (NINDS); National Institutes of Health (NIH); Office of Disease Prevention and Health Promotion (ODPHP); U.S. Department of Agriculture (USDA); U.S. Department of Health and Human Services (HHS); U.S. Department of Homeland Security (DHS); and U.S. Food and Drug Administration (FDA).

It may also contain original material produced by Omnigraphics and reviewed by medical consultants.

The photograph on the front cover is © Dragon Images/Shutterstock.

About the *Health Reference Series*

The *Health Reference Series* is designed to provide basic medical information for patients, families, caregivers, and the general public. Each volume concentrates on a particular topic and provides comprehensive coverage. This is especially important for people who may be dealing with a newly diagnosed disease or a chronic disorder in themselves or a family member. People looking for preventive guidance, information about disease warning signs, medical statistics, and risk factors for health problems will also find answers to their questions in the *Health Reference Series*. The *Series*, however, is not intended to serve as a tool for diagnosing illness, in prescribing treatments, or as a substitute for the physician–patient relationship. All people concerned about medical symptoms or the possibility of disease are encouraged to seek professional care from an appropriate healthcare provider.

A Note about Spelling and Style

Health Reference Series editors use *Stedman's Medical Dictionary* as an authority for questions related to the spelling of medical terms and *The Chicago Manual of Style* for questions related to grammatical structures, punctuation, and other editorial concerns. Consistent adherence is not always possible, however, because the individual volumes within the *Series* include many documents from a wide variety of different producers, and the editor's primary goal is to present material from each source as accurately as is possible. This sometimes means that information in different chapters or sections may follow other guidelines and alternate spelling authorities. For example, occasionally a copyright holder may require that eponymous terms be shown in possessive forms (Crohn's disease vs. Crohn disease) or that British spelling norms be retained (leukaemia vs. leukemia).

Medical Review

Omnigraphics contracts with a team of qualified, senior medical professionals who serve as medical consultants for the *Health Reference*

Series. As necessary, medical consultants review reprinted and originally written material for currency and accuracy. Citations including the phrase "Reviewed (month, year)" indicate material reviewed by this team. Medical consultation services are provided to the *Health Reference Series* editors by:

Dr. Vijayalakshmi, MBBS, DGO, MD

Dr. Senthil Selvan, MBBS, DCH, MD

Dr. K. Sivanandham, MBBS, DCH, MS (Research), PhD

Our Advisory Board

We would like to thank the following board members for providing initial guidance on the development of this series:

- Dr. Lynda Baker, Associate Professor of Library and Information Science, Wayne State University, Detroit, MI
- Nancy Bulgarelli, William Beaumont Hospital Library, Royal Oak, MI
- Karen Imarisio, Bloomfield Township Public Library, Bloomfield Township, MI
- Karen Morgan, Mardigian Library, University of Michigan-Dearborn, Dearborn, MI
- Rosemary Orlando, St. Clair Shores Public Library, St. Clair Shores, MI

Health Reference Series Update Policy

The inaugural book in the *Health Reference Series* was the first edition of *Cancer Sourcebook* published in 1989. Since then, the *Series* has been enthusiastically received by librarians and in the medical community. In order to maintain the standard of providing high-quality health information for the layperson the editorial staff at Omnigraphics felt it was necessary to implement a policy of updating volumes when warranted.

Medical researchers have been making tremendous strides, and it is the purpose of the *Health Reference Series* to stay current with the most recent advances. Each decision to update a volume is made on an individual basis. Some of the considerations include how much new information is available and the feedback we receive from people who use the books. If there is a topic you would like to see added to the update list, or an area of medical concern you feel has not been adequately addressed, please write to:

Managing Editor
Health Reference Series
Omnigraphics
615 Griswold St., Ste. 520
Detroit, MI 48226

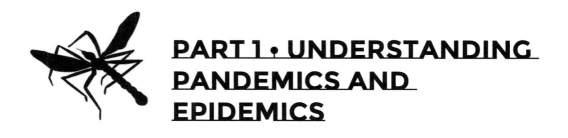

PART 1 • UNDERSTANDING PANDEMICS AND EPIDEMICS

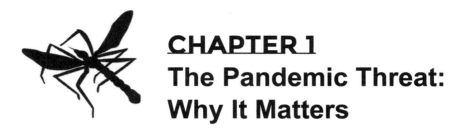

CHAPTER 1
The Pandemic Threat: Why It Matters

While one cannot predict exactly when or where the next epidemic or pandemic will begin, everyone knows that one is coming. Global health security is how outbreaks can be stopped from becoming widespread pandemics that threaten us all.

Global-health threats include:

- Infectious disease outbreaks such as influenza or Ebola viruses
- Chronic illnesses, such as heart disease, cancer, or diabetes
- Environmental disasters, such as hurricanes, mudslides, or earthquakes
- Humanitarian emergencies such as war or famine
- Biological or chemical terrorism

National Security at Risk

Outbreaks take hold in the world's most vulnerable areas—countries with few resources to stem the tide of infection before it reaches our shores. When a pathogen can travel from a remote village to major cities on all continents in 36 hours, the threat to the country's national security is greater than ever.

This chapter includes text excerpted from "Why It Matters: The Pandemic Threat," Centers for Disease Control and Prevention (CDC), April 30, 2019.

Why Is It Risky for Everyone When Local Outbreaks Turn into Global Pandemics?

Many challenges exist worldwide that increase the risk that outbreaks will occur and spread rapidly, including:

- Increased risk of infectious pathogens "spilling over" from animals to humans
- Development of antimicrobial resistance
- Spread of infectious diseases through global travel and trade
- Acts of bioterrorism
- Weak public-health infrastructures

How Global Outbreaks Impact the Country's Economy

A global infectious disease outbreak can have a catastrophic impact on the U.S. economy—even if the disease never reaches the United States.

Jobs

In 2015, the United States exported over $300 billion in material goods and services to 49 health-security priority countries. These exports supported over 1.6 million jobs across America in sectors such as agriculture, manufacturing, and natural resource extraction.

Travel and Trade

Fear of contagion can impact travel, tourism, and imports, especially if cases occur in the United States, as they did with the 2014–2016 West Africa Ebola outbreak.

Cost

Estimates show that pandemics are likely to cost over $6 trillion in the next century, with an annualized expected loss of more than $60 billion for potential pandemics. However, investing $4.5 billion per year in building global capacities could avert these catastrophic costs.

How Potential Pandemics Can Be Stopped from Spreading

The global-health security work focuses on building public-health systems that work hand-in-hand to help countries detect and contain public-health threats:

- **Surveillance** systems to rapidly detect and report cases
- **Laboratory** networks to accurately identify the cause of illness
- **A trained workforce** to identify, track, and contain outbreaks
- **Emergency management systems** to coordinate an effective response

Did You Know?

In 2017, stronger public-health systems meant faster, smarter responses to contain potential pandemics and threats of international importance in partner countries of the United States:

- **January 2017:** Uganda's emergency operations center (EOC) responds to the first cases of highly pathogenic avian influenza in the country.
- **February 2017:** Guinea's EOC coordinates rapid response to a measles outbreak.
- **March 2017:** Cameroon's EOC responds in a record time of under 24 hours to contain a meningitis outbreak.
- **April 2017:** Liberia's new EOC and Field Epidemiology Training Program (FETP) respond to a deadly meningococcal disease outbreak.
- **May 2017:** Democratic Republic of Congo's FETP-trained disease detectives help rapidly contain Ebola.
- **June 2017:** Nigeria's EOC helps contain a widespread meningitis outbreak.
- **July 2017:** Guatemala's hospital surveillance systems identify two outbreaks of Dengue.
- **August 2017:** Kenya's new mobile surveillance system detects an anthrax outbreak.
- **September 2017:** Georgia's FETP-trained disease detectives help contain a measles outbreak.

- **October 2017:** Kenya's Indigenous Movement for Peace Advancement and Conflict Transformation (IMPACT) fellows respond to an outbreak of cholera.
- **November 2017:** Uganda's EOC coordinates rapid response to a deadly Marburg virus outbreak.
- **December 2017:** Bangladesh's FETP-trained disease detectives respond to a diphtheria outbreak.

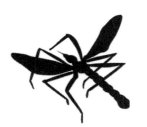

CHAPTER 2
Outbreaks, Epidemics, and Pandemics

Level of Disease

The amount of a particular disease that is usually present in a community is referred to as the "baseline" or "endemic" level of the disease. This level is not necessarily the desired level, which may, in fact, be zero, but rather is the observed level. In the absence of intervention and assuming that the level is not high enough to deplete the pool of susceptible persons, the disease may continue to occur at this level indefinitely. Thus, the baseline level is often regarded as the expected level of the disease.

While some diseases are so rare in a given population that a single case warrants an epidemiologic investigation (e.g., rabies, plague, polio), other diseases occur more commonly so that only deviations from the norm warrant investigation. "Sporadic" refers to a disease that occurs infrequently and irregularly. "Endemic" refers to the constant presence and/or usual prevalence of a disease or infectious agent in a population within a geographic area. "Hyperendemic" refers to persistent, high levels of disease occurrence.

Occasionally, the amount of disease in a community rises above the expected level. "Epidemic" refers to an increase, often sudden, in the number of cases of a disease above what is normally expected in

This chapter includes text excerpted from "Principles of Epidemiology in Public Health Practice," Centers for Disease Control and Prevention (CDC), May 18, 2012. Reviewed January 2020.

that population in that area. Outbreak carries the same definition of the epidemic but is often used for a more limited geographic area. A "cluster" refers to an aggregation of cases grouped in place and time that are suspected to be greater than the number expected, even though the expected number may not be known. "Pandemic" refers to an epidemic that has spread over several countries or continents, usually affecting a large number of people.

Epidemics occur when an agent and susceptible hosts are present in adequate numbers, and the agent can be effectively conveyed from a source to the susceptible hosts. More specifically, an epidemic may result from:

- A recent increase in amount or virulence of the agent
- The recent introduction of the agent into a setting where it has not been before
- An enhanced mode of transmission so that more susceptible persons are exposed
- A change in the susceptibility of the host response to the agent
- Factors that increase host exposure or involve introduction through new portals of entry

Epidemic Patterns

Epidemics can be classified according to their manner of spread through a population:

- Common-source
  - Point
  - Continuous
  - Intermittent
- Propagated
- Mixed
- Other

A common-source outbreak is one in which a group of persons is all exposed to an infectious agent or a toxin from the same source.

If the group is exposed over a relatively brief period, so that everyone who becomes ill does so within one incubation period, then the common-source outbreak is further classified as a point-source outbreak.

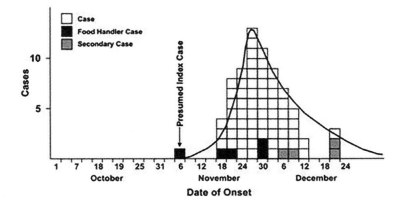

Figure 2.1. Hepatitis A Cases by Date of Onset, November to December 1978

The epidemic of leukemia cases in Hiroshima following the atomic bomb blast and the epidemic of hepatitis A among patrons of the Pennsylvania restaurant who ate green onions each had a point source of exposure. If the number of cases during an epidemic were plotted over time, the resulting graph, called an "epidemic curve," would typically have a steep upslope and a more gradual downslope (a so-called log-normal distribution).

In some common-source outbreaks, case-patients may have been exposed over a period of days, weeks, or longer. In a continuous common-source outbreak, the range of exposures and range of incubation periods tend to flatten and widen the peaks of the epidemic curve (Figure 2.2). The epidemic curve of an intermittent common-source outbreak often has a pattern reflecting the intermittent nature of the exposure.

A propagated outbreak results from transmission from one person to another. Usually, the transmission is by direct person-to-person contact, as with syphilis. Transmission may also be vehicle-borne (e.g., the transmission of hepatitis B or human immunodeficiency virus (HIV) by sharing needles) or vector-borne (e.g., the transmission of yellow fever by mosquitoes). In propagated outbreaks, cases occur over more than one incubation period. In Figure 2.3, note the peaks occurring about 11 days apart, consistent with the incubation period for measles. The epidemic usually wanes after a few generations, either because the number of susceptible persons falls below

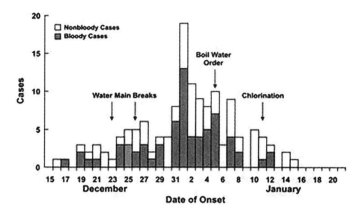

Figure 2.2. Diarrheal Illness in City Residents by Date of Onset and Character of Stool, December 1989 to January 1990

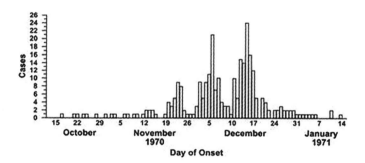

Figure 2.3. Measles Cases by Date of Onset, October 15, 1970 to January 16, 1971

some critical level required to sustain transmission, or because intervention measures become effective.

Some epidemics have features of both common-source epidemics and propagated epidemics. The pattern of a common-source outbreak followed by secondary person-to-person spread is not uncommon. These are called "mixed epidemics." For example, a common-source epidemic of shigellosis occurred among a group of 3,000 women attending a national music festival (Figure 2.4). Many developed symptoms after returning home. Over the next few weeks, several state health departments detected subsequent

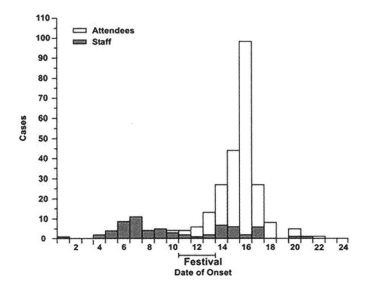

Figure 2.4. Shigella Cases at a Music Festival by Day of Onset, August 1988

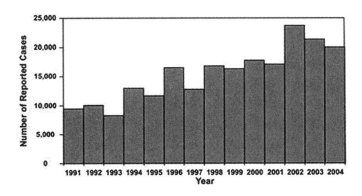

Figure 2.5. The number of Reported Cases of Lyme Disease by Year—the United States, 1992–2003

generations of Shigella cases propagated by person-to-person transmission from festival attendees.

Finally, some epidemics are neither common-source in its usual sense nor propagated from person to person. Outbreaks of the zoonotic (animal to human) or vector-borne (arthropods such as mosquitoes, ticks, and fleas,

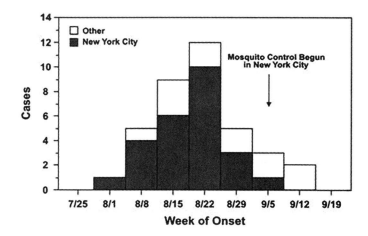

Figure 2.6. Number of Reported Cases of West Nile Encephalitis—New York City, 1999

to humans) disease may result from a sufficient prevalence of infection in host species, sufficient presence of vectors, and sufficient human-vector interaction. Examples (Figures 1.5 and 1.6) include the epidemic of Lyme disease that emerged in the northeastern United States in the late 1980s (spread from deer to humans by deer ticks) and the outbreak of West Nile encephalitis in the Queens section of New York City in 1999 (spread from birds to humans by mosquitoes).

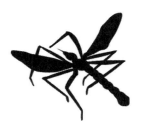

CHAPTER 3
Concepts of Occurrence, Progression, and Spectrum of Disease

Concepts of Disease Occurrence

A critical premise of epidemiology is that disease and other health events do not occur randomly in a population, but are more likely to occur in some members of the population than others because of risk factors that may not be distributed randomly in the population. One important use of epidemiology is to identify the factors that place some members at greater risk than others.

Causation

A number of models of disease causation have been proposed. Among the simplest of these is the epidemiologic triad or triangle, the traditional model for infectious disease. The triad consists of an external agent, a susceptible host, and an environment that brings the host and agent together. In this model, the disease results from the interaction between the agent and the susceptible host in an environment that supports the transmission of the agent from a source to that host.

Agent, host, and environmental factors interrelate in a variety of complex ways to produce disease. Different diseases require different balances and interactions of these three components. The development of appropriate,

This chapter includes text excerpted from "Principles of Epidemiology in Public Health Practice," Centers for Disease Control and Prevention (CDC), May 18, 2012. Reviewed January 2020.

practical, and effective public-health measures to control or prevent disease usually requires an assessment of all three components and their interactions.

Agent originally referred to an infectious microorganism or pathogen: a virus, bacterium, parasite, or other microbes. Generally, the agent must be present for the disease to occur; however, the presence of that agent alone is not always sufficient to cause disease. A variety of factors influence whether exposure to an organism will result in disease, including the organism's pathogenicity (ability to cause disease) and dose.

Over time, the concept of agent has been broadened to include chemical and physical causes of disease or injury. These include chemical contaminants (such as the L-tryptophan contaminant responsible for eosinophilia-myalgia syndrome (EMS)), as well as physical forces (such as repetitive mechanical forces associated with carpal tunnel syndrome (CTS)). While the epidemiologic triad serves as a useful model for many diseases, it has proven inadequate for cardiovascular disease (CVD), cancer, and other diseases that appear to have multiple contributing causes without a single necessary one.

"Host" refers to the human who can get the disease. A variety of factors intrinsic to the host, sometimes called "risk factors," can influence an individual's exposure, susceptibility, or response to a causative agent. Opportunities for exposure are often influenced by behaviors, such as sexual practices, hygiene, and other personal choices as well as by age and sex. Susceptibility and response to an agent are influenced by factors, such as genetic composition, nutritional and immunologic status, anatomic structure, presence of disease, or medications, and psychological makeup.

"Environment" refers to extrinsic factors that affect the agent and the opportunity for exposure. Environmental factors include physical factors, such as geology and climate, biological factors such as insects that transmit the agent, and socioeconomic factors such as crowding, sanitation, and the availability of health services.

Component Causes and Causal Pies

Because the agent-host-environment model did not work well for many noninfectious diseases, several other models that attempt to account for the multifactorial nature of causation have been proposed. One such model was proposed by Rothman in 1976, and has come to be known as the "Causal Pies." An individual factor that contributes to cause disease is shown as a piece of a pie. After all the pieces of a pie fall into place, the pie is complete — and disease occurs. The individual factors are called "component causes." The complete pie, which might be considered a causal pathway, is called a "sufficient cause." A disease may have more than one sufficient cause, with each sufficient cause being composed of several component causes that may or may not overlap. A component that appears in every pie or pathway is called a "necessary cause" because, without it, the disease does not occur.

The component causes may include intrinsic host factors as well as the agent and the environmental factors of the agent-host-environment triad. A single component cause is rarely a sufficient cause by itself. For example, even exposure to a highly infectious agent, such as measles virus does not invariably result in measles disease. Host susceptibility and other host factors also may play a role.

As the model indicates, a particular disease may result from a variety of different sufficient causes or pathways. For example, lung cancer may result from a sufficient cause that includes smoking as a component cause. Smoking is not a sufficient cause by itself, however, because not all smokers develop lung cancer. Neither is smoking a necessary cause because a small fraction of lung cancer victims have never smoked. Suppose Component Cause B is smoking and Component Cause C is asbestos. Sufficient Cause I includes both smoking (B) and asbestos (C). Sufficient Cause II includes smoking without asbestos, and Sufficient Cause III includes asbestos without smoking. But, because lung cancer can develop in people who have never been exposed to either smoking or asbestos, a proper model for lung cancer would have to show at least one more Sufficient Cause Pie that does not include either component B or component C.

Note that public-health action does not depend on the identification of every component cause. Disease prevention can be accomplished by blocking any single component of a sufficient cause, at least through that pathway. For example, elimination of smoking (component B) would prevent lung cancer from sufficient causes I and II, although some lung cancer would still occur through sufficient cause III.

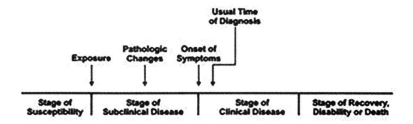

Figure 3.1. Natural History of Disease Timeline *(Source: Centers for Disease Control and Prevention (CDC), Principles of epidemiology, 2nd ed. Atlanta: U.S. Department of Health and Human Services (HSS);1992)*

Natural History and Spectrum of Disease

The "natural history of the disease" refers to the progression of a disease process in an individual over time, in the absence of treatment. For example, untreated infection with human immunodeficiency virus (HIV) causes a spectrum of clinical problems beginning at the time of seroconversion (primary HIV) and terminating with acquired immunodeficiency syndrome (AIDS) and usually death. It is now recognized that it may take 10 years or more for AIDS to develop after seroconversion. Many, if not most, diseases have a characteristic natural history, although the time frame and specific manifestations of the disease may vary from individual to individual and are influenced by preventive and therapeutic measures.

The process begins with the appropriate exposure to or accumulation of factors sufficient for the disease process to begin in a susceptible host. For infectious diseases, exposure is a microorganism. For cancer, the exposure may be a factor that initiates the process, such as asbestos fibers or components in tobacco smoke (for lung cancer), or one that promotes the process, such as estrogen (for endometrial cancer).

After the disease process has been triggered, pathological changes then occur without the individual being aware of them. This stage of subclinical disease, extending from the time of exposure to onset of disease symptoms, is usually called the "incubation period" for infectious diseases, and the latency period for chronic diseases. During this stage, the disease is said to be asymptomatic (no symptoms) or inapparent. This period may be as brief as seconds for hypersensitivity and toxic reactions to as long as decades for certain chronic diseases. Even for a single disease, the characteristic incubation period has a range. For example, the typical incubation period for hepatitis A is as long as 7 weeks. The latency period for leukemia to become evident among survivors of the atomic bomb blast in Hiroshima ranged from 2 to 12 years, peaking at 6 to 7 years. Incubation periods of selected exposures and diseases varying from minutes to decades are displayed in Table 3.1.

The onset of symptoms marks the transition from subclinical to clinical disease. Most diagnoses are made during the stage of clinical disease. In some people, however, the disease process may never progress to clinically apparent illness. In others, the disease process may result in illness that ranges from mild to severe or fatal. This range is called the "spectrum of disease." Ultimately, the disease process ends either in recovery, disability, or death. Although the disease is not apparent during the incubation period, some pathologic changes may be detectable with laboratory, radiographic, or other screening methods. Most screening programs attempt to identify the disease process during this phase of its natural history since intervention at this early stage is likely to be more effective than treatment given after the disease has progressed and become symptomatic.

For an infectious agent, "infectivity" refers to the proportion of exposed persons who become infected. "Pathogenicity" refers to the proportion of infected individuals who develop the clinically apparent disease. Virulence refers to the proportion of clinically apparent cases that are severe or fatal. Because the spectrum of disease can include asymptomatic and mild cases, the cases of illness diagnosed by clinicians in the community often represent only the tip of the iceberg. Many additional cases may be too early to diagnose or may never progress to the clinical stage. Unfortunately, persons with inapparent or undiagnosed infections may nonetheless be able to transmit the infection to others. Such persons who are infectious but have the subclinical disease are called "carriers." Frequently, carriers are persons with incubating disease or inapparent infection. Persons with measles, hepatitis A, and several other diseases become infectious a few days before the onset of symptoms. However, carriers may also be persons who appear to have recovered from their clinical illness but remain infectious, such

Table 3.1. Incubation Periods of Selected Exposures and Diseases

Exposure	Clinical Effect	Incubation/Latency Period
Saxitoxin and similar toxins from shellfish	Paralytic shellfish poisoning (tingling, numbness around lips and fingertips, giddiness, incoherent speech, respiratory paralysis, sometimes death)	Few minutes to 30 minutes
Organophosphorus ingestion	Nausea, vomiting, cramps, headache, nervousness, blurred vision, chest pain, confusion, twitching, convulsions	Few minutes to few hours
Salmonella	Diarrhea, often with fever and cramps	Usually 6 to 48 hours
Sars-associated coronavirus	Severe acute respiratory syndrome (SARS)	3 to 10 days, usually 4 to 6 days
Varicella-zoster virus	Chickenpox	10 to 21 days, usually 14 to 16 days
Treponema pallidum	Syphilis	10 to 90 days, usually 3 weeks
Hepatitis A virus	Hepatitis	14 to 50 days, average 4 weeks
Hepatitis B virus	Hepatitis	50 to 180 days, usually 2 to 3 months
Human immunodeficiency virus (HIV)	Acquired immunodeficiency syndrome (AIDS)	<1 to 15+ years
Atomic bomb radiation (Japan)	Leukemia	2 to 12 years
Radiation (Japan, Chernobyl)	Thyroid cancer	3 to 20+ years
Radium (watch-dial painters)	Bone cancer	8 to 40 years

as chronic carriers of hepatitis B virus, or persons who never exhibited symptoms. The challenge to public-health workers is that these carriers, unaware that they are infected and infectious to others, are sometimes more likely to unwittingly spread infection than are people with an obvious illness.

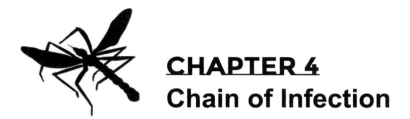

CHAPTER 4
Chain of Infection

The traditional epidemiologic triad model holds that infectious diseases result from the interaction of agent, host, and environment. More specifically, transmission occurs when the agent leaves its reservoir or host through a portal of exit, is conveyed by some mode of transmission, and enters through an appropriate portal of entry to infect a susceptible host. This sequence is sometimes called the "chain of infection."

Reservoir

The reservoir of an infectious agent is the habitat in which the agent normally lives, grows, and multiplies. Reservoirs include humans, animals, and the environment. The reservoir may or may not be the source from which an agent is transferred to a host. For example, the reservoir of *Clostridium botulinum* is soil, but the source of most botulism infections is improperly canned food containing *C. botulinum* spores.

Human Reservoirs

Many common infectious diseases have human reservoirs. Diseases that are transmitted from person to person without intermediaries include sexually

This chapter includes text excerpted from "Principles of Epidemiology in Public Health Practice," Centers for Disease Control and Prevention (CDC), May 18, 2012. Reviewed January 2020.

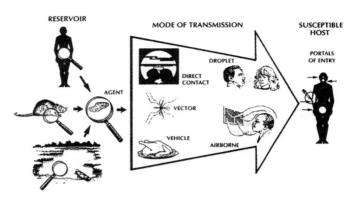

Figure 4.1. Chain of Infection *(Source: Centers for Disease Control and Prevention (CDC). Principles of Epidemiology, 2nd Ed. Atlanta: U.S. Department of Health and Human Services (HHS); 1992)*

transmitted diseases (STDs), measles, mumps, streptococcal infection, and many respiratory pathogens. Because humans were the only reservoir for the smallpox virus, naturally occurring smallpox was eradicated after the last human case was identified and isolated.

Human reservoirs may or may not show the effects of illness. A carrier is a person with an inapparent infection who is capable of transmitting the pathogen to others. Asymptomatic or passive or healthy carriers are those who never experience symptoms despite being infected. Incubatory carriers are those who can transmit the agent during the incubation period before clinical illness begins. Convalescent carriers are those who have recovered from their illness but remain capable of transmitting to others. Chronic carriers are those who continue to harbor a pathogen such as hepatitis B virus or *Salmonella* Typhi, the causative agent of typhoid fever, for months or even years after their initial infection. One notorious carrier is Mary Mallon, or Typhoid Mary, who was an asymptomatic chronic carrier of *Salmonella* Typhi. As a cook in New York City and New Jersey in the early 1900s, she unintentionally infected dozens of people until she was placed in isolation on an island in the East River, where she died 23 years later.

Carriers commonly transmit the disease because they do not realize they are infected, and consequently take no special precautions to prevent transmission. Symptomatic persons who are aware of their illness, on the other hand, may be less likely to transmit infection because they are either too sick to be out and about, take precautions to reduce transmission or receive treatment that limits the disease.

Animal Reservoirs

Humans are also subject to diseases that have animal reservoirs. Many of these diseases are transmitted from animal to animal, with humans as incidental hosts. The term "zoonosis" refers to an infectious disease that is transmissible under natural conditions from vertebrate animals to humans. Long recognized zoonotic diseases include brucellosis (cows and pigs), anthrax (sheep), plague (rodents), trichinellosis/trichinosis (swine), tularemia (rabbits), and rabies (bats, raccoons, dogs, and other mammals). Zoonoses newly emergent in North America include West Nile encephalitis (birds), and monkeypox (prairie dogs). Many infectious diseases in humans, including human immunodeficiency virus (HIV)/acquired immunodeficiency syndrome (AIDS), Ebola infection, and severe acute respiratory syndrome (SARS), are thought to have emerged from animal hosts, although those hosts have not yet been identified.

Environmental Reservoirs

Plants, soil, and water in the environment are also reservoirs for some infectious agents. Many fungal agents, such as those that cause histoplasmosis, live and multiply in the soil. Outbreaks of Legionnaires disease are often traced to water supplies in cooling towers and evaporative condensers, reservoirs for the causative organism *Legionella pneumophila*.

Portal of Exit

A portal of exit is the path by which a pathogen leaves its host. It usually corresponds to the site where the pathogen is localized. For example, influenza viruses and *Mycobacterium tuberculosis* exit through the respiratory tract, schistosomes through urine, *cholera vibrios* in feces, and *Sarcoptes scabiei* in scabies skin lesions. Some blood-borne agents can exit by crossing the placenta from mother to fetus (rubella, syphilis, toxoplasmosis), while others exit through cuts or needles in the skin (hepatitis B) or blood-sucking arthropods (malaria).

Modes of Transmission

An infectious agent may be transmitted from its natural reservoir to a susceptible host in different ways. There are different classifications for modes of transmission. Here is one of them:

- Direct
  - Direct contact
  - Droplet spread
- Indirect
  - Airborne
  - Vehicle-borne
  - Vector-borne (mechanical or biologic)

Indirect transmission, an infectious agent, is transferred from a reservoir to a susceptible host by direct contact or droplet spread.

Direct Contact

Direct contact occurs through skin-to-skin contact, kissing, and sexual intercourse. "Direct contact" also refers to contact with soil or vegetation harboring infectious organisms. Thus, infectious mononucleosis ("kissing disease") and gonorrhea are spread from person to person by direct contact. Hookworm is spread by direct contact with contaminated soil.

Droplet Spread

"Droplet spread" refers to spray with relatively large, short-range aerosols produced by sneezing, coughing, or even talking. Droplet spread is classified as direct because transmission is by direct spray over a few feet before the droplets fall to the ground. Pertussis and meningococcal infection are examples of diseases transmitted from an infectious patient to a susceptible host by droplet spread.

Indirect Transmission

"Indirect transmission" refers to the transfer of an infectious agent from a reservoir to a host by suspended air particles, inanimate objects (vehicles), or animate intermediaries (vectors).

Airborne Transmission

Airborne transmission occurs when infectious agents are carried by dust or droplet nuclei suspended in the air. Airborne dust includes material that has settled on surfaces and become resuspended by air currents as well as infectious particles blown from the soil by the wind. Droplet nuclei are dried residue of fewer than five microns in size. In contrast to droplets that fall to the ground within a few feet, droplet nuclei may remain suspended in the air for long periods and may be blown over great distances. Measles, for example, has occurred in children who came into a physician's office after a child with measles had left, because the measles virus remained suspended in the air.

Vehicles

Vehicles that may indirectly transmit an infectious agent include food, water, biological products (blood), and fomites (inanimate objects, such as handkerchiefs, bedding, or surgical scalpels). A vehicle may passively carry a pathogen—as food or water may carry the hepatitis A virus. Alternatively, the vehicle may provide an environment in which the agent grows, multiplies, or produces toxin—as improperly canned foods provide an environment that supports the production of botulinum toxin by *Clostridium botulinum*.

Vectors, such as mosquitoes, fleas, and ticks, may carry an infectious agent through purely mechanical means or may support growth or changes in the agent. Examples of mechanical transmission are flies carrying Shigella on their appendages and fleas carrying *Yersinia pestis*, the causative agent of plague, in their gut. In contrast, in biological transmission, the causative agent of malaria or guinea worm disease undergoes maturation in an intermediate host before it can be transmitted to humans (Figure 3.2).

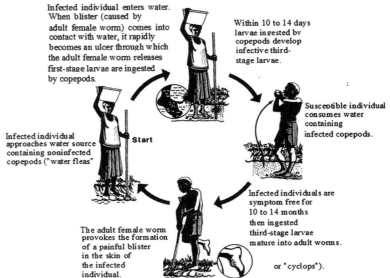

The agent, *Dracunculus* develops in the intermediate host (fresh water copepod). Man acquires the infection by ingesting infected copepods in drinking water.

Figure 4.2. Complex Life Cycle of *Dracunculus medinensis* (Guinea Worm) *(Source: Centers for Disease Control and Prevention (CDC). Principles of Epidemiology, 2nd Ed. Atlanta: U.S. Department of Health and Human Services (HHS); 1992)*

Portal of Entry

The "portal of entry" refers to the manner in which a pathogen enters a susceptible host. The portal of entry must provide access to tissues in which the pathogen can multiply or a toxin can act. Often, infectious agents use the same portal to enter a new host that they used to exit the source host. For example, the influenza virus exits the respiratory tract of the source host and enters the respiratory tract of the new host. In contrast, many pathogens that cause gastroenteritis to follow a so-called fecal-oral route because they exit the source host in feces, are carried on inadequately washed hands to a vehicle, such as food, water, or utensils, and enter a new host through the mouth. Other portals of entry include the skin (hookworm), mucous membranes (syphilis), and blood (hepatitis B, HIV).

Host

The final link in the chain of infection is a susceptible host. Susceptibility of a host depends on genetic or constitutional factors, specific immunity, and nonspecific factors that affect an individual's ability to resist infection or to limit pathogenicity. An individual's genetic makeup may either increase or decrease susceptibility. For example, persons with sickle cell trait seem to be at least partially protected from a particular type of malaria. "Specific immunity" refers to protective antibodies that are directed against a specific agent. Such antibodies may develop in response to infection, vaccine, or toxoid (a toxin that has been deactivated but retains its capacity to stimulate the production of toxin antibodies) or may be acquired by transplacental transfer from mother to fetus or by injection of antitoxin or immune globulin. Nonspecific factors that defend against infection include the skin, mucous membranes, gastric acidity, cilia in the respiratory tract, the cough reflex, and nonspecific immune response. Factors that may increase susceptibility to infection by disrupting host defenses include malnutrition, alcoholism, and disease or therapy that impairs the nonspecific immune response.

Implications for Public Health

Knowledge of the portals of exit and entry and modes of transmission provides a basis for determining appropriate control measures. In general, control measures are usually directed against the segment in the infection chain that is most susceptible to intervention, unless practical issues dictate otherwise.

For some diseases, the most appropriate intervention may be directed at controlling or eliminating the agent at its source. A patient sick with a communicable disease may be treated with antibiotics to eliminate the infection. An asymptomatic but infected person may be treated both to clear the infection and to reduce the risk of transmission to others. In the community, the soil may be decontaminated or covered to prevent the escape of the agent.

Some interventions are directed at the mode of transmission. Interruption of direct transmission may be accomplished by isolation of someone with the infection, or counseling persons to avoid the specific type of contact associated with transmission. Vehicle-borne transmission may be interrupted by the elimination or decontamination of the vehicle. To prevent fecal-oral transmission, efforts often focus on rearranging the environment to reduce the risk of contamination in the future and on changing behaviors, such as promoting handwashing. For airborne diseases, strategies may be directed at modifying ventilation or air pressure, and filtering or treating the air. To interrupt vector-borne transmission, measures may be directed toward controlling the vector population, such as spraying to reduce the mosquito population.

Some strategies that protect the portals of entry are simple and effective. For example, bed nets are used to protect sleeping persons from being bitten by mosquitoes that may transmit malaria. A dentist's mask and gloves are intended to protect the dentist from a patient's blood, secretions, and droplets, as well as to protect the patient from the dentist. Wearing long pants and sleeves and the use of insect repellent is recommended to reduce the risk of Lyme disease and West Nile virus (WNV) infection, which are transmitted by the bite of ticks and mosquitoes, respectively.

Some interventions aim to increase the host's defenses. Vaccinations promote the development of specific antibodies that protect against infection. On the other hand, prophylactic use of antimalarial drugs, recommended for visitors to malaria-endemic areas, does not prevent exposure through mosquito bites but does prevent infection from taking root.

Finally, some interventions attempt to prevent a pathogen from encountering a susceptible host. The concept of herd immunity suggests that if a high enough proportion of individuals in a population are resistant to an agent, then those few who are susceptible will be protected by the resistant majority since the pathogen will be unlikely to "find" those few susceptible individuals. The degree of herd immunity necessary to prevent or interrupt an outbreak varies by disease. In theory, herd immunity means that not everyone in a community needs to be resistant (immune) to prevent disease spread and the occurrence of an outbreak. In practice, herd immunity has not prevented outbreaks of measles and rubella in populations with immunization levels as high as 85 to 90 percent. One problem is that, in highly immunized populations, the relatively few susceptible persons are often clustered in subgroups defined by socioeconomic or cultural factors. If the pathogen is introduced into one of these subgroups, an outbreak may occur.

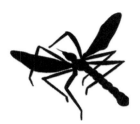

CHAPTER 5
Deadliest Outbreaks and Pandemics in History

The terms "epidemics" and "pandemics" are used to describe the spread of infectious diseases over a relatively large geographical area at a rapid pace. When the spread of disease is confined to a particular country or region, it is considered an "epidemic." But, when it goes beyond national boundaries involving multiple continents or worldwide, it is called a "pandemic." Widespread outbreaks of infectious diseases have proven to be disastrous throughout the history of humankind. Outbreaks of these diseases have caused millions of deaths and some continue to pose a threat to human life. This chapter identifies some of the deadliest epidemics and pandemics in human history.

Smallpox

Smallpox is an old disease whose origin dates back to ancient Egypt. In the 16th century, the disease was introduced to colonial America by European settlers—some of whom engaged in early biological warfare by giving smallpox-infested blankets and handkerchiefs to native American dignitaries as gifts. Since Native Americans had not developed a natural immunity to this foreign disease, smallpox wiped out almost the entire

"Deadliest Outbreaks and Pandemics in History," © 2020 Omnigraphics. Reviewed January 2020.

population of indigenous people. The death toll is estimated to be around 90 million.

The European continent also had an outbreak of smallpox in the 18th century with an estimated death of 60 million people. The smallpox vaccine was developed by Edward Jenner in 1796.

Typhus

Typhus is also called "camp fever." This disease typically spreads among people living in close quarters. The speed at which it spreads is attributed to unsanitary living conditions. In the 17th century, the disease originated in the crowded cities of Europe, spread across the continent, and is believed to have killed over 10 million people. Another outbreak occurred during World War II (WWII) and claimed the lives of Polish, Romanian, and Russian soldiers.

Yellow Fever

Yellow fever is a lethal viral, hemorrhagic disease that is spread by mosquitoes. It generally occurs during the hot summer months in places with high humidity. In the summer of 1793, Caribbean refugees brought the disease to the United States, and an epidemic broke out in Philadelphia. This outbreak claimed approximately 2,000 lives. Yellow fever continues to exist in several lower-income countries and causes approximately 30,000 deaths each year.

Cholera

Cholera was prevalent in India centuries ago. In 1817, the disease was spread to other south Asian countries by merchants traveling along the Ganges River. By 1832, the disease had spread to North America and Europe. To date, the world has faced seven deadly epidemics of cholera since the 19th century. The 1821 cholera outbreak in Iraq is considered to be the most severe of these outbreaks, with over 18,000 deaths occurring. Cholera outbreaks continue today and the World Health Organization (WHO) reports that 3 to 5 million people are affected by the disease each year.

Asiatic Flu or Russian Flu

The outbreak of Asiatic Flu, also known as "Russian flu," happened in May 1889 and lasted until 1890. Researchers once believed that the disease was caused by the H2N2 subtype of the Influenza A virus. But, more recent research revealed that the H3N8 subtype of Influenza A is what actually caused the disease. Initially, the outbreak was reported in three different parts of the world: Athabasca (Canada), Bukhara (Turkestan), and Greenland. This flu later spread across the globe and claimed over a million lives.

Polio

Paralytic poliomyelitis, commonly known as "polio," is a viral disease that affects the central nervous system (CNS); the infection can lead to paralysis or death. The polio-causing virus has been around for thousands of years, but it caused a frenzy across Europe, North America, New Zealand, and Australia in the 1940s and 1950s. In 1894, first outbreak of polio in epidemic form occurred in Vermont with 132 cases. In 1908, Karl Landsteiner and Erwin Popper identified a virus as the cause of polio by transmitting to a monkey. The disease was first reported in 1912, but reached its peak in 1952 when it claimed the lives of around 6,000 people in the United States. American physician Jonas Salk developed the first polio vaccine in 1950 and his vaccine made America polio-free by 1979. Albert Sabin introduced an oral vaccine in the 1960s that replaced Salk's. Medical researchers believe that the disease can be eradicated across the world in the near future with appropriate vaccinations.

Spanish Flu

Spanish flu is considered to be one of the deadliest global pandemics involving H1N1 influenza virus ever recorded in history. It struck in 1918 and killed tens of millions of people in the span of one year. The major reason for the massive outbreak was the return of World War I (WWI) soldiers, many of whom were severely affected by the disease during the war, to their homelands. Medical researchers believe that more people were killed by this outbreak of Spanish flu than were killed in the war.

Hong Kong Flu

The Hong Kong flu is a flu pandemic caused by the H3N2 strain of the Influenza A virus. It hit Hong Kong in 1968 and spread to Singapore, Vietnam, India, the Philippines, Europe, Australia, and the United States. The outbreak killed around 15 percent of the total population of Hong Kong.

HIV/AIDS

Human immunodeficiency virus (HIV)/acquired immunodeficiency syndrome (AIDS) is a sexually transmitted disease (STD) that was first reported in 1981. The disease has claimed more than 36 million lives around the world. It is estimated that around 31 to 35 million people are living with HIV, and the vast majority of them live in Sub-Saharan Africa. Although there is no proven cure for the disease, medicines and treatments are available to manage its symptoms.

Severe Acute Respiratory Syndrome

Severe acute respiratory syndrome (SARS) originated in Asia (appearing in 2002 in China). It is spread through the bodily fluids—mucus and saliva, etc.—of an infected person. In 2003, the disease infected 12 different countries, affecting around 8,000 people and claiming the lives of 774 people. As of now, there is no known cure for SARS.

Ebola

Ebola is a virus that is initially transmitted through human contact with wild animals and later spread from human to human. The pandemic that occurred in 2014 is considered to be one of the worst Ebola pandemics in human history. By November 2015, the disease had caused 11,314 fatalities. Ebola still exists in central and western African countries where healthcare is scarce and insufficient.

References

1. "Outbreak: 10 of the Worst Pandemics in History," MPHonline, November 3, 2014.

2. Barnato, Katy. "History's Deadliest Pandemics," Consumer News and Business Channel (CNBC), July 23, 2015.

3. "The Five Deadliest Outbreaks and Pandemics in History," Robert Wood Johnson Foundation (RWJF), December 16, 2013.

4. Jacoby, Ariel. "10 of the Deadliest Epidemics from History to Modern Day," Medelita, May 11, 2018.

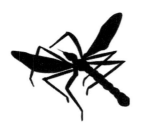

CHAPTER 6
Factors in the Emergence of Infectious Diseases

Infectious diseases emerging throughout history have included some of the most feared plagues of the past. New infections continue to emerge today, while many of the old plagues are with us still. These are global problems, William Foege, director of the Carter Center, calls them "global infectious disease threats." Under suitable circumstances, a new infection first appearing anywhere in the world could traverse entire continents within days or weeks.

The term "emerging infections" can be defined as those infections that have newly appeared in the population, or have existed but are rapidly increasing in incidence or geographic range. Examples of emerging diseases in various parts of the world include human immunodeficiency virus (HIV), acquired immunodeficiency syndrome (AIDS), classic cholera in South America and Africa, cholera due to *Vibrio cholerae* O139, Rift Valley fever (RVF), hantavirus pulmonary syndrome (HPS), Lyme disease, and hemolytic uremic syndrome (HUS), a food-borne infection caused by certain strains of *Escherichia coli* (*E. coli*) (in the United States, serotype O157: H7).

Although these occurrences may appear inexplicable, rarely if ever do emerging infections appear without reason. Specific factors responsible for

This chapter includes text excerpted from "Factors in the Emergence of Infectious Diseases," Centers for Disease Control and Prevention (CDC), June 8, 2011. Reviewed January 2020.

disease emergence can be identified in virtually all cases studied. Table 5.1 summarizes the known causes of a number of infections that have emerged recently. Infectious disease emergence can be viewed operationally as a two-step process:

- Introduction of the agent into a new host population (whether the pathogen originated in the environment, possibly in another species, or as a variant of an existing human infection)
- Establishment and further dissemination within the new host population (adoption)

Whatever its origin, the infection emerges when it reaches a new population. Factors that promote one or both of these steps will, therefore, tend to precipitate disease emergence. Most emerging infections, and even antibiotic-resistant strains of common bacterial pathogens, usually originate in one geographic location and then disseminate to new places.

Regarding the introduction step, the numerous examples of infections originating as zoonoses suggest that the zoonotic pool introductions of infections from other species is an important and potentially rich source of emerging diseases; periodic discoveries of new zoonoses suggest that the zoonotic pool appears by no means exhausted. Once introduced, an infection might then be disseminated through other factors, although the rapid course and high mortality combined with low transmissibility, are often limiting. However, even if a zoonotic agent is not able to spread readily from person to person and establish itself, other factors (e.g., nosocomial, or hospital-acquired, infection) might transmit the infection. Additionally, if the reservoir host or vector becomes more widely disseminated, the microbe can appear in new places. Bubonic plague transmitted by rodent fleas and rat-borne hantavirus infections is an example.

Most emerging infections appear to be caused by pathogens already present in the environment, brought out of obscurity or given a selective advantage by changing conditions and afforded an opportunity to infect new host populations (on rare occasions, a new variant may also evolve and cause a new disease). The process by which infectious agents may transfer from animals to humans or disseminate from isolated groups into new populations can be called "microbial traffic." A number of activities increase

Table 6.1. Emerging Infections and Probable Factors in Their Emergence

Infection or Agent	Factor(s) Contributing to Emergence
Viral	
Argentine, Bolivian hemorrhagic fever (BHF)	Changes in agriculture favoring rodent host
Bovine spongiform encephalopathy (BSE) (cattle)	Changes in rendering processes
Dengue, dengue hemorrhagic fever (DHF)	Transportation, travel, and migration; urbanization
Ebola, Marburg	Unknown (in Europe and the United States, importation of monkeys)
Hantaviruses	Ecological or environmental changes increasing contact with rodent hosts
Hepatitis B, C	Transfusions, organ transplants, contaminated hypodermic apparatus, sexual transmission, vertical spread from infected mother to child
Human immunodeficiency virus (HIV)	Migration to cities and travel; after introduction, sexual transmission, vertical spread from infected mother to child, contaminated hypodermic apparatus (including during intravenous drug use, transfusions, organ transplants
Human T-cell leukemia virus (HTLV)	Contaminated hypodermic apparatus, other
Influenza (pandemic)	Possibly pig-duck agriculture, facilitating reassortment of avian and mammalian influenza viruses*
Lassa fever	Urbanization favoring rodent host, increasing exposure (usually in homes)
Rift Valley fever (RVF)	Dam building, agriculture, irrigation; possibly change in virulence or pathogenicity of the virus
Yellow fever (in new areas)	Conditions favoring mosquito vector
Bacterial	
Brazilian purpuric fever (BPF) (*Haemophilus influenzae, biotype aegyptius*)	Probably new strain

Table 6.1. Continued

Infection or Agent	Factor(s) Contributing to Emergence
Cholera	In recent epidemic in South America, probably introduced from Asia by ship, with spread facilitated by reduced water chlorination; a new strain (type O139) from Asia recently disseminated by travel (similarly to past introductions of classic cholera)
Helicobacter pylori (*H. pylori*) (associated with gastric ulcers, possibly other)	Probably long widespread, now recognized (associated with gastric ulcers, possibly other gastrointestinal (GI) disease)
Hemolytic uremic syndrome (HUS) (*Escherichia coli* (*E. coli*) O157: H7)	Mass food processing technology allowing contamination of meat
Legionella (Legionnaires' disease)	Cooling and plumbing systems (organism grows in biofilms that form on water storage tanks and in stagnant plumbing)
Lyme borreliosis (*Borrelia burgdorferi*)	Reforestation around homes and other conditions favoring tick vector and deer (a secondary reservoir host)
Streptococcus, group A (invasive; necrotizing)	Uncertain
Toxic shock syndrome (TSS) (*Staphylococcus aureus*)	Ultra-absorbency tampons
Parasitic	
Cryptosporidium, other waterborne pathogens	Contaminated surface water, faulty water purification
Malaria (in "new" areas)	Travel or migration
Schistosomiasis	Dam building

Reappearances of influenza are due to two distinct mechanisms: Annual or biennial epidemics involving new variants due to antigenic drift (point mutations, primarily in the gene for the surface protein, hemagglutinin) and pandemic strains, arising from antigenic shift (genetic reassortment, generally between avian and mammalian influenza strains.)

microbial traffic and as a result promote emergence and epidemics. In some cases, including many of the most novel infections, the agents are zoonotic, crossing from their natural hosts into the human population. In other cases, pathogens already present in geographically isolated populations are given an opportunity to disseminate further. Surprisingly often, disease emergence is caused by human actions, however, inadvertently; natural causes, such as changes in climate, can also be responsible.

Table 6.2 summarizes the underlying factors responsible for emergence. Any categorization of the factors is, of course, somewhat arbitrary but should be representative of the underlying processes that cause emergence. Researchers have essentially adopted the categories developed in the Institute of Medicine's (IOM) report on emerging infections, with additional definitions from the Centers for Disease Control and Prevention's (CDC) emerging infections plan. Responsible factors include ecological changes, such as those due to agricultural or economic development or to anomalies in climate; human demographic changes and behavior; travel and commerce; technology and industry; microbial adaptation and change; and a breakdown of public-health measures. Each of these has been considered in turn.

Examples of infections originating as zoonoses suggest that the zoonotic pool introductions of infections from other species is an important and potentially rich source of emerging diseases; periodic discoveries of new zoonoses suggest that the zoonotic pool appears by no means exhausted.

Once introduced, an infection might then be disseminated through other factors, although the rapid course and high mortality combined with low transmissibility, are often limiting. However, even if a zoonotic agent is not able to spread readily from person to person and establish itself, other factors (e.g., nosocomial infection) might transmit the infection. Additionally, if the reservoir host or vector becomes more widely disseminated, the microbe can appear in new places. Bubonic plague transmitted by rodent fleas and rat-borne hantavirus infections is an example.

Ecological interactions can be complex, with several factors often working together or in sequence. For example, population movement from rural areas to cities can spread a once-localized infection. The strain on infrastructure in the overcrowded and rapidly growing cities may disrupt or slow public-health measures, perhaps allowing the establishment of the newly introduced infection. Finally, the city may also provide a gateway for further dissemination of the infection. Most successful emerging infections, including HIV, cholera, and dengue, have followed this route.

Table 6.2. Factors in Infectious Disease Emergence

Factor	Examples of Specific Factors	Examples of Diseases
Ecological changes (including those due to economic development and land use)	Agriculture; dams, changes in water ecosystems; deforestation/ reforestation; flood/drought; famine; climate changes	Schistosomiasis (dams); Rift Valley fever (RVF) (dams, irrigation); Argentine hemorrhagic fever (AHF) (agriculture); Hantaan (Korean hemorrhagic fever (KHF)) (agriculture); hantavirus pulmonary syndrome (HPS), southwestern U.S., 1993 (weather anomalies)
Human demographics, behavior	Societal events: Population growth and migration (movement from rural areas to cities); war or civil conflict; urban decay; sexual behavior; intravenous drug use; use of high-density facilities	Introduction of the human immunodeficiency virus (HIV); spread of dengue; spread of HIV and other sexually transmitted diseases (STDs)
International travel commerce	The worldwide movement of goods and people; air travel	"Airport" malaria; dissemination of mosquito vectors; rat-borne hantaviruses; introduction of cholera into South America; dissemination of O139 V. cholerae
Technology and industry	Globalization of food supplies; changes in food processing and packaging; organ or tissue transplantation; drugs causing immunosuppression; widespread use of antibiotics	Hemolytic uremic syndrome (HUS) (*E.coli* contamination of hamburger meat), bovine spongiform encephalopathy; transfusion-associated hepatitis (hepatitis B, C), opportunistic infections in immunosuppressed patients, Creutzfeldt-Jakob disease (CJD) from contaminated batches of human growth hormone (medical technology)

Table 6.2. Continued

Factor	Examples of Specific Factors	Examples of Diseases
Microbial adaptation and change	Microbial evolution, response to selection in the environment	Antibiotic-resistant bacteria, "antigenic drift" in influenza virus
Breakdown in public-health measures	Curtailment or reduction in prevention programs; inadequate sanitation and vector control measures	The resurgence of tuberculosis (TB) in the United States; cholera in refugee camps in Africa; the resurgence of diphtheria in the former Soviet Union

Consider HIV as an example. Although the precise ancestry of HIV-1 is still uncertain, it appears to have had a zoonotic origin. Ecological factors that would have allowed human exposure to a natural host carrying the virus that was the precursor to HIV-1 were, therefore, instrumental in the introduction of the virus into humans. This probably occurred in a rural area. A plausible scenario is suggested by the identification of an HIV-2-infected man in a rural area of Liberia whose virus strain resembled viruses isolated from the sooty mangabey monkey (an animal widely hunted for food in rural areas and the putative source of HIV-2) more closely than it did strains circulating in the city. Such findings suggest that zoonotic introductions of this sort may occur on occasion in isolated populations but may well go unnoticed so long as the recipients remain isolated. But with increasing movement from rural areas to cities, such isolation is increasingly rare. After its likely first move from a rural area into a city, HIV-1 spread regionally along highways, then by long-distance routes, including air travel, to more distant places. This last step was critical for HIV and facilitated the global pandemic. Social changes that allowed the virus to reach a larger population and to be transmitted despite its relatively low natural transmissibility were instrumental in the success of the virus in its newfound human host. For HIV, the long duration of infectivity allowed this normally poorly transmissible virus many opportunities to be transmitted and to take advantage of such factors as human behavior (sexual transmission, intravenous drug use) and changing technology (early spread through blood transfusions and blood products) (Table 5.1).

Ecological Changes and Agricultural Development

Ecological changes, including those due to agricultural or economic development, are among the most frequently identified factors in emergence. They are especially frequent as factors in outbreaks of previously unrecognized diseases with high case-fatality rates, which often turn out to be zoonotic introductions. Ecological factors usually precipitate emergence of the disease by placing people in contact with a natural reservoir or host for an infection hitherto unfamiliar but usually already present (often a zoonotic or arthropod-borne infection), either by increasing proximity or, often, also by changing conditions so as to favor an increased population of the microbe or its natural host. The emergence of Lyme disease in the United States and Europe was probably due largely to reforestation, which increased the population of deer and the deer tick, the vector of Lyme disease. The movement of people into these areas placed a larger population in close proximity to the vector.

Agricultural development, one of the most common ways in which people alter and interpose themselves into the environment, is often a factor (Table 5.2). Hantaan virus, the cause of Korean hemorrhagic fever (KHF), causes over 100,000 cases a year in China and has been known in Asia for centuries. The virus is a natural infection of the field mouse *Apodemus agrarius*. The rodent flourishes in rice fields; people usually contract the disease during the rice harvest from contact with infected rodents. Junin virus (JUNV), the cause of Argentine hemorrhagic fever (AHF), is an unrelated virus with a history remarkably similar to that of the Hantaan virus. Conversion of grassland to maize cultivation favored a rodent that was the natural host for this virus, and human cases increased in proportion to the expansion of maize agriculture. Other examples, in addition to those already known, are likely to appear as new areas are placed under cultivation.

Perhaps most surprisingly, pandemic influenza appears to have an agricultural origin: integrated pig-duck farming in China. Strains causing the frequent annual or biennial epidemics generally result from mutation (antigenic drift), but pandemic influenza viruses do not generally arise by this process. Instead, gene segments from two influenza strains resort to producing a new virus that can infect humans. Evidence amassed by researchers indicates that waterfowl, such as ducks, are major reservoirs of influenza and that pigs can serve as mixing vessels for new mammalian influenza strains. Pandemic influenza viruses have generally come from China. Researchers Scholtissek and Naylor suggested that integrated pig-duck agriculture, an extremely efficient food production system traditionally practiced in certain parts of China for several centuries, puts these two species in contact and provides a natural laboratory for making new influenza recombinants. One of the researchers has suggested that, with high-intensity agriculture and movement of livestock across borders, suitable conditions may now also be found in Europe.

Water is also frequently associated with disease emergence. Infections transmitted by mosquitoes or other arthropods, which include some of the most serious and widespread diseases, are often stimulated by the expansion of standing water, simply because many of the mosquito vectors breed in water. There are many cases of diseases transmitted by water-breeding vectors, most involving dams, water for irrigation, or stored drinking water in cities. The incidence of Japanese encephalitis, another mosquito-borne disease that accounts for almost 30,000 human cases and approximately 7,000 deaths annually in Asia, is closely associated with flooding of fields for rice growing. Outbreaks of Rift Valley fever in some parts of Africa have been associated with dam building as well as with periods of heavy rainfall. In the outbreaks of Rift Valley fever in Mauritania in 1987, the human cases occurred in villages near dams on the Senegal River. The same effect has been documented with other infections that have aquatic hosts, such as schistosomiasis.

Because humans are important agents of ecological and environmental change, many of these factors are anthropogenic (or, the result of human activity that causes environmental pollution and pollutants). Of course, this is not always the case, and natural environmental changes, such as climate or weather anomalies, can have the same effect. The outbreak of hantavirus pulmonary syndrome (HPS) in the southwestern United States in 1993 is one example. It is likely that the virus has long been present in mouse populations but an unusually mild and wet winter and spring in that area led to an increased rodent population in the spring and summer and thus to greater opportunities for people to come in contact with infected rodents (and, hence, with the virus); it has been suggested that the weather anomaly was due to large-scale climatic effects. The same causes may have been responsible for outbreaks of hantaviral disease in Europe at approximately the same time. With cholera, it has been suggested that certain organisms in marine environments are natural reservoirs for cholera vibrios and that large-scale effects on ocean currents may cause local increases in the reservoir organism with consequent flare-ups of cholera.

Changes in Human Demographics and Behavior

Human population movements, or upheavals, caused by migration or war, are often important factors in disease emergence. In many parts of the world, economic conditions are encouraging the mass movement of workers from rural areas to cities. The United Nations has estimated that, largely as a result of continuing migration, by the year 2025, 65 percent of the world population (also expected to be larger in absolute numbers), including 61 percent of the population in developing regions, will live in cities. As discussed above for HIV, rural urbanization allows infections arising in isolated rural areas, which may once have remained obscure and localized, to reach larger populations. Once in a city, the newly introduced infection would have the opportunity to spread locally among the population and could also spread further along highways and interurban transport routes and by airplane. HIV has been, and in Asia is becoming, the best-known beneficiary of this dynamic, but many other diseases, such as dengue, stand to benefit. The frequency of the most severe form, dengue hemorrhagic fever (DHF), which is thought to occur when a person is sequentially infected by two types of dengue virus, is increasing as different dengue viruses have extended their range and now overlap. Dengue hemorrhagic fever is now common in some cities in Asia, where the high prevalence of infection is attributed to the proliferation of open containers needed for water storage (which also provide breeding grounds for the mosquito vector) as the population size exceeds the infrastructure. In urban environments, rain-filled tires or plastic bottles are often breeding grounds of choice for mosquito vectors. The resulting mosquito population boom is complemented by the high human population density in such situations, increasing the chances of stable transmission cycles between infected and susceptible persons. Even in industrialized countries, e.g., the United States, infections, such as tuberculosis (TB) can spread through high-population density settings (e.g., daycare centers or prisons.)

Human behavior can have important effects on disease dissemination. The best-known examples are sexually transmitted diseases (STDs), and the ways in which such human behavior as sex or intravenous drug use have contributed to the emergence of HIV are now well known. Other factors responsible for disease emergence are influenced by a variety of human actions, so human behavior in the broader sense is also very important. Motivating appropriate individual behavior and constructive action, both locally and in a larger scale, will be essential for controlling emerging infections. Ironically, as AIDS prevention efforts have demonstrated, human behavior remains one of the weakest links in our scientific knowledge.

International Travel and Commerce

The dissemination of HIV through travel has already been mentioned. In the past, an infection introduced into people in a geographically isolated area might, on occasion, be brought to a new place through travel, commerce, or war. Trade between Asia and Europe, perhaps beginning with the silk route and continuing with the Crusades, brought the rat and one of its infections, the bubonic plague, to Europe. Beginning in the 16th and 17th centuries, ships bringing slaves from West Africa to the New World also brought yellow fever and its mosquito vector, *Aedes aegypti*, to the new territories. Similarly, smallpox escaped its Old World origins to wreak new havoc in the New World. In the 19th century, cholera had similar opportunities to spread from its probable origin in the Ganges plain to the Middle East and, from there, to Europe and much of the remaining world.

Each of these infections had once been localized and took advantage of opportunities to be carried to previously unfamiliar parts of the world.

Similar histories are being repeated nowadays, but opportunities in recent years have become far richer and more numerous, reflecting the increasing volume, scope, and speed of traffic in an increasingly mobile world. Rats have carried hantaviruses virtually worldwide. *Aedes albopictus* (the Asian tiger mosquito) was introduced into the United States, Brazil, and parts of Africa in shipments of used tires from Asia. Since its introduction in 1982, this mosquito has established itself in at least 18 states of the United States and has acquired local viruses including Eastern equine encephalomyelitis, a cause of serious disease. Another mosquito-borne disease, malaria, is one of the most frequently imported diseases in nonendemic disease areas, and cases of airport malaria are occasionally identified.

A classic bacterial disease, cholera, recently entered both South America (for the first time this century) and Africa. Molecular typing shows the South American isolates to be of the current pandemic strain, supporting the suggestion that the organism was introduced in contaminated bilge water from an Asian freighter. Other evidence indicates that cholera was only one of many organisms to travel in ballast water; dozens, perhaps hundreds, of species have been exchanged between distant places through this means of transport alone. New bacterial strains, such as the recently identified *Vibrio cholerae* O139, or an epidemic strain of *Neisseria meningitidis* (also examples of microbial adaptation and change) have disseminated rapidly along routes of trade and travel, as have antibiotic-resistant bacteria.

Technology and Industry

High-volume rapid movement characterizes not only travel but also other industries in modern society. In operations, including food production, that process or use products of biological origin, modern production methods yield increased efficiency and reduced costs but can increase the chances of accidental contamination and amplify the effects of such contamination. The problem is further compounded by globalization, allowing the opportunity to introduce agents from far away. A pathogen present in some of the raw material may find its way into a large batch of the final product, as happened with the contamination of hamburger meat by *E. coli* strains to cause hemolytic uremic syndrome. In the United States, the implicated *E. coli* strains are serotype O157: H7; additional serotypes have been identified in other countries. Bovine spongiform encephalopathy (BSE), which emerged in Britain within the last few years, was likely an interspecies transfer of scrapie from sheep to cattle that occurred when changes in rendering processes led to incomplete inactivation of scrapie agent in sheep byproducts fed to cattle.

The concentrating effects that occur with blood and tissue products have inadvertently disseminated infections unrecognized at the time, such as HIV and hepatitis B and C. Medical settings are also at the front line of exposure to new diseases, and a number of infections, including many emerging infections, have spread nosocomially in healthcare settings (Table 6.2). Among the numerous examples, in outbreaks of Ebola fever in Africa many of the secondary cases were hospital-acquired, most transmitted to other patients through contaminated hypodermic apparatus, and some to the healthcare staff by contact. Transmission of Lassa fever (LF) to healthcare workers has also been documented.

On the positive side, advances in diagnostic technology can also lead to a new recognition of agents that are already widespread. When such agents are newly recognized, they may at first often be labeled, in some cases incorrectly, as emerging infections. Human herpesvirus 6 (HHV-6) was identified only a few years ago, but the virus appears to be extremely widespread and has been implicated as the cause of roseola (exanthem subitum), a very common childhood disease. Because roseola has been known since at least 1910, HHV-6 is likely to have been common for decades and probably much longer. Another example is the bacterium *Helicobacter pylori* (*H. pylori*), a probable cause of gastric ulcers and some cancers. Humankind has lived with these diseases for a long time without knowing their cause. Recognition of the agent is often advantageous, offering a new promise of controlling a previously intractable disease, such as treating gastric ulcers with specific antimicrobial therapy.

Microbial Adaptation and Change

Just like other living things, Microbes are constantly evolving. The emergence of antibiotic-resistant bacteria as a result of the ubiquity of antimicrobials in the environment is an evolutionary lesson on microbial adaptation, as well as a demonstration of the power of natural selection. Selection for antibiotic-resistant bacteria and drug-resistant parasites has become frequent, driven by the wide and sometimes inappropriate use of antimicrobial drugs in a variety of applications. Pathogens can also acquire new antibiotic resistance genes from other, often nonpathogenic, species in the environment, selected or perhaps even driven by the selection pressure of antibiotics.

Many viruses show a high mutation rate and can rapidly evolve to yield new variants. A classic example is an influenza. Regular annual epidemics are caused by antigenic drift in a previously circulating influenza strain. A change in an antigenic site of a surface protein, usually the hemagglutinin (H) protein, allows the new variant to reinfect previously infected persons because the altered antigen is not immediately recognized by the immune system.

On rare occasions, perhaps more often with nonviral pathogens than with viruses, the evolution of a new variant may result in a new expression of disease. The epidemic of Brazilian purpuric fever (BPF) in 1990, associated with a newly emerged clonal variant of *Hemophilus influenzae*, biogroup *aegyptius*, may fall into this category. It is possible, but not yet clear, that some recently described manifestations of disease by group A *Streptococcus*, such as rapidly invasive infection or necrotizing fasciitis, may also fall into this category.

Breakdown of Public-Health Measures and Deficiencies in Public-Health Infrastructure

Classical public-health and sanitation measures have long served to minimize dissemination and human exposure to many pathogens spread by traditional routes such as water or preventable by immunization or vector control. The pathogens themselves often still remain, albeit in reduced numbers, in reservoir hosts or in the environment, or in small pockets of infection and, therefore, are often able to take advantage of the opportunity to reemerge if there are breakdowns in preventive measures.

Reemerging diseases are those, such as cholera, that were once decreasing but are now rapidly increasing again. These are often conventionally understood and well recognized public-health threats for which (in most cases) previously active public-health measures had been allowed to lapse, a situation that unfortunately now applies all too often in both developing countries and the inner cities of the industrialized world. The appearance of reemerging diseases may, therefore, often be a sign of the breakdown of public-health measures and should be a warning against complacency in the war against infectious diseases.

Cholera, for example, has been raging in South America (for the first time in this century) and Africa. The rapid spread of cholera in South America may have been abetted by recent reductions in chlorine levels used to treat water supplies. The success of cholera and other enteric diseases is often due to the lack of a reliable water supply. These problems are more severe in developing countries but are not confined to these areas. The United States outbreak of water-borne *Cryptosporidium* infection in Milwaukee, Wisconsin, in the spring of 1993, with over 400,000 estimated cases, was in part due to a nonfunctioning water filtration plant; similar deficiencies in water purification have been found in other cities in the United States.

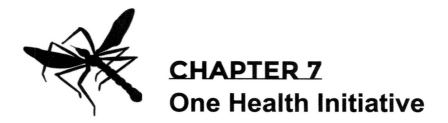

CHAPTER 7
One Health Initiative

What Is One Health?

"One Health" has been defined in many ways. At its core, One Health fosters a collaborative approach to issues that intersect human, animal, and environmental health.

Although One Health is not a new concept, it has gained importance over the years. Interactions among people, animals, and the environment continue to change. The expansion of human and animal populations, changes in climate and land use, and increased international travel and trade provide opportunities for disease spread. Approximately 75 percent of emerging infectious diseases affecting humans are diseases of animal origin; approximately 60 percent of all human pathogens are zoonotic.

Zoonotic diseases are those that are spread between people and animals.

One Health obviously includes health professionals. But, it also includes wildlife specialists, anthropologists, economists, environmentalists, behavioral scientists, and sociologists, among others. One Health embraces the idea that complex problems at the human-animal-environmental interface can best be solved through multidisciplinary communication, cooperation, and collaboration.

This chapter includes text excerpted from "What Is One Health?" U.S. Department of Agriculture (USDA), February 16, 2017.

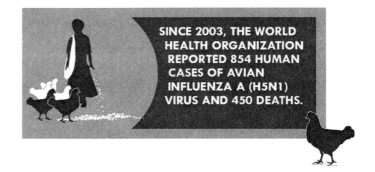

Figure 7.1. Avian Influenza *(Source: "One Health," Centers for Disease Control and Prevention (CDC))*

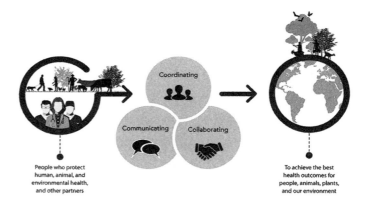

Figure 7.2. Outcomes of One Health *(Source: "One Health Basics," Centers for Disease Control and Prevention (CDC))*

One Health is increasingly being acknowledged by national and international institutions as the most constructive approach to address complex issues at the animal-human-environmental interface.

The History of One Health

A German scholar from the mid-1800s, Rudolf Virchow, who came from a farming family, was an early proponent of One Health. He said, "Between animal and human medicine there is no dividing line—nor should there be.

The object is different but the experience obtained constitutes the basis of all medicine."

During the past 3 decades, approximately 75 percent of emerging infectious diseases among humans have been zoonotic diseases, which can be transmitted from animals to people. This has encouraged the modern proponents of One Health. In the 1980s, epidemiologist Calvin Schwabe called for a unified human and veterinary approach to combat zoonotic diseases, providing the modern foundation for One Health.

The concept was advanced further when, in 2004, the Wildlife Conservation Society (WCS) hosted a symposium that brought together an international group of human and animal-health experts to discuss shared diseases among humans, wild animals, and domestic animal populations. This symposium introduced a set of priorities for an international and interdisciplinary approach to combat joint threats to human and animal health.

In 2007, The American Veterinary Medical Association (AVMA) and the American Medical Association (AMA) adopted a vision supporting the concept of One Health and formed the One Health Initiative task force. The task force brought together the U.S. human and animal-health agencies, medical doctors, and veterinarians. In addition, the National Strategy for Pandemic Influenza (NSPI) and its Implementation Plan led to several International Ministerial Conferences. In 2008, the Food and Agriculture Organization (FAO) of the United Nations (UN), the World Health Organization (WHO), the World Organization for Animal Health (OIE), the United Nations Children's Fund (UNICEF), the World Bank, and the United Nations System Influenza Coordination (UNSIC) came together to develop a document titled, "Contributing to One World, One Health™—A Strategic Framework for Reducing Risks of Infectious Diseases at the Animal-Human Ecosystems Interface."

In 2010, the UN and the World Bank recommended the adoption of One Health approaches in the document "Fifth Global Progress Report on Animal and Pandemic Influenza." The 1st International One Health Congress was held in Melbourne, Australia, in February 2011. Representing a range of disciplines, more than 650 people from 60 countries gathered to discuss the benefits of working together to promote a One

Health approach. Going beyond the importance of understanding the interdependence of human, animal, and environmental health, attendees supported the inclusion of disciplines, such as economics, social behavior, and food security and safety. The first One Health Summit, sponsored by the Global Risk Forum (GRF), was held in Davos, Switzerland in February 2012.

One Health has also gained ground throughout the U.S. government, led by the President's new initiatives for coordination and collaboration on the Global Health Security Agenda (GHSA). The Centers for Disease Control and Prevention (CDC) established its One Health office in 2009. The U.S. Department of Agriculture's (USDA) Animal and Plant Health Inspection Service (APHIS) established its One Health Coordination Center in 2012.

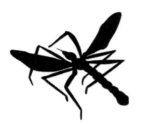

CHAPTER 8
Notable Pseudopandemics of the Last Century

Extreme Intrasubtypic Antigenic Variation and the Pseudopandemic of 1947 (H1N1)

In late 1946, an outbreak of influenza (the flu) occurred in Japan and Korea in American troops. It spread in 1947 to other military bases in the United States, including Fort Monmouth, New Jersey, where the prototype FM-1 strain was isolated. The epidemic was notable because of the initial difficulty in establishing its cause as an influenza A virus because of its considerable antigenic difference from previous influenza A viruses. Indeed, for a time it was identified as "influenza A prime." The 1947 epidemic has been thought of as a mild pandemic because the disease, although globally distributed, caused relatively few deaths. However, the fact was that there was nothing mild about the illness in young recruits in whom signs and symptoms closely matched those of earlier descriptions of influenza.

Most remarkable was the total failure of vaccine containing a 1943 H1N1 strain (effective in 1943 to 1944 and 1944 to 1945 seasons) to protect a large number of U.S. military personnel who were vaccinated. Previously, antigenic variation had been noted but never had it been of a sufficient degree to compromise vaccine-induced immunity. Years later, extensive characterization

This chapter includes text excerpted from "Influenza Pandemics of the 20th Century," Centers for Disease Control and Prevention (CDC), February 16, 2012. Reviewed January 2020.

of hemagglutinin (HA) and neuraminidase (NA) antigens of the 1943 and 1947 viruses and comparison of their nucleotide and amino acid sequences showed marked differences in the viruses isolated in these 2 years; studies in a mouse model also showed that the 1943 vaccine afforded no protection to the 1947 virus challenge. Studies in the Fort Monmouth epidemic also documented, by serial bacterial cultures, for the first time the long-suspected relationship of influenza to group A streptococcal carriage and disease.

1976: Abortive, Potentially Pandemic, Swine Influenza Virus Epidemic, Fort Dix, New Jersey (H1N1)

In 1976 on February 13, influenza viruses isolated from patients at Fort Dix, New Jersey, a few days earlier and provisionally identified as swine influenza viruses were tested in a laboratory in New York City. A high-yield (6:2) genetic reassortant virus (X-53) was produced and later used as a vaccine in a clinical trial in 3,000 people. An even higher-yielding HA mutant virus, X-53a, was selected from X-53 and subsequently used in the mass vaccination of 43,000,000 people. When no cases were found outside Fort Dix in subsequent months and the neurologic complication of Guillain-Barré syndrome occurred in association with administration of swine influenza vaccine, the National Immunization Program (NIP) was abandoned, and the entire effort was assailed as a fiasco and disaster.

Experience had shown a decrease or even disappearance of epidemic viruses in the summer. However, they return in winter to produce disease in conditions favoring transmission: indoor crowding and decreased relative humidity. None of these facts was noted by critics of the program.

1977: Russian Flu, a Juvenile, Age-Restricted Pandemic, and the Return of Human H1N1 Virus

An obsession with geographic eponyms for a disease of worldwide distribution is best illustrated by Russian, or later red influenza or red flu, which first came to attention in November 1977, in the Soviet Union. However, it was later reported as having first occurred in northeastern China in May of that year. It quickly became apparent that this rapidly spreading epidemic was almost entirely restricted to persons <25 years of age and that, in general, the disease was mild, although characterized by typical symptoms of influenza. The age distribution was attributed to the absence of H1N1 viruses in humans after 1957 and the subsequent successive dominance of the H2N2 and H3N2 subtypes.

When antigenic and molecular characterization of this virus showed that both the HA and NA antigens were remarkably similar to those of the 1950s, this finding had profound implications. Where had the virus been that it was relatively unchanged after 20 years? If serially (and cryptically) transmitted in humans, antigenic drift should have led to many changes after 2 decades. Reactivation of a long-dormant infection was a possibility, but the idea conflicts with all we know of the biology of the virus in which a latent phase has not been found. Had the virus been in a deep freeze? This was a disturbing thought because it implied concealed experimentation with live virus, perhaps in a vaccine. Delayed mutation and consequent evolutionary stasis in an animal host are not unreasonable, but in what host? And if a full-blown epidemic did originate, it would be the first to do so in the history of modern virology and a situation quite unlike the contemporary situation with H5N1 and its protracted epizootic phase. Thus, the final answer to the 1977 epidemic is not yet known.

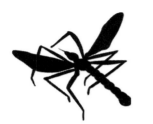

CHAPTER 9
Bioterrorism and the Pandemic Potential

Chapter Contents

Section 9.1
Bioterrorism Basics

This section includes text excerpted from "Biodefense and Bioterrorism," MedlinePlus, National Institutes of Health (NIH), April 7, 2017.

What Is Bioterrorism?

A bioterrorism attack is the deliberate release of viruses, bacteria, or other germs to cause illness or death. These germs are often found in nature. But, they can sometimes be made more harmful by increasing their ability to cause disease, spread, or resist medical treatment.

What Are Biological Agents?*

Biological agents are organisms or toxins that can kill or incapacitate people, livestock, and crops.

There are three basic groups of biological agents that could likely be used as weapons: bacteria, viruses, and toxins. Biological agents can be dispersed by spraying them into the air, person-to-person contact, infecting animals that carry the disease to humans and by contaminating food and water.

Text excerpted from "Bioterrorism," Ready, U.S. Department of Homeland Security (DHS), July 31, 2017

Biological agents do not cause illness for several hours or days.

Scientists worry that anthrax, botulism, Ebola and other hemorrhagic fever viruses (HFV), plague, or smallpox could be used as biological agents.

Potential List of Biological Agents**

Category A. The U.S. public-health system and primary-healthcare providers must be prepared to address various biological agents, including pathogens that are rarely seen in the United States. High-priority agents include organisms that pose a risk to national security because they can:

- Can be easily disseminated or transmitted from person to person
- Result in high mortality rates and have the potential for major public-health impact
- Might cause public panic and social disruption
- Require special action for public-health preparedness

Agents and diseases under this category include anthrax (*Bacillus anthracis*), botulism (*Clostridium botulinum toxin*), plague (*Yersinia pestis*), smallpox (variola major), tularemia (*Francisella tularensis*), viral hemorrhagic fevers (VHF), including filoviruses (Ebola, Marburg) and arenaviruses (Lassa, Machupo)

Category B. Second highest priority agents include those that:

- Are moderately easy to disseminate
- Result in moderate morbidity rates and low mortality rates
- Require specific enhancements of the Centers for Disease Control and Prevention's (CDC) diagnostic capacity and enhanced disease surveillance

Agents and diseases under this category include brucellosis (*Brucella species*), Epsilon toxin of Clostridium perfringens, food safety threats (*Salmonella species, Escherichia coli O157: H7, Shigella*), glanders (*Burkholderia mallei*), melioidosis (*Burkholderia pseudomallei*), psittacosis (*Chlamydia psittaci*), Q fever (*Coxiella burnetii*), ricin toxin from Ricinus communis (*castor beans*), Staphylococcal enterotoxin B, typhus fever (*Rickettsia prowazekii*), viral encephalitis (alphaviruses, such as eastern equine encephalitis, Venezuelan equine encephalitis (VEE), and western equine encephalitis (WEE)), and water safety threats (*Vibrio cholerae, Cryptosporidium parvum*).

Category C. Third highest priority agents include emerging pathogens that could be engineered for mass dissemination in the future because of:

- Availability
- Ease of production and dissemination
- Potential for high morbidity and mortality rates and major health impact

Agents under this category include emerging infectious diseases such as Nipah virus and hantavirus.

**Text excerpted from "Bioterrorism Agents/Diseases," Centers for Disease Control and Prevention (CDC), April 4, 2018

How Bioterrorism Can Be Countered

Biodefense uses medical measures to protect people against bioterrorism. This includes medicines and vaccinations. It also includes medical research and preparations to defend against bioterrorist attacks.

Section 9.2

Potential Biological Agents

This section contains text excerpted from the following sources:
Text under the heading "Anthrax" is excerpted from "Anthrax," Centers for Disease Control and Prevention (CDC), January 31, 2017; Text under the heading "Smallpox" is excerpted from "Smallpox," Centers for Disease Control and Prevention (CDC), July 12, 2017; Text under the heading "Glanders" is excerpted from "Glanders," Centers for Disease Control and Prevention (CDC), October 31, 2017; Text under the heading "Melioidosis" is excerpted from "Melioidosis," Centers for Disease Control and Prevention (CDC), August 8, 2017.

Anthrax

Anthrax is a serious infectious disease caused by gram-positive, rod-shaped bacteria known as *"Bacillus anthracis."* Although it is rare, people can get sick with anthrax if they come in contact with infected animals or contaminated animal products.

Why Would Anthrax Be Used as a Weapon?

If a bioterrorist attack were to happen, *Bacillus anthracis*, the bacteria that causes anthrax, would be one of the biological agents most likely to be used.

Figure 9.1. Potential
Risks of Anthrax

The type of illness a person develops depends on how anthrax spores enter the body. All types of anthrax can cause death if they are not treated with antibiotics.

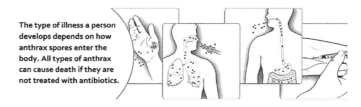

Biological agents are germs that can sicken or kill people, livestock, or crops. Anthrax is one of the most likely agents to be used because:

- Anthrax spores are easily found in nature, can be produced in a lab, and can last for a long time in the environment.
- Anthrax makes a good weapon because it can be released quietly and without anyone knowing. The microscopic spores could be put into powders, sprays, food, and water. Because they are so small, you may not be able to see, smell, or taste them.
- Anthrax has been used as a weapon before.

Anthrax has been used as a weapon around the world for nearly a century. In 2001, powdered anthrax spores were deliberately put into letters that were mailed through the U.S. postal system. It was reported that 22 people, including 12 mail handlers, got anthrax, and 5 of them died.

How Dangerous Is Anthrax?

A subset of select agents and toxins have been designated as Tier 1 because these biological agents and toxins present the greatest risk of deliberate misuse with significant potential for mass casualties or devastating effects to the economy, critical infrastructure, or public confidence, and pose a severe threat to public health and safety. *Bacillus anthracis* is a Tier 1 agent.

B. anthracis is a select agent. The possession, use, or transfer of *B. anthracis* is regulated by the Division of Select Agents and Toxins (DSAT), located in the Centers for Disease Control and Prevention's (CDC) Office of Public Health Preparedness and Response (OPHPR).

What Might an Anthrax Attack Look Like?

An anthrax attack could take many forms. For example, it could be placed in letters and mailed, as was done in 2001, or it could be put into food or water. Anthrax also could be released into the air from a truck, building, or plane. This type of attack would mean the anthrax spores could easily be blown around by the wind or carried on people's clothes, shoes, and other objects. It only takes a small amount of anthrax to infect a large number of people.

If anthrax spores were released into the air, people could breathe them in and get sick with anthrax. Inhalation anthrax is the most serious form and can kill quickly if not treated immediately. If the attack were not detected by one of the monitoring systems in place in the United States, it might go unnoticed until doctors begin to see unusual patterns of illness among sick people showing up in emergency rooms.

Smallpox

Thousands of years ago, the variola virus (smallpox virus) emerged and began causing illness and deaths in human populations, with smallpox outbreaks occurring from time to time. Thanks to the success of vaccination, the last natural outbreak of smallpox in the United States, occurred in 1949. In 1980, the World Health Assembly (WHA) declared smallpox eradicated (eliminated), and no cases of naturally occurring smallpox have happened since.

Smallpox research in the United States continues and focuses on the development of vaccines, drugs, and diagnostic tests to protect people against smallpox in the event that it is used as an agent of bioterrorism. There is no immediate, direct threat of a bioterrorist attack using smallpox. No bioterrorist attack using smallpox has happened in modern times. Throughout history, though, some people have used smallpox to their advantage by deliberately infecting their enemies with the disease.

Why Is Smallpox a Concern?

Public-health authorities are concerned about smallpox because it is a serious—even deadly—disease. Nowadays, there are only two labs in the world that are approved to have the smallpox virus for research: the CDC in the United States and the Russian State Centre for Research on Virology and Biotechnology in the Russian Federation. There is a credible concern that in the past some countries made the virus into weapons, which may have fallen into the hands of terrorists or other people with criminal intentions.

The last natural outbreak of smallpox in the United States happened in 1949. The last naturally spread case in the entire world happened in 1977. The WHA declared smallpox eradicated in 1980. Even a single confirmed case of smallpox today would be considered an emergency.

If the virus that causes smallpox were used in a bioterrorist attack, people who come into contact with the virus would be at risk of getting sick. By 1972, the smallpox vaccine was no longer given routinely in the United States. As a result, most people born in the United States after 1972 have not been vaccinated against the disease. Some people have been vaccinated through the military or because they were part of Smallpox Response Teams that were formed after the 9/11 terrorist attacks. These vaccination efforts are part of the larger plan to prepare for a bioterrorist attack. However, the vaccine does not give lifelong immunity, and people who have been vaccinated against smallpox before may still need to be revaccinated in a smallpox emergency.

What Might a Bioterrorist Attack with Smallpox Look Like?

Most likely, if smallpox is released into the United States as a bioterrorist attack, public-health authorities will find out once the first person sick with the disease goes to a hospital for treatment of an unknown illness. Doctors will examine the person and use tools developed by the CDC to figure out if the person's signs and symptoms are similar to those of smallpox. If doctors suspect the person has smallpox, they will care for the person and isolate them in the hospital so that others do not come in contact with the smallpox virus. The medical staff at the hospital will contact local public-health authorities to let them know they have a patient who might have smallpox.

Local public-health authorities would then alert public-health officials at the state and federal levels, such as the CDC, to help diagnose the disease. If experts confirm the illness is smallpox, then the CDC, along with state and local public-health authorities, will put into place their plans to respond to a bioterrorist attack with smallpox.

Glanders

Glanders is an infectious disease that is caused by the bacterium Burkholderia mallei. While people can get the disease, glanders is primarily a disease affecting horses. It also affects donkeys and mules and can be naturally contracted by other mammals such as goats, dogs, and cats.

Why Might Glanders Be Used as a Weapon?

If people or groups wanted to use germs as a weapon, they might use the germs that cause glanders because they:

- Can cause a disease that could make people very sick. Without prompt treatment with specific antibiotics, people sick with glanders can die.
- Can cause a disease that is rare and not well-known, which might make it more difficult for healthcare providers to diagnose a person with glanders quickly and accurately
- Have been used as a biological weapon in the past

How Dangerous Is Glanders?

Glanders can be a serious disease. Without treatment with specific antibiotics, as many as 9 of every 10 people who get it die. When people with glanders get treatment with the correct antibiotics, up to 5 of 10 people die.

People sick with glanders often need to be hospitalized for treatment. Even after they are well enough to go home, people who have had glanders need to take antibiotics for several months. This long period of treatment makes sure the antibiotics kill all the glanders germs in the person's body and prevent the disease from coming back.

It can also be difficult to diagnose glanders quickly. The symptoms of glanders are the same as more common diseases, such as community-acquired pneumonia (CAP), the flu, or tuberculosis (TB). Only a few people are diagnosed with glanders each year in the entire world. Because glanders in humans is so rare, most doctors are unfamiliar with the disease.

What Might an Attack with Glanders Look Like?

A biological attack that releases glanders germs into the air, water, or food supply might put many people at risk of getting sick. For example, if the germs that cause glanders were released into the air in a crowded place, many people might inhale them. Or, if the germs were put into food, people who eat the contaminated food would eat the germs, too. Anyone who comes into contact with these germs is in danger of getting sick with glanders.

It might not be known right away that there had been an attack because you cannot see, smell, or taste the germs. An attack might not be noticed until doctors begin to see many people sick with fevers and respiratory illnesses. Once doctors diagnose patients with glanders, they will work with public-health authorities to find out how the patients came into contact with the glanders germs.

Could My Pets or Livestock Get Sick with Glanders?

Because glanders has been eradicated (eliminated) from the United States since the 1940s, it is extremely unlikely that pets or livestock will get the disease naturally. However, if there were ever a biological attack that released the germs that cause glanders into the air or into an animal's food or water supply, certain kinds of animals could get sick. Animals that are likely to get glanders after coming into contact with these germs are:

- Livestock and farm animals
  - Horses, donkeys, and mules
  - Goats
- Household pets
  - Dogs
  - Cats
  - Rabbits
  - Guinea pigs
  - Hamsters

Of note, cattle, swine, and chickens appear to be resistant to glanders.

If a biological attack with glanders germs ever happens, public-health authorities and veterinarians will give more information about what to do if you think your pets or livestock might have glanders.

Melioidosis

Melioidosis, also called "Whitmore disease," is an infectious disease that can infect humans or animals. The disease is caused by the bacterium *Burkholderia pseudomallei*.

It is predominantly a disease of tropical climates, especially in Southeast Asia and northern Australia, where it is widespread. The bacteria causing melioidosis are found in contaminated water and soil. It is spread to humans and animals through direct contact with the contaminated source.

Why Might Germs That Cause Melioidosis Be Used as a Weapon?

If people or groups wanted to use germs as a weapon, they might use the germs that cause melioidosis because:

- They are found in nature in certain parts of the world
- They cause a disease that can make people very sick. Without prompt treatment with specific antibiotics, people sick with melioidosis can die.
- In the past, some countries that have used bioweapons during the war have used germs closely related to the one that causes melioidosis

How Dangerous Is Melioidosis?

Melioidosis can be a serious disease. Melioidosis germs are naturally resistant to many commonly used antibiotics, which makes the disease difficult to treat. There are a few antibiotics that are effective, though. Without treatment, up to 9 out of every 10 people who get it die. When people with melioidosis get treatment with the correct antibiotics, fewer than 4 out of 10 people die. Medical treatment in an intensive care facility can decrease deaths even more. Only 2 out of 10 people die when they get this level of medical treatment.

People with certain medical conditions are more likely than others to get melioidosis if they come into contact with the germs that cause it. Some of these conditions are diabetes, heavy alcohol use, chronic lung disease, chronic kidney disease (CKD), and others that affect the immune system.

People sick with melioidosis frequently need to be hospitalized for treatment. Even after they are well enough to go home, people who have had melioidosis need to take antibiotics for several months. This long period of treatment makes sure the antibiotics kill all the melioidosis germs in the person's body and prevent the disease from coming back.

It can also be hard to diagnose melioidosis quickly. The symptoms of melioidosis are the same as more common diseases, such as CAP, flu, or TB. There are only a few people diagnosed with melioidosis each year in the United States. Those who get melioidosis usually come into contact with the germs that cause it when they are traveling or living in a country where it is found naturally. Because there are so few people in the United States who get melioidosis, most doctors are unfamiliar with the disease.

What Might an Attack with Germs That Cause Melioidosis Look Like?

A biological attack that releases germs that cause melioidosis into the air, water, or food might put many people at risk of getting sick. For example, if the germs were released into the air in a crowded place, many people might inhale them. Or, if the germs were put into food, people who eat the contaminated food would eat the germs, too. Anyone who comes into contact with these germs is in danger of getting sick with melioidosis.

You cannot see, smell, or taste the germs, so people might not know right away if there had been an attack. An attack might not be noticed until doctors begin to see many people sick with fevers and respiratory illnesses. Once doctors diagnose patients with melioidosis, they will work with public-health authorities to find out how the patients came into contact with the melioidosis germs.

Section 9.3

Before, during, and after a Biological Threat

This section includes text excerpted from "Bioterrorism," Ready, U.S. Department of Homeland Security (DHS), July 31, 2017.

Before a Biological Threat

A biological attack may or may not be immediately obvious. In most cases, local healthcare workers will report a pattern of unusual illness or there will be a wave of sick people seeking emergency medical attention. The public would be alerted through an emergency radio or television broadcast, or some other signal used in your community, such as a telephone call or a home visit from an emergency response worker.

The following are things you can do to protect yourself, your family, and your property from the effects of a biological threat:

- Build an emergency supply kit
- Make a family emergency plan
- Check with your doctor to ensure all required or suggested immunizations are up to date for yourself, your children and elderly family members.
- Consider installing a high-efficiency particulate air (HEPA) filter in your furnace return duct, which will filter out most biological agents that may enter your house

During a Biological Threat

The first evidence of an attack may be when you notice symptoms of the disease caused by exposure to an agent. In the event of a biological attack, public-health officials may not immediately be able to provide information on what you should do. It will take time to determine exactly what the illness is, how it should be treated, and who is in danger.

Follow these guidelines during a biological threat:

- Watch TV, listen to the radio, or check the Internet for official news and information including signs and symptoms of the disease, areas in danger, if medications or vaccinations are being distributed and where you should seek medical attention if you become ill.
- If you become aware of an unusual and suspicious substance, quickly get away.
- Cover your mouth and nose with layers of fabric that can filter the air but still allow breathing. Examples include two to three layers of cotton such as a t-shirt, handkerchief or towel.
- Depending on the situation, wear a face mask to reduce inhaling or spreading germs.
- If you have been exposed to a biological agent, remove and bag your clothes and personal items. Follow official instructions for the disposal of contaminated items.
- Wash with soap and water and put on clean clothes.
- Contact authorities and seek medical assistance. You may be advised to stay away from others or even quarantined.
- If your symptoms match those described and you are in the group considered at risk, immediately seek emergency medical attention.
- Follow the instructions of doctors and other public-health officials.
- If the disease is contagious expect to receive medical evaluation and treatment.
- For noncontagious diseases, expect to receive medical evaluation and treatment.
- In a declared biological emergency or developing epidemic avoid crowds.
- Wash your hands with soap and water frequently.
- Do not share food or utensils.

After a Biological Threat

Pay close attention to all official warnings and instructions on how to proceed. The delivery of medical services for a biological event may be handled differently to respond to increased demand.

The basic public-health procedures and medical protocols for handling exposure to biological agents are the same as for any infectious disease. It is important for you to pay attention to official instructions via radio, television, and emergency alert systems.

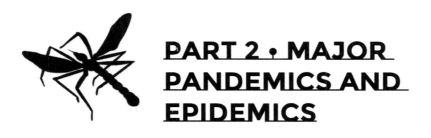

PART 2 • MAJOR PANDEMICS AND EPIDEMICS

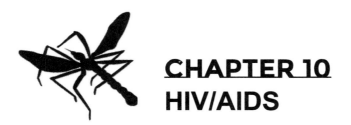

CHAPTER 10
HIV/AIDS

Chapter Contents

HIV/AIDS Basics

This section contains text excerpted from the following sources: Text in this section begins with excerpts from "About HIV/AIDS," Centers for Disease Control and Prevention (CDC), December 2, 2019; Text beginning with the heading "What Is HIV/AIDS?" is excerpted from "HIV/AIDS: The Basics," AIDS*info*, U.S. Department of Health and Human Services (HHS), July 3, 2019.

Human immunodeficiency virus (HIV) is a virus spread through certain body fluids that attacks the body's immune system, specifically the CD4 cells, often called "T cells." Over time, HIV can destroy so many of these cells that the body cannot fight off infections and disease. These special cells help the immune system fight off infections. Untreated, HIV reduces the number of CD4 cells (T cells) in the body. This damage to the immune system makes it harder and harder for the body to fight off infections and some other diseases. Opportunistic infections or cancers take advantage of a very weak immune system and signal that the person has acquired immunodeficiency syndrome (AIDS).

Scientists identified a type of chimpanzee in Central Africa as the source of HIV infection in humans. They believe that the chimpanzee version of the immunodeficiency virus (called "simian immunodeficiency virus," or "SIV") most likely was transmitted to humans and mutated into HIV when humans hunted these chimpanzees for meat and came into contact with their infected blood. Studies show that HIV may have jumped from apes to humans as far back as the late 1800s. Over the decades, the virus slowly spread across Africa and later into other parts of the world.

What Is HIV/AIDS?

HIV stands for "human immunodeficiency virus," which is the virus that causes HIV infection. The abbreviation "HIV" can refer to the virus or to HIV infection.

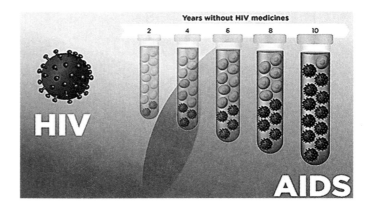

Figure 10.1. HIV and AIDS

AIDS stands for "acquired immunodeficiency syndrome." AIDS is the most advanced stage of HIV infection.

Human immunodeficiency virus attacks and destroys the infection-fighting cluster of differentiation 4 (CD4) cells (T cells) of the immune system. The loss of CD4 cells makes it difficult for the body to fight off infections and certain cancers. Without treatment, HIV can gradually destroy the immune system and advance to AIDS.

How Is HIV Spread?

The spread of HIV from person to person is called "HIV transmission." HIV spreads only in certain body fluids from a person who has HIV. These body fluids include:
- Blood
- Semen
- Preseminal fluid
- Vaginal fluids
- Rectal fluids
- Breast milk

Human immunodeficiency virus transmission is only possible through contact with HIV-infected body fluids. In the United States, HIV is spread mainly by:

————— HIV IS NOT TRANSMITTED BY —————

Air or Water

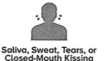
Saliva, Sweat, Tears, or
Closed-Mouth Kissing

Insects or Pets

Sharing Toilets,
Food, or Drinks

Figure 10.2. Facts about HIV Transmission *(Source: "HIV Transmission,"
Centers for Disease Control and Prevention (CDC))*

- Having anal or vaginal sex with someone who has HIV without using a condom or taking medicines to prevent or treat HIV
- Sharing injection-drug equipment (works), such as needles, with someone who has HIV

The spread of HIV from a woman with HIV to her child during pregnancy, childbirth, or breastfeeding is called "mother-to-child transmission of HIV."

You cannot get HIV by shaking hands or hugging a person who has HIV. You also cannot get HIV from contact with objects, such as dishes, toilet seats, or doorknobs used by a person with HIV. HIV is not spread through the air or in water or by mosquitoes, ticks, or other blood-sucking insects.

How Can You Reduce Your Risk of Getting HIV?

To reduce your risk of HIV infection, use condoms correctly every time you have sex, limit your number of sexual partners, and never share injection-drug equipment.

Also, talk to your healthcare provider about pre-exposure prophylaxis (PrEP). PrEP is an HIV prevention option for people who do not have HIV but who are at high risk of becoming infected with HIV. PrEP involves taking a specific HIV medicine every day.

Human immunodeficiency virus medicines, given to women with HIV during pregnancy and childbirth and to their babies after birth, reduce the risk of mother-to-child transmission of HIV. In addition, because HIV can be transmitted in breast milk, women with HIV should not breastfeed their babies. Baby formula is a safe and healthy alternative to breast milk.

What Are the Symptoms of HIV/AIDS?

Within two to four weeks after infection with HIV, some people may have flu-like symptoms, such as fever, chills, or rash. The symptoms may last for a few days to several weeks. During this earliest stage of HIV infection, the virus multiplies rapidly.

After the initial stage of infection, HIV continues to multiply but at very low levels. More severe symptoms of HIV infection, such as signs of opportunistic infections (infections that are more severe in people with weakened immune systems), generally do not appear for many years.

Without treatment with HIV medicines, HIV infection usually advances to AIDS in 10 years or longer, though it may advance faster in some people.

Human immunodeficiency virus transmission is possible at any stage of HIV infection—even if a person with HIV has no symptoms of HIV.

How Is AIDS Diagnosed?

Symptoms, such as fever, weakness, and weight loss may be a sign that a person's HIV has advanced to AIDS. However, a diagnosis of AIDS is based on the following criteria:

- A drop in CD4 count to less than 200 cells/mm. A CD4 count measures the number of CD4 cells in a sample of blood, or
- The presence of certain opportunistic infections

Although an AIDS diagnosis indicates severe damage to the immune system, HIV medicines can still help people at this stage of HIV infection.

What Is the Treatment for HIV?

Antiretroviral therapy (ART) is the use of HIV medicines to treat HIV infection. People on ART take a combination of HIV medicines (called an "HIV treatment regimen") every day.

Antiretroviral therapy is recommended for everyone who has HIV. ART prevents HIV from multiplying, which reduces the amount of HIV in the body (called the "viral load"). Having less HIV in the body protects the immune system and prevents HIV infection from advancing to AIDS. ART cannot cure HIV, but HIV medicines help people with HIV live longer, healthier lives. ART also reduces the risk of HIV transmission. The main goal of ART is to reduce a person's viral load to an undetectable level. An undetectable viral load means that the level of HIV in the blood is too low to be detected by a viral load test. People with HIV who maintain an undetectable viral load have effectively no risk of transmitting HIV to their HIV-negative partner through sex.

Section 10.2
Global Impact of HIV

This section includes text excerpted from "Global HIV/AIDS Overview," HIV.gov, U.S. Department of Health and Human Services (HHS), July 31, 2019.

The Global HIV/AIDS Epidemic

Human immunodeficiency virus (HIV), the virus that causes acquired immunodeficiency syndrome (AIDS), is one of the world's most serious public-health challenges. But there is a global commitment to stopping new HIV infections and ensuring that everyone with HIV has access to HIV treatment.

Number of People with HIV

There were approximately 37.9 million people across the globe, with HIV/AIDS in 2018. Of these, 36.2 million were adults, and 1.7 million were children (<15 years old).

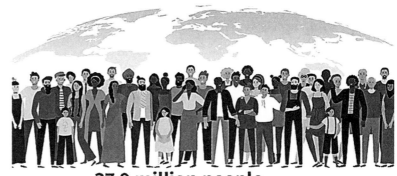

37.9 million people worldwide are currently living with HIV or AIDS.

Figure 10.3. Global Impact of HIV/AIDS

New HIV Infections

An estimated 1.7 million individuals worldwide became newly infected with HIV in 2018. ("New HIV infections" or "HIV incidence" refers to the estimated number of people who newly acquired HIV during a year, which is different from the number of people diagnosed with HIV during a year. Some people may have HIV but not know it.) Of these new infections:

- 1.6 million infections were among people ages 15 and older
- 160,000 infections were among children ages 0 to 14

HIV Testing

Approximately 79 percent of people with HIV globally knew their HIV status in 2018. The remaining 21 percent (about 8.1 million people) still need access to HIV testing services. HIV testing is an essential gateway to HIV prevention, treatment, care, and support services.

HIV Treatment Access

In 2018, 23.3 million people with HIV (62%) were accessing antiretroviral therapy (ART) globally, an increase of 1.6 million since 2017, and up from 8 million in 2010. HIV treatment access is key to the global effort to

Almost **80%** of people with HIV worldwide have been tested and **know their HIV status.**

Testing is the essential **first step** to accessing treatment.

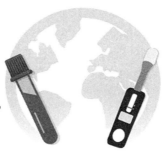

Figure 10.4. HIV Testing across the Globe

end AIDS as a public-health threat. People with HIV, who are aware of their status, take ART daily as prescribed, and keep an undetectable viral load, can live long, healthy lives, and have effectively no risk of sexually transmitting HIV to their HIV-negative partners.

HIV Care Continuum

The term "HIV care continuum" refers to the sequence of steps a person with HIV takes from diagnosis through receiving treatment until her or his viral load is suppressed to undetectable levels. Each step in the continuum is marked by an assessment of the number of people who have reached that stage. The stages include; being diagnosed with HIV, being linked to medical care, starting ART, adhering to the treatment regimen; and, finally, having HIV suppressed to undetectable levels in the blood. The Joint United Nations Program on HIV/AIDS (UNAIDS) 90-90-90 goals set as targets that by 2020, 90 percent of all people with HIV will know their HIV status; 90 percent of all people who know their status will be on ART; and 90 percent of all people receiving ART will have viral suppression. Tracking progress toward those goals, UNAIDS reports that in 2018, of all people with HIV worldwide:

- 79 percent knew their HIV status
- 78 percent of all people who knew their status were accessing ART
- 86 percent of all people receiving ART had viral suppression

Mother-to-Child Transmission

In 2018, 92 percent of pregnant women with HIV received ART to prevent transmitting HIV to their babies during pregnancy and childbirth and to protect their health. This is compared to 49 percent in 2010.

AIDS-Related Deaths

Acquired immunodeficiency syndrome-related deaths have been reduced by more than 55 percent since its peak in 2004. In 2018, around 770,000 people died from AIDS-related illnesses worldwide, compared to 1.2 million in 2010 and 1.7 million in 2004.

Regional Impact

The vast majority of people with HIV are in low- and middle-income countries. In 2018, there were 20.6 million people with HIV (57%) in eastern and southern Africa, 5.0 million (13%) in western and central Africa, 5.9 million (16%) in Asia and the Pacific, and 2.2 million (6%) in western and central Europe and North America.

Challenges and Progress

Despite advances in our scientific understanding of HIV and its prevention and treatment as well as years of significant effort by the global-health community and leading government and civil society organizations, too many people with HIV or at risk for HIV still do not have access to prevention, care, and treatment, and there is still no cure. Further, the HIV epidemic not only affects the health of individuals, but it also impacts households, communities, and the development and economic growth of nations. Many of the countries hardest hit by HIV also suffer from other infectious diseases, food insecurity, and other serious problems.

Despite these challenges, there have been successes and promising signs. New global efforts have been mounted to address the epidemic, particularly in the last decade. The number of people newly infected with HIV has declined over the years. In addition, the number of people with HIV receiving treatment in resource-poor countries has dramatically increased in the past decade and dramatic progress has been made in preventing mother-to-child transmission of HIV and keeping mothers alive.

However, despite the availability of a widening array of effective HIV prevention tools and methods and a massive scale-up of HIV treatment in recent years, UNAIDS cautions that the pace of progress in reducing new HIV infections, increasing access to treatment, and ending AIDS-related deaths is slowing down, with some countries making impressive gains while others are experiencing rises in new HIV infections and AIDS-related deaths.

The United States' Response to the Global Epidemic

The U.S. President's Emergency Plan for AIDS Relief (PEPFAR) is the U.S. Government's response to the global HIV/AIDS epidemic and represents the largest commitment by any nation to address a single disease in history. Through PEPFAR, the U.S. has supported a world safer and more secure from infectious disease threats. It has demonstrably strengthened the global capacity to prevent, detect, and respond to new and existing risks—which ultimately enhances global-health security and protects America's borders.

In addition, the National Institutes of Health (NIH) represents the largest public investment in HIV/AIDS research in the world. NIH is engaged in research around the globe to understand, diagnose, treat, and prevent HIV infection and its many associated conditions, and to find a cure.

Section 10.3

Ending the HIV Epidemic: A Plan for America

This section includes text excerpted from "What Is 'Ending the HIV Epidemic: A Plan for America'?" HIV.gov, U.S. Department of Health and Human Services (HHS), September 3, 2019.

In the State of the Union Address on February 5, 2019, President Donald J. Trump announced his Administration's goal to end the human immunodeficiency virus (HIV) epidemic in the United States within 10 years. To achieve this goal and address the ongoing public-health crisis of HIV, the proposed Ending the HIV Epidemic: A Plan for America will leverage the powerful data and tools now available to reduce new HIV infections in the United States by 75 percent in 5 years and by 90 percent by 2030.

Background

Human immunodeficiency virus has cost America too much for too long and remains a significant public-health issue:

- More than 700,000 American lives have been lost to HIV since 1981.
- More than 1.1 million Americans are currently living with HIV and many more are at risk of HIV infection.
- While new HIV diagnoses have declined significantly from their peak, progress on further reducing them has stalled with an estimated 40,000 Americans being newly diagnosed each year. Without intervention another 400,000 Americans will be newly diagnosed over 10 years despite the available tools to prevent infections.
- The U.S. government spends $20 billion in annual direct health expenditures for HIV prevention and care.
- There is a real risk of an HIV resurgence due to several factors, including injection-drug use and diagnostic complacency among healthcare providers.

Goal

The new initiative seeks to reduce the number of new HIV infections in the United States by 75 percent within 5 years, and then by at least 90 percent within 10 years, for an estimated 250,000 total HIV infections averted.

Right Leadership

This initiative will leverage critical scientific advances in HIV prevention, diagnosis, treatment, and care by coordinating the highly successful programs, resources, and infrastructure of many U.S. Department of Health and Human Services (HHS) agencies and offices, including the:

- Centers for Disease Control and Prevention (CDC)
- Health Resources and Services Administration (HRSA)
- Indian Health Service (IHS)
- National Institutes of Health (NIH)
- Office of the HHS Assistant Secretary for Health
- Substance Abuse and Mental Health Services Administration (SAMHSA)

The HHS Office of the Assistant Secretary for Health (OASH) is coordinating this cross-agency Plan.

Right Data and Right Tools

Nowadays, there are tools available to end the HIV epidemic. Landmark biomedical and scientific research advances have led to the development of many successful HIV treatment regimens, prevention strategies, and improved care for persons living with HIV.

- Data reveals that most new infections occur in a limited number of counties and among specific populations.
- Thanks to advances in antiretroviral therapy (ART), the medicine used to treat HIV, individuals with HIV who take their medicine as prescribed and, as a result, maintain an undetectable viral load can live long, healthy lives and have effectively no risk of sexually transmitting HIV to a partner.

- There are proven models of effective HIV care and prevention based on over two decades of experience engaging and retaining patients in effective care. Pre-exposure prophylaxis (PrEP), a daily regimen of two oral antiretroviral drugs in a single pill, has proven to be highly effective in preventing HIV infection for individuals at high risk, reducing the risk of acquiring HIV by up to 97 percent.
- New laboratory and epidemiological techniques help to pinpoint where HIV infections are spreading most rapidly so health officials can respond swiftly with resources to stop further spread of new infections.

With these powerful data and tools, the Administration sees a once-in-a-generation opportunity to end the epidemic.

Whole-of-Society Initiative

In addition to the coordination of federal agencies, key components for the success of this initiative will be active partnerships with city, county, tribal, and state public-health departments, local and regional clinics, and healthcare facilities, clinicians, providers of medication-assisted treatment for opioid-use disorder (OUD), professional associations, advocates, community- and faith-based organizations, and academic and research institutions.

Budget Request

President Trump proposed $291 million in the FY2020 HHS budget to begin his administration's multiyear initiative focused on ending the HIV epidemic in America by 2030.

Phase I: Geographic Focus

Most new HIV infections in the United States are highly concentrated in certain geographic hotspots. More than 50 percent of new HIV diagnoses in 2016 and 2017 occurred in 48 counties, Washington, DC, and San Juan, Puerto Rico. It is also known that 7 states have a disproportionate occurrence of HIV in rural areas. For the first 5 years (Phase I), the initiative will focus on a rapid infusion of new resources, expertise, and technology into those parts of the country which are most impacted by HIV.

Phases II and III

In Phase II, efforts will be even more widely disseminated across the nation to reduce new infections by 90 percent by 2030. In Phase III, intensive case management will be implemented to maintain the number of new infections at fewer than 3,000 per year.

Challenges

Despite the game-changing developments in HIV prevention and treatment tools, not everyone is benefiting equally from these advances. New infections are highly concentrated among men who have sex with men; minorities, especially African Americans, Hispanics/Latinx, and American Indians and Alaska Natives; and those who live in the southern United States.

Further, analysis from the CDC shows the vast majority (about 80%) of new HIV infections in the United States in 2016 were transmitted from the nearly 40 percent of people with HIV who either did not know they had HIV or who had been diagnosed but were not receiving HIV care. These data underscore the impact of undiagnosed and untreated HIV in the nation and also the critical need to expand HIV testing and treatment in the United States.

And stigma—which can be a debilitating barrier preventing people from living with, or at risk for, HIV from receiving the healthcare, services, and respect they need and deserve—still tragically surrounds HIV. Responding to HIV is not just a biomedical issue, but a social challenge, too.

Effective interventions have driven the number of new HIV infections down to approximately 40,000 per year—the lowest level ever. However, the data show that the country's progress in reducing the number of new HIV infections has plateaued. Now there are new threats to the progress made, the most significant being the opioid crisis: 1 in 10 new HIV infections occur among people who inject drugs.

Key Strategies in the Plan

Ending the HIV Epidemic is a plan for America which will provide the hardest-hit communities with the additional expertise, technology, and resources required to address the HIV epidemic locally.

The plan's major areas of action include:

- **Increasing investments** in geographic hotspots through our existing, effective programs, such as the Ryan White HIV/AIDS Program, as well as a new program through community health centers that will provide PrEP to protect people at the highest risk for getting HIV.
- **Using data** to identify where HIV is spreading most rapidly and guide decision-making to address prevention, care, and treatment needs at the local level.
- **Supporting** the jurisdictions to establish local teams committed to the success of the Initiative and expand HIV prevention and treatment services.

The efforts will focus on four key strategies that together can end the HIV epidemic in the United States: diagnose, treat, prevent, and respond.

Diagnose all individuals with HIV as early as possible. Approximately 165,000 Americans are living with HIV but do not know they have it. Early detection is critical and can lead to quicker results in treatment and prevent transmission to others. Using the latest diagnostics and advanced automation systems will make HIV testing simple, accessible, and routine. And the diagnosis of infection early will become possible which in turn will help connect people with HIV immediately to care.

Treat people with HIV rapidly and effectively to reach sustained viral suppression. People with HIV who take medication as prescribed and stay virally suppressed can live long, healthy lives and have effectively no risk of sexually transmitting HIV to a partner. Eighty percent of annual new infections are transmitted by those living with HIV who are not receiving HIV care and treatment. Efforts will be made to establish and expand programs to follow up with people with HIV no longer receiving care— and provide the resources needed to reengage them with effective HIV care and treatment. The Ryan White HIV/AIDS Program has achieved a

Diagnose all people with HIV as early as possible.

Treat people with HIV rapidly and effectively to reach sustained viral suppression.

 Prevent new HIV transmissions by using proven interventions, including pre-exposure prophylaxis (PrEP) and syringe services programs (SSPs).

Respond quickly to potential HIV outbreaks to get needed prevention and treatment services to people who need them.

Figure 10.5. Key Strategies to End HIV Epidemic

viral suppression rate of nearly 86 percent. Plans are there to leverage the program's comprehensive system of care and treatment to increase viral suppression around the country to 90 percent.

Prevent new HIV transmissions by using proven interventions, including PrEP and syringe-services programs (SSPs). Of the estimated 1 million Americans at substantial risk for HIV and who could benefit from PrEP, less than 1 in 4 are actually using this medication. In May 2019, HHS and Gilead Sciences announced that the pharmaceutical company has agreed to donate PrEP medication for up to 200,000 individuals each year for up to 11 years. HHS will make the medication available to individuals who are at risk for HIV and who are uninsured and might otherwise not be able to access or afford this powerful HIV prevention tool. In addition, SSPs are an effective component of a comprehensive, integrated approach to HIV prevention among people who inject drugs. Nearly 30 years of research has shown that comprehensive SSPs are safe, effective, and cost-saving, do not increase illegal-drug use or crime and play an important role in reducing the transmission of viral hepatitis, HIV, and other infections.

Respond quickly to potential HIV outbreaks to get needed prevention and treatment services to people who need them. New laboratory methods and epidemiological techniques allow seeing where HIV may be spreading most rapidly, thereby allowing the CDC and other partners to quickly develop and implement strategies to stop ongoing transmission. Working with impacted communities will ensure that they have the technology, personnel, and prevention resources to follow up on all HIV cases and to intervene to stop chains of transmission, and to get those impacted into appropriate care and treatment.

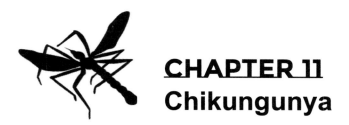

CHAPTER 11
Chikungunya

Chikungunya virus is spread to people by the bite of an infected mosquito. The most common symptoms of infection are fever and joint pain. Other symptoms may include headache, muscle pain, joint swelling, or rash. Outbreaks have occurred in countries in Africa, Asia, Europe, and the Indian and Pacific Oceans.

In late 2013, the chikungunya virus was found for the first time in the Americas on islands in the Caribbean. There is a risk that the virus will be imported to new areas by infected travelers. There is no vaccine to prevent or medicine to treat chikungunya virus infection. Travelers can protect themselves by preventing mosquito bites. When traveling to countries with chikungunya virus, use insect repellent, wear long sleeves and pants, and stay in places with air conditioning or that use window and door screens.

Symptoms of Chikungunya

Most people infected with the chikungunya virus will develop some symptoms. Symptoms usually begin three to seven days after being bitten by an infected mosquito. The most common symptoms are fever and joint pain. Other symptoms may include headache, muscle pain, joint swelling, or rash.

This chapter includes text excerpted from "Chikungunya Virus," Centers for Disease Control and Prevention (CDC), September 19, 2019.

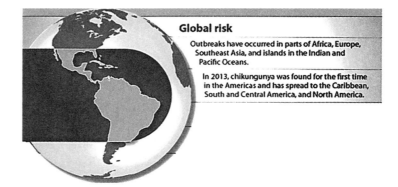

Figure 11.1. Chikungunya: A Global Risk *(Source: "Chikungunya Virus: What You Need to Know," Centers for Disease Control and Prevention (CDC))*

Chikungunya disease does not often result in death, but the symptoms can be severe and disabling. Most patients feel better within a week. In some people, joint pain may persist for months.

People at risk for more severe disease include newborns infected around the time of birth, older adults (≥65 years), and people with medical conditions, such as high blood pressure, diabetes, or heart disease.

Once a person has been infected, she or he is likely to be protected from future infections.

Diagnosis of Chikungunya

The symptoms of chikungunya are similar to those of dengue and Zika.

See your healthcare provider if you develop the symptoms described above and have visited an area where chikungunya is found. If you have recently traveled, tell your healthcare provider when and where you traveled. Your healthcare provider may order blood tests to look for chikungunya or other similar viruses such as dengue and Zika.

Treatment of Chikungunya

There is no vaccine to prevent or medicine to treat chikungunya virus. However, you can treat the symptoms:

- Get plenty of rest.
- Drink fluids to prevent dehydration.
- Take medicine such as acetaminophen (Tylenol®) or paracetamol to reduce fever and pain.
- Do not take aspirin and other nonsteroidal anti-inflammatory drugs (NSAIDs) until dengue can be ruled out to reduce the risk of bleeding.
- If you are taking medicine for another medical condition, talk to your healthcare provider before taking additional medication.

If you have chikungunya, prevent mosquito bites for the first week of your illness.
- During the first week of infection, the chikungunya virus can be found in the blood and passed from an infected person to a mosquito through mosquito bites.
- An infected mosquito can then spread the virus to other people.

Transmission of Chikungunya
Through Mosquito Bites
Chikungunya virus is transmitted to people through mosquito bites. Mosquitoes become infected when they feed on a person already infected with the virus. Infected mosquitoes can then spread the virus to other people through bites.

Chikungunya virus is most often spread to people by *Aedes aegypti* and *Aedes albopictus* mosquitoes. These are the same mosquitoes that transmit the dengue virus. They bite during the day and at night.

Mother to Child
Chikungunya virus is transmitted rarely from mother to newborn around the time of birth.

To date, no infants have been found to be infected with the chikungunya virus through breastfeeding. Because of the benefits of breastfeeding, mothers are encouraged to breastfeed even in areas where the chikungunya virus is circulating.

Infected Blood

In theory, the virus could be spread through a blood transfusion. To date, there are no known reports of this happening.

Prevention of Chikungunya

The most effective way to prevent infection from the chikungunya virus is to prevent mosquito bites. Mosquitoes bite during the day and night. Use insect repellent, wear long-sleeved shirts and pants, treat clothing and gear, and take steps to control mosquitoes indoors and outdoors.

Protect Yourself and Your Family from Mosquito Bites
Use Insect Repellent

Use the U.S. Environmental Protection Agency (EPA)-registered insect repellent with one of the active ingredients listed below.

- DEET
- Picaridin (known as "KBR 3023" and "icaridin outside the U.S.")
- IR3535
- Oil of lemon eucalyptus (OLE)
- Para-menthane-diol (PMD)
- 2-undercanone

When used as directed, EPA-registered insect repellents are proven safe and effective, even for pregnant and breastfeeding women.

Tips for Babies and Children

Dress your child in clothing that covers arms and legs. Cover strollers and baby carriers with mosquito netting.

When using insect repellent on your child:
- Always follow label instructions.
- Do not use products containing oil of lemon eucalyptus (OLE) or para-menthane-diol (PMD) on children under 3 years old.
- Do not apply insect repellent to a child's hands, eyes, mouth, cuts, or irritated skin.

- Adults: Spray insect repellent onto your hands and then apply to a child's face.

Tips for Everyone
Always follow the product label instructions.

Reapply insect repellent as directed.

- Do not spray repellent on the skin under clothing.
- If you are also using sunscreen, first apply sunscreen followed by insect repellent.

Natural Insect Repellents
Not much is known about the effectiveness of non-EPA registered insect repellents, including some natural repellents. To protect yourself against diseases spread by mosquitoes, the CDC and EPA recommend using an EPA-registered insect repellent. Choosing an EPA-registered repellent ensures that the product has been evaluated for its effectiveness.

Wear Long-Sleeved Shirts and Long Pants
When treating clothing and gear use permethrin to treat clothing and gear (such as boots, pants, socks, and tents) or buy permethrin-treated clothing and gear. Permethrin is an insecticide that kills or repels mosquitoes. Permethrin-treated clothing provides protection after washing multiple times. Read product information to find out how long the protection will last. If treating items yourself, follow the product instructions. Note, do not use permethrin products directly on the skin.

Take Steps to Control Mosquitoes Indoors and Outdoors
Use screens on windows and doors. Repair holes in screens to keep mosquitoes outdoors.

Use air conditioning, if available.

Stop mosquitoes from laying eggs in or near water.

- Once a week, empty and scrub, turn over, cover, or throw out items that hold water, such as tires, buckets, planters, toys, pools, birdbaths, flowerpots, or trash containers.
- Check indoors and outdoors.

Prevent Mosquito Bites When Traveling Overseas

Choose a hotel or lodging with air conditioning or screens on windows and doors. Sleep under a mosquito bed net if you are outside or in a room that does not have screens. Buy a bed net at your local outdoor store or online before traveling overseas.

Choose a World Health Organization Pesticide Evaluation Scheme (WHOPES)-approved bed net: compact, white, rectangular, with 156 holes per square inch, and long enough to tuck under the mattress.

Permethrin-treated bed nets provide more protection than untreated nets.

Do not wash bed nets or expose them to sunlight. This will break down the insecticide more quickly.

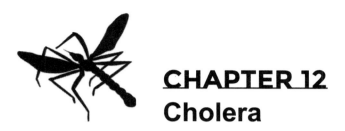

CHAPTER 12
Cholera

Cholera, caused by the bacteria *Vibrio cholerae*, is rare in the United States and other industrialized nations. However, globally, cholera cases have increased steadily since 2005 and the disease still occurs in many places including Africa, Southeast Asia, and Haiti.

Cholera can be life-threatening but it is easily prevented and treated. Travelers, public health and medical professionals, and outbreak responders should be aware of areas with high rates of cholera, know how the disease spreads, and what to do to prevent it.

What Is Cholera?

Cholera is an acute, diarrheal illness caused by infection of the intestine with the toxigenic bacterium *Vibrio cholerae* serogroup O1 or O139. An estimated 2.9 million cases and 95,000 deaths occur each year around the world.

Where Is Cholera Found?

The cholera bacterium is usually found in water or food sources that have been contaminated by feces (poop) from a person infected with cholera.

This chapter includes text excerpted from "Cholera-*Vibrio Cholerae* Infection," Centers for Disease Control and Prevention (CDC), May 3, 2018.

Cholera is most likely to be found and spread in places with inadequate water treatment, poor sanitation, and inadequate hygiene.

The cholera bacterium may also live in the environment in brackish rivers and coastal waters. Shellfish eaten raw have been a source of cholera, and a few persons in the United States have contracted cholera after eating raw or undercooked shellfish from the Gulf of Mexico.

How Does a Person Get Cholera?

A person can get cholera by drinking water or eating food contaminated with the cholera bacterium. In an epidemic, the source of the contamination is usually the feces of an infected person that contaminates water and/or food. The disease can spread rapidly in areas with inadequate treatment of sewage and drinking water. The disease is not likely to spread directly from one person to another; therefore, casual contact with an infected person is not a risk for becoming ill.

What Are the Symptoms of Cholera?

Cholera infection is often mild or without symptoms, but can sometimes be severe. Approximately one in ten (10%) infected persons will have severe disease characterized by profuse watery diarrhea, vomiting, and leg cramps. In these people, the rapid loss of body fluids leads to dehydration and shock. Without treatment, death can occur within hours.

It can take anywhere from a few hours to five days for symptoms to appear after infection. Symptoms typically appear in two-three days.

Who Is Most Likely to Get Cholera?

Individuals living in places with unsafe drinking water, poor sanitation, and inadequate hygiene are at a greater risk for cholera.

How Is Cholera Diagnosed?

To test for cholera, doctors must take a stool sample or a rectal swab and send it to a laboratory to look for the cholera bacterium.

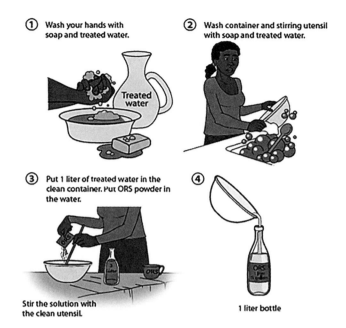

① Wash your hands with soap and treated water.

Treated water

② Wash container and stirring utensil with soap and treated water.

③ Put 1 liter of treated water in the clean container. Put ORS powder in the water.

④

Stir the solution with the clean utensil.

1 liter bottle

Figure 12.1. How to Prepare Oral Rehydration Solution *(Source: "How to Make Oral Rehydration Solution (ORS)," Centers for Disease Control and Prevention (CDC))*

What Is the Treatment for Cholera?

Cholera can be simply and successfully treated by immediate replacement of the fluid and salts lost through diarrhea. Patients can be treated with oral rehydration solution (ORS), a prepackaged mixture of sugar and salts to be mixed with one liter of water and drunk in large amounts. This solution is used throughout the world to treat diarrhea. Severe cases also require intravenous (IV) fluid replacement.

With prompt appropriate rehydration, fewer than one percent of cholera patients die.

Antibiotics shorten the course and diminish the severity of the illness, but they are not as important as receiving rehydration. Persons who develop severe diarrhea and vomiting in countries where cholera occurs should seek medical attention promptly.

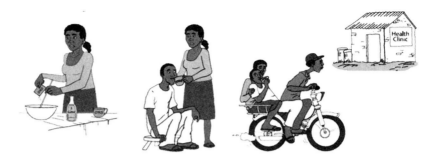

Figure 12.2. If You or Your Family Get Cholera *(Source: "If You or Your Family Get Cholera (Adult), Centers for Disease Control and Prevention (CDC))*

What Should You Do If You Think a Family Member or You Have Cholera?

If you think you or a member of your family may have cholera, seek medical attention immediately. Dehydration can be rapid so fluid replacement is essential. If you have an ORS, the ill person should start taking it immediately; it can save a life. She or he should continue to drink ORS at home and during travel to get medical treatment. If you have an infant who has watery diarrhea, continue to breastfeed.

Should You Be Worried about Getting Cholera from Others

The disease is not likely to spread directly from one person to another; therefore, casual contact with an infected person is not a risk for becoming ill.

How Can You Avoid Getting Cholera?

The risk for cholera is very low for people visiting areas with epidemic cholera. When simple precautions are observed, contracting the disease is unlikely.

All people (visitors or residents) in areas where cholera is occurring or has occurred should observe the following recommendations:

- Drink only bottled, boiled, or chemically treated water and bottled or canned carbonated beverages. When using bottled drinks, make sure that the seal has not been broken.
  - To disinfect your own water: boil for 1 minute or filter the water and add 2 drops of household bleach or ½ an iodine tablet per liter of water.
  - Avoid tap water, fountain drinks, and ice cubes.
- Wash your hands often with soap and clean water.
- If no water and soap are available, use an alcohol-based hand cleaner (with at least 60% alcohol).
  - Clean your hands, especially before eating or preparing food and after using the bathroom.
- Use bottled, boiled, or chemically treated water to wash dishes, brush your teeth, wash and prepare food, or make ice.
- Eat foods that are packaged or that are freshly cooked and served hot.
  - Do not eat raw or undercooked meats and seafood, or raw or undercooked fruits and vegetables unless they are peeled.
- Dispose of feces in a sanitary manner to prevent contamination of water and food sources.

Is There a Vaccine Available to Prevent Cholera?

The U.S. Food and Drug Administration (FDA) approved a single-dose live oral cholera vaccine called "Vaxchora®" (lyophilized CVD 103-HgR) for adults 18 to 64 years old who are traveling to an area of active cholera transmission with toxigenic *Vibrio cholerae* O1 (the bacteria strain that most commonly causes cholera). The vaccine is not routinely recommended for most travelers from the United States, as most people do not visit areas of active cholera transmission. Three other oral inactivated, or nonlive cholera vaccines, Dukoral®, ShanChol®, and Euvichol-Plus®/Euvichol® are World Health Organization (WHO) prequalified, but these vaccines are not available in the United States. No cholera vaccine is 100 percent protective and vaccination against cholera is not a substitute for standard prevention and control measures, including precautions for food and water as outlined above.

What Is the Risk for Cholera in the United States?

In the United States, cholera was prevalent in the 1800s but the water-related spread has been eliminated by modern water and sewage treatment systems. Very rarely, persons in the United States acquire cholera from shellfish consumed raw or inadequately cooked.

However, U.S. travelers to areas with epidemic cholera (for example, parts of Africa, Asia, or Latin America) may be exposed to the cholera bacterium. In addition, travelers may bring contaminated seafood back to the U.S. food-borne outbreaks of cholera have been caused by contaminated seafood brought into the United States by travelers.

What Is the U.S. Government Doing to Combat Cholera?

The U.S. and international public health authorities are working to enhance surveillance for cholera, investigate cholera outbreaks, and design and implement preventive measures across the globe. The Centers for Disease Control and Prevention (CDC) investigates epidemic cholera wherever it occurs at the invitation of the affected country and trains laboratory workers in proper techniques for identification of *Vibrio cholerae*. In addition, the CDC provides information on diagnosis, treatment, and prevention of cholera to public health officials and educates the public about effective preventive measures. The U.S. Agency for International Development sponsors some of the international U.S. government activities and provides medical supplies, and water, sanitation and hygiene supplies to affected countries.

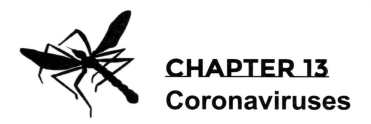

CHAPTER 13
Coronaviruses

Chapter Contents

Human Coronavirus Types

This section includes text excerpted from "Human Coronavirus Types," Centers for Disease Control and Prevention (CDC), January 10, 2020.

Coronaviruses are named for the crown-like spikes on their surface. There are four main subgroupings of coronaviruses, known as "alpha," "beta," "gamma," and "delta."

Human coronaviruses were first identified in the mid-1960s. The seven coronaviruses that can infect people are:

Common Human Coronaviruses
- 229E (alpha coronavirus)
- NL63 (alpha coronavirus)
- OC43 (beta coronavirus)
- HKU1 (beta coronavirus)

Other Human Coronaviruses
- SARS-CoV (the beta coronavirus that causes severe acute respiratory syndrome, or SARS)
- MERS-CoV (the beta coronavirus that causes Middle East Respiratory Syndrome, or MERS)
- 2019 Novel Coronavirus (2019-nCoV)

Sometimes coronaviruses that infect animals can evolve and make people sick and become a new human coronavirus. Three recent examples of this are 2019-nCoV, SARS-CoV, and MERS-CoV.

Section 13.2
SARS Coronavirus

This chapter includes text excerpted from "About
Severe Acute Respiratory Syndrome (SARS)," Centers
for Disease Control and Prevention (CDC), February
20, 2013. Reviewed January 2020.

Severe acute respiratory syndrome (SARS) is a viral-respiratory illness
caused by a coronavirus called "SARS-associated coronavirus" (SARS-
CoV). SARS was first reported in Asia in February 2003. The illness
spread to more than two dozen countries in North America, South
America, Europe, and Asia before the SARS global outbreak of 2003 was
contained.

There is no known SARS transmission anywhere in the world. The
human cases of SARS-CoV infection were reported in China in April
2004 in an outbreak resulting from laboratory-acquired infections (LAIs).
The Centers for Disease Control and Prevention (CDC) and its partners,
including the World Health Organization (WHO), continue to monitor
the SARS situation globally. Any new updates on disease transmission and
SARS preparedness activities will be posted on the CDC's website.

Signs and Symptoms of Severe Acute Respiratory Syndrome

The illness usually begins with a high fever (measured temperature
greater than 100.4°F (greater than 38.0°C)). The fever is sometimes
associated with chills or other symptoms, including headache, a general
feeling of discomfort, and body aches. Some people also experience mild
respiratory symptoms at the outset. Diarrhea is seen in approximately 10
to 20 percent of patients. After 2 to 7 days, SARS patients may develop
a dry, nonproductive cough that might be accompanied by or progress to
a condition in which the oxygen levels in the blood are low (hypoxia). In

10 to 20 percent of cases, patients require mechanical ventilation. Most patients develop pneumonia.

Causes of Severe Acute Respiratory Syndrome

A severe acute respiratory syndrome is caused by a previously unrecognized coronavirus SARS-CoV. It is possible that other infectious agents might have a role in some cases of SARS.

How Severe Acute Respiratory Syndrome Spread

The primary way that SARS appears to spread is by close person-to-person contact. SARS-CoV is thought to be transmitted most readily by respiratory droplets (droplet spread) produced when an infected person coughs or sneezes. Droplet spread can happen when droplets from the cough or sneeze of an infected person have propelled a short distance (generally up to 3 feet) through the air and deposited on the mucous membranes of the mouth, nose, or eyes of people who are nearby. The virus also can spread when a person touches a surface or object contaminated with infectious droplets and then touches her or his mouth, nose, or eye(s). In addition, it is possible that SARS-CoV might be spread more broadly through the air (airborne spread) or by other ways that are not now known.

Close Contact

"Close contact" is defined as having cared for or lived with a person known to have SARS or having a high likelihood of direct contact with respiratory secretions and/or body fluids of a patient known to have SARS. Examples include kissing or embracing, sharing eating or drinking utensils, close conversation (within 3 feet), physical examination, and any other direct physical contact between people. Close contact does not include activities such as walking by a person or briefly sitting across a waiting room or office.

Exposure to SARS-Associated Coronavirus

The time between exposure to SARS-CoV and the onset of symptoms is called the "incubation period." The incubation period for SARS is typically 2 to 7 days, although in some cases it may be as long as 10 days. In a very small proportion of cases, incubation periods of up to 14 days have been reported.

How Long a Person with Severe Acute Respiratory Syndrome Is Infectious to Others

People with SARS are most likely to be contagious only when they have symptoms, such as a fever or cough. Patients are most contagious during the second week of illness. However, as a precaution against spreading the disease, the CDC recommends that people with SARS limit their interactions outside the home (for example, by not going to work or to school) until 10 days after their fever has gone away and their respiratory (breathing) symptoms have gotten better.

Is a Person with Severe Acute Respiratory Syndrome Contagious before Symptoms Appear?

To date, no cases of SARS have been reported among people who were exposed to a SARS patient before the onset of the patient's symptoms.

Treatment for Patients with Severe Acute Respiratory Syndrome

The CDC recommends that patients with SARS receive the same treatment that would be used for a patient with any serious community-acquired atypical pneumonia. SARS-CoV is being tested against various antiviral drugs to see if effective treatment can be found.

How to Protect Yourself from an Outbreak of Severe Acute Respiratory Syndrome

If transmission of SARS-CoV recurs, there are some common-sense precautions that you can take that apply to many infectious diseases. The most important is frequent handwashing with soap and water or use of an alcohol-based hand rub. You should also avoid touching your eyes, nose, and mouth with unclean hands and encourage people around you to cover their nose and mouth with a tissue when coughing or sneezing.

Outbreaks of Severe Acute Respiratory Syndrome in the Past
Global Severe Acute Respiratory Syndrome Outbreak, 2003

From November 2002 through July 2003, a total of 8,098 people worldwide became sick with SARS that was accompanied by either pneumonia or respiratory distress syndrome (RDS) (probable cases), according to the WHO. Of these, 774 died. By late July 2003, no new cases were being reported, and the WHO declared the global outbreak to be over.

In the United States, only eight people were laboratory-confirmed as SARS cases. There were no SARS-related deaths in the United States. All of the eight people with laboratory-confirmed SARS had traveled to areas where SARS-CoV transmission was occurring.

Severe Acute Respiratory Syndrome Situation, 2004

In April 2004, the Chinese Ministry of Health reported several new cases of possible SARS in Beijing and in Anhui Province, which is located in east-central China. As of April 26, the Ministry of Health had reported eight possible SARS cases: six in Beijing and two in Anhui Province. One of the patients in Anhui Province died. Nearly 1,000 contacts of these patients with possible SARS were under medical observation, including 640 in Beijing and 353 in Anhui.

In addition, health authorities reported that two doctors who treated one of the patients during her hospitalization in Anhui developed a fever. A person in close contact with one of the doctors also developed a fever.

Severe Acute Respiratory Syndrome-Associated Coronavirus

Coronaviruses are a group of viruses that have a halo or crown-like (corona) appearance when viewed under a microscope. Until recently, these viruses were a common cause of mild to moderate upper-respiratory illness in humans and remain associated with respiratory, gastrointestinal, liver and neurologic disease in animals.

There is not enough information about the new virus to determine the full range of illnesses that it might cause. Coronaviruses have occasionally been linked to pneumonia in humans, especially people with weakened immune systems. The viruses also can cause severe disease in animals, including cats, dogs, pigs, mice, and birds.

Preliminary studies in some research laboratories suggest that the virus may survive in the environment for several days. The length of time that the virus survives likely depends on a number of factors. These factors could include the type of material or body fluid containing the virus and various environmental conditions, such as temperature or humidity. Researchers at the CDC and other institutions are designing standardized experiments to measure how long SARS-CoV can survive in situations that simulate natural environmental conditions.

Section 13.3

MERS Coronavirus

This section includes text excerpted from "Middle East Respiratory Syndrome (MERS)," Centers for Disease Control and Prevention (CDC), August 2, 2019.

About Middle East Respiratory Syndrome

Middle East Respiratory Syndrome (MERS) is an illness caused by a virus (more specifically, a coronavirus) called "Middle East Respiratory Syndrome Coronavirus" (MERS-CoV). Most MERS patients developed severe respiratory illness with symptoms of fever, cough, and shortness of breath. About 3 or 4 out of every 10 patients reported with MERS have died.

All cases are linked to the Arabian Peninsula. Health officials first reported the disease in Saudi Arabia in September 2012. Through retrospective (backward-looking) investigations, they later identified that the first known cases of MERS occurred in Jordan in April 2012. So far, all cases of MERS have been linked through travel to, or residence in, countries in and near the Arabian Peninsula. The largest known outbreak of MERS outside the Arabian Peninsula occurred in the Republic of Korea in 2015. The outbreak was associated with a traveler returning from the Arabian Peninsula.

People with MERS can spread it to others. MERS-CoV has spread from ill people to others through close contact, such as caring for or living with an infected person.

MERS can affect anyone. MERS patients have ranged in age from younger than 1 to 99 years old.

The CDC continues to closely monitor the MERS situation globally. The CDC is working with partners to better understand the risks of this virus, including the source, how it spreads, and how to prevent infections. The CDC recognizes the potential for MERS-CoV to spread further and cause more cases globally and in the U.S. The CDC has provided information for travelers and is working with health departments, hospitals, and other partners to prepare for this possibility.

Symptoms and Complications of Middle East Respiratory Syndrome

Most people confirmed to have MERS-CoV infection have had severe respiratory illness with symptoms of:

- Fever
- Cough
- Shortness of breath

Some people also had diarrhea and nausea/vomiting. For many people with MERS, more severe complications, such as pneumonia and kidney failure, followed. About 3 or 4 out of every 10 people reported with MERS have died. Most of the people who died had a preexisting medical condition that weakened their immune system, or an underlying medical condition that had not yet been discovered. Medical conditions sometimes weaken people's immune systems and make them more likely to get sick or have severe illness.

Preexisting conditions among people who got MERS have included:
- Diabetes
- Cancer
- Chronic lung disease
- Chronic heart disease
- Chronic kidney disease

Some infected people had mild symptoms (such as cold-like symptoms) or no symptoms at all.

The symptoms of MERS start to appear about 5 or 6 days after a person is exposed, but can range from 2 to 14 days.

Transmission of Middle East Respiratory Syndrome

MERS-CoV, like other coronaviruses, likely spreads from an infected person's respiratory secretions, such as through coughing. However, the CDC does not fully understand the precise ways that it spreads.

MERS-CoV has spread from ill people to others through close contact, such as caring for or living with an infected person. Infected people have spread MERS-CoV to others in healthcare settings, such as hospitals. Researchers studying MERS have not seen any ongoing spreading of MERS-CoV in the community.

All reported cases have been linked to countries in and near the Arabian Peninsula. Most infected people either lived on the Arabian Peninsula or recently traveled from the Arabian Peninsula before they became ill. A few people have gotten MERS after having close contact with an infected person who had recently traveled from the Arabian Peninsula. The largest known outbreak of MERS outside the Arabian Peninsula occurred in the Republic of Korea in 2015 and was associated with a traveler returning from the Arabian Peninsula.

Public-health agencies continue to investigate clusters of cases in several countries to better understand how MERS-CoV spreads from person to person.

Treatment

There is no specific antiviral treatment recommended for MERS-CoV infection. Individuals with MERS often receive medical care to help relieve symptoms. For severe cases, current treatment includes care to support vital organ functions.

Prevention of Middle East Respiratory Syndrome

There is currently no vaccine to protect people against MERS. But, scientists are working to develop one.

You can help reduce your risk of getting respiratory illnesses:

- Wash your hands often with soap and water for at least 20 seconds, and help young children do the same. If soap and water are not available, use an alcohol-based hand sanitizer.
- Cover your nose and mouth with a tissue when you cough or sneeze, then throw the tissue in the trash.
- Avoid touching your eyes, nose, and mouth with unwashed hands.
- Avoid personal contact, such as kissing, or sharing cups or eating utensils, with sick people.
- Clean and disinfect frequently touched surfaces and objects, such as doorknobs.

If you are caring for or living with a person confirmed to have, or being evaluated for, MERS-CoV infection, see the CDC's interim guidance for Preventing MERS-CoV from Spreading to Others in Homes and Communities at cdc.gov/coronavirus/mers/hcp/home-care-patient.html.

People Who May Be at Increased Risk for Middle East Respiratory Syndrome
Recent Travelers from the Arabian Peninsula

If you develop a fever* and symptoms of respiratory illness, such as cough or shortness of breath, within 14 days after traveling from countries in or near the Arabian Peninsula**, you should call a healthcare provider and mention your recent travel.

Close Contacts of an Ill Traveler from the Arabian Peninsula

If you have had close contact*** with someone within 14 days after they traveled from a country in or near the Arabian Peninsula**, and the traveler has/had fever* and symptoms of respiratory illness, such as cough or shortness of breath, you should monitor your health for 14 days, starting from the day you were last exposed to the ill person.

If you develop a fever* and symptoms of respiratory illness, such as cough or shortness of breath, you should call a healthcare provider and mention your recent contact with the traveler.

Close Contacts of a Confirmed Case of MERS

If you have had close contact*** with someone who has a confirmed MERS-CoV infection, you should contact a healthcare provider for an evaluation. Your healthcare provider may request laboratory testing and outline additional recommendations, depending on the findings of your evaluation and whether you have symptoms. You most likely will be asked to monitor your health for 14 days, starting from the day you were last exposed to the ill person. Watch for these symptoms:

- Fever*. Take your temperature twice a day.
- Coughing
- Shortness of breath
- Other early symptoms to watch for are chills, body aches, sore throat, headache, diarrhea, nausea/vomiting, and runny nose.

If you develop symptoms, call your healthcare provider as soon as possible and tell them about your possible exposure to MERS-CoV so the office can take steps to keep other people from getting infected. Ask your healthcare provider to call the local or state health department.

Healthcare Personnel Not Using Recommended Infection-Control Precautions

Healthcare personnel should adhere to recommended infection-control measures, including standard, contact, and airborne precautions, while managing symptomatic close contacts, patients under investigation, and patients who have probable or confirmed MERS-CoV infections. They should also use recommended infection-control precautions when collecting specimens.

Healthcare personnel who had close contact*** with a confirmed case of MERS while the patient was ill, if not using recommended infection control precautions (e.g., appropriate use of personal protective equipment), are at increased risk of developing a MERS-CoV infection. These individuals should be evaluated and monitored by a healthcare professional with a higher index of suspicion.

People with Exposure to Camels

Direct contact with camels is a risk factor for human infection with MERS-CoV.

The World Health Organization (WHO) has posted a general precaution for anyone visiting farms, markets, barns, or other places where animals are present. Travelers should practice general hygiene measures, including regular handwashing before and after touching animals, and avoiding contact with sick animals. Travelers should also avoid consumption of raw or undercooked animal products.

The World Health Organization considers certain groups to be at high risk for severe MERS. These groups include people with diabetes, kidney failure, or chronic lung disease, and people who have weakened immune systems. The WHO recommends that these groups take additional precautions:

- Avoid contact with camels.
- Do not drink raw camel milk or raw camel urine.
- Do not eat undercooked meat, particularly camel meat.

Fever may not be present in some patients, such as those who are very young, elderly, immunosuppressed, or taking certain medications.

Countries considered in and near the Arabian Peninsula include: Bahrain; Iraq; Iran; Israel, the West Bank, and Gaza; Jordan; Kuwait; Lebanon; Oman; Qatar; Saudi Arabia; Syria; the United Arab Emirates (UAE); and Yemen.

✻✻✻*Close contact is defined as (a) being within approximately 6 feet (2 meters), or within the room or care area, of a confirmed MERS case for a prolonged period of time (such as caring for, living with, visiting, or sharing a healthcare waiting area or room with, a confirmed MERS case) while not wearing recommended personal protective equipment or PPE (e.g., gowns, gloves, NIOSH-certified disposable N95 respirator, eye protection); or (b) having direct contact with infectious secretions of a confirmed MERS case (e.g., being coughed on) while not wearing recommended personal protective equipment. See the CDC's Interim Infection Prevention and Control Recommendations for Hospitalized Patients with MERS at cdc.gov/ coronavirus/mers/infection-prevention-control. Data to inform the definition of close contact are limited; considerations when assessing close contact include the duration of exposure (e.g., longer exposure time likely increases exposure risk) and the clinical symptoms of the person with MERS (e.g., coughing likely increases exposure risk). Special consideration should be given to those exposed in healthcare settings. For detailed information regarding healthcare personnel (HCP) please review CDC's Interim U.S. Guidance for Monitoring and Movement of Persons with Potential Middle East Respiratory Syndrome (MERS-CoV) Exposure at cdc. gov/coronavirus/mers/hcp/monitoring-movement-guidance. Transient interactions, such as walking by a person with MERS, are not thought to constitute an exposure; however, final determination should be made in consultation with public-health authorities.*

Frequently Asked Questions and Answers
What Is Middle East Respiratory Syndrome?

Middle East Respiratory Syndrome (MERS) is a viral respiratory illness

Why Is It Sometimes Called MERS-CoV?

"MERS-CoV" is the acronym for Middle East Respiratory Syndrome Coronavirus, the virus that causes MERS. When referring to the virus and not the illness, the CDC uses "MERS-CoV." When referring to the illness, the CDC uses "MERS." The virus was first reported in 2012 in Saudi Arabia. It is different from any other coronavirus that researchers have found in people before.

What Is the Source of MERS-CoV?

MERS-CoV likely came from an animal source in the Arabian Peninsula. Researchers have found MERS-CoV in camels from several countries. Studies have shown that direct contact with camels is a risk factor for human infection with MERS-CoV. But, we need more information to understand the interactions between humans and camels that are important for transmission.

Has Anyone in the United States Gotten Infected?

Yes, two patients in the U.S. tested positive for MERS-CoV infection, both in May 2014. Get the most up-to-date information about MERS in the United States at cdc.gov/coronavirus/mers/index.

What Is the Centers for Disease Control and Prevention Doing about MERS?

The Centers for Disease Control and Prevention (CDC) works 24/7 to protect people's health. It is the CDC's job to be concerned and move quickly whenever there is a potential public-health problem. The CDC continues to closely monitor the MERS situation globally. The CDC is working with the WHO and other partners to better understand the virus, how it spreads, the source, and risks to the public's health. The CDC recognizes the potential for MERS-CoV to spread further and cause more cases in the United States and globally. In preparation for this, the CDC has:

- Increased lab testing capacity in states to detect cases
- Developed guidance and tools for health departments to conduct public-health investigations when MERS cases are suspected or confirmed
- Provided recommendations for healthcare infection control and other measures to prevent disease spread
- Provided guidance for flight crews, Emergency Medical Service (EMS) units at airports, and U.S. Customs and Border Protection (CPB) officers about reporting ill travelers to the CDC

- Disseminated up-to-date information to the general public, international travelers, and public-health partners
- Used Advanced Molecular Detection (AMD) methods to sequence the complete virus genome on specimens from cases to help evaluate and further describe the characteristics of MERS-CoV
- Continues to collaborate with international partners on epidemiologic and laboratory studies to better understand MERS

Am I at Risk for MERS-CoV Infection in the United States?

The MERS situation in the U.S. represents a very low risk to the general public in this country. Only two patients in the U.S. have tested positive for MERS-CoV infection—both in May 2014 after recently traveling from Saudi Arabia—while more than 1,300 have tested negative. The CDC continues to closely monitor the situation.

What Should I Do If I Had Close Contact with Someone Who Has MERS?

If you have had close contact with a confirmed MERS case within the last 14 days without using the recommended infection control precautions, you should contact a healthcare provider for an evaluation. Person-to-person spread of MERS-CoV, usually after close and prolonged contact, such as caring for or living with an infected person, has been well documented.

It is important to note, however, that most people who had close contact with someone who had MERS did not get infected or become ill.

Can I Still Travel to the Arabian Peninsula or Neighboring Countries Where MERS Cases Have Occurred?

Yes, there are currently no travel restrictions for the Arabian Peninsula.

What Should I Do If I Had Close Contact with a Recent Traveler from the Arabian Peninsula?

If you have had close contact with someone within 14 days after they traveled from a country in or near the Arabian Peninsula, and the traveler has/had a fever and symptoms of respiratory illness, such as a cough or shortness of breath, you should monitor your health for 14 days, starting from the day you were last exposed to the ill person. If you develop a fever and symptoms of respiratory illness, such as a cough or shortness of breath, you should call a healthcare provider and mention your recent contact with the traveler.

Does the U.S. Detain Arriving Travelers Whom They Believe Have MERS?

The CDC may detain individuals arriving in the U.S. or traveling between states whom they believe are infected with a quarantinable disease, including MERS, as of July 31, 2014, per amended U.S. Executive Order 13295. "Isolation" is used to separate ill people who have a contagious disease from those who are healthy; "quarantine" is used to separate and restrict the movement of well people who may have been exposed to a contagious disease to see if they become ill.

Is There a Vaccine?

Currently, there is no vaccine available to protect against MERS.

Should I Be Tested for Middle East Respiratory Syndrome?

If you develop a fever and symptoms of respiratory illness, such as a cough or shortness of breath, within 14 days after travel from a country in or near the Arabian Peninsula, you should call a healthcare provider and mention your recent travel or close contact. If you have had close contact with someone showing these symptoms who has recently traveled from this area, you should call a healthcare provider and mention your recent travel or close contact. Your healthcare provider will work with your state's public health department to test you for MERS.

How Do You Test a Person for Middle East Respiratory Syndrome?

There are two main ways to determine if a person is, or has been, infected with MERS-CoV.

- One type of test, conducted by state and CDC labs, is called "PCR," or "polymerase chain reaction," assays:
  - PCR assays are done with respiratory, serum, or stool samples and can quickly indicate if a person has an active infection with MERS-CoV.
- A second type of test, conducted by the CDC lab, is called "serology testing."
  - Serology testing uses serum samples and is designed to look for antibodies to MERS-CoV that would indicate a person had been previously infected with the virus and developed an immune response or has an active MERS-CoV infection for approximately 14 or more days.
  - Serology for MERS-CoV often includes two separate tests–(1) a screening test called "ELISA," or "enzyme-linked immunosorbent assay," and (2) a more definitive confirmatory test called the "neutralizing antibody assay."

Is MERS-CoV the Same as the SARS Virus?

No. MERS-CoV is not the same coronavirus that caused severe acute respiratory syndrome (SARS) in 2003. However, like the SARS virus, MERS-CoV is most similar to coronaviruses found in bats. The CDC is still learning about MERS.

- Close contact is defined as (a) being within approximately 6 feet (2 meters), or within the room or care area, of a confirmed MERS case for a prolonged period of time (such as caring for, living with, visiting, or sharing a healthcare waiting area or room with a confirmed MERS case) while not wearing recommended personal protective equipment, or PPE (e.g., gowns, gloves, NIOSH-certified disposable N95 respirator, eye protection); or (b) having direct contact with infectious secretions of a confirmed MERS case (e.g., being coughed on) while not wearing recommended personal protective equipment. Data to inform the definition of close contact are limited; considerations when assessing close contact include the duration of exposure (e.g., longer exposure time likely increases exposure risk) and the clinical symptoms of the person with MERS (e.g., coughing likely increases exposure risk). Special consideration should be given to those exposed in healthcare settings. Transient interactions, such as walking by a person with MERS, are not thought to constitute an exposure; however, final determination should be made in consultation with public health authorities.

- Countries considered in the Arabian Peninsula and neighboring include: Bahrain; Iraq; Iran; Israel, the West Bank, and Gaza; Jordan; Kuwait; Lebanon; Oman; Qatar, Saudi Arabia; Syria; the United Arab Emirates (UAE); and Yemen.
- Fever may not be present in some patients, such as those who are very young, elderly, immunosuppressed, or taking certain medications.

Middle East Respiratory Syndrome in the United States

MERS represents a very low risk to the general public in this country. Only two patients in the United States have ever tested positive for MERS-CoV infection—both in May 2014—while more than 1,300 have tested negative. The CDC continues to closely monitor the situation.

In May 2014, the CDC confirmed 2 unlinked imported cases of MERS in the United States—one to Indiana, the other to Florida. Both cases were among healthcare providers who lived and worked in Saudi Arabia. Both traveled to the U.S. from Saudi Arabia, where scientists believe they were infected. Both were hospitalized in the U.S. and later discharged after fully recovering.

The CDC and other public-health partners continue to closely monitor the MERS situation. The CDC recognizes the potential for MERS-CoV to spread further and cause more cases in the United States and globally. In preparation for this, the CDC continues to

- Collaborate with international partners on epidemiologic and laboratory studies to better understand MERS
- Improve the way it collects data about MERS cases
- Increase lab testing capacity in states to detect cases
- Develop guidance and tools for health departments to conduct public-health investigations when MERS cases are suspected or confirmed

- Provide recommendations for healthcare infection control and other measures to prevent disease spread
- Provide guidance for flight crews, Emergency Medical Service (EMS) units at airports, and U.S. Customs and Border Protection (CPB) officers about reporting ill travelers to the CDC
- Disseminate up-to-date information to the general public, international travelers, and public-health partners
- Use advanced molecular detection (AMD) methods to sequence the complete virus genome on specimens from the two U.S. MERS cases to help evaluate and further describe the characteristics of MERS-CoV.

Section 13.4

2019 Novel Coronavirus

This section contains text excerpted from the following sources: Text in this section begins with excerpts from "Update and Interim Guidance on Outbreak of 2019 Novel Coronavirus (2019-nCoV) in Wuhan, China," Centers for Disease Control and Prevention (CDC), January 15, 2020; Text under the heading "Situation Summary" is excerpted from "2019 Novel Coronavirus (2019-nCoV), Wuhan, China," Centers for Disease Control and Prevention (CDC), January 29, 2020; Text beginning with the heading "Symptoms of 2019 Novel Coronavirus" is excerpted from "2019 Novel Coronavirus," Centers for Disease Control and Prevention (CDC), January 28, 2020; Text under the heading "Prevention of Spreading 2019-nCoV in Homes and Communities" is excerpted from "Interim Guidance for Preventing 2019 Novel Coronavirus (2019-nCoV) from Spreading to Others in Homes and Communities," Centers for Disease Control and Prevention (CDC), January 29, 2020; Text under the headin "Traveler's Guide" is excerpted from "Travelers from China Arriving in the United States," Centers for Disease Control and Prevention (CDC), January 26, 2020.

The Centers for Disease Control and Prevention (CDC) continues to closely monitor an outbreak of a 2019 novel coronavirus (2019-nCoV) in Wuhan City, Hubei Province, China, that began in December 2019. The CDC has established an Incident Management System to coordinate a domestic and international public-health response.

Coronaviruses are a large family of viruses. Some cause illness in people; numerous other coronaviruses circulate among animals, including camels, cats, and bats. Rarely, animal coronaviruses can evolve and infect people and then spread between people such as has been seen with Middle Eastern Respiratory Syndrome Coronavirus (MERS-CoV) (www.cdc.gov/coronavirus/mers/index.html) and Severe Acute Respiratory Syndrome Coronavirus (SARS-CoV) (www.cdc.gov/sars/index.html).

Chinese authorities report most patients in the Wuhan City outbreak have been epidemiologically linked to a large seafood and animal market, suggesting a possible zoonotic (animal-to-human) origin to the outbreak. Chinese authorities additionally report that they are monitoring several hundred healthcare workers who are caring for outbreak patients; no spread of this virus from patients to healthcare personnel has been reported to date. Chinese authorities are reporting no ongoing spread of this virus in the community, but they cannot rule out that some limited person-to-person spread may be occurring. China has reported that two of the patients have died, including one with preexisting medical conditions. Chinese health officials publicly posted the genetic sequence of the 2019-nCoV on January 12, 2020. This will facilitate identification of infections with this virus and development of specific diagnostic tests.

Thailand and Japan have confirmed additional cases of 2019-nCoV in travelers from Wuhan, China. It is possible that more cases will be identified in the coming days. This is an ongoing investigation and given previous experience with MERS-CoV and SARS-CoV, it is possible that person-to-person spread may occur. There is much more to learn about the transmissibility, severity, and other features associated with 2019-nCoV as the investigations in China, Thailand, and Japan continue. Additional information about this novel virus is needed to better inform population risk.

This health alert network (HAN) Update provides a situational update and guidance to state and local health departments and healthcare providers that supersedes guidance in the CDC's HAN Advisory 424 distributed on January 8, 2020. This HAN Update adds guidance for evaluation of patients under investigation (PUI) for 2019-nCoV, prevention and infection control guidance, including the addition of an eye protection recommendation, and additional information on specimen collection.

Background

An outbreak of pneumonia of unknown etiology in Wuhan City was initially reported to World Health Organization (WHO) on December 31, 2019. Chinese health authorities have confirmed more than 40 infections with a novel coronavirus as the cause of the outbreak. Reportedly, most patients had epidemiological links to a large seafood and animal market. The market was closed on January 1, 2020. Currently, Chinese health authorities report no community spread of this virus, and no transmission among healthcare personnel caring for outbreak patients. No additional cases of infection with 2019-nCoV have been identified in China since January 3, 2020.

On January 13, 2020 public-health officials in Thailand confirmed detection of a human infection with 2019-nCoV in a traveler from Wuhan, China. This was the first confirmed case of 2019-nCoV documented outside China. On January 17, 2020 a second case was confirmed in Thailand, also in a returned traveler from Wuhan City. On January 15, 2020 health officials in Japan confirmed 2019-nCoV infection in a returned traveler from Wuhan City. These persons had onset dates after January 3, 2020. These cases did not report visiting the large seafood and animal market to which many cases in China have been linked.

Situation Summary
Source and Spread of the Virus

Chinese health authorities were the first to post the full genome of the 2019-nCoV in GenBank, the National Institutes of Health (NIH) genetic sequence database, and in the Global Initiative on Sharing All Influenza Data (GISAID) portal, an action which has facilitated detection of this virus. The CDC posted the full genome of the 2019-nCoV virus detected in the first and second U.S. patients to GenBank.

2019-nCoV is a betacoronavirus, such as MERS and SARs, all of which have their origins in bats. The sequences from U.S. patients are similar to the one that China initially posted, suggesting a likely single, recent emergence of this virus from an animal reservoir.

Early on, many of the patients in the outbreak of respiratory illness caused by 2019-nCov in Wuhan, China had some link to a large seafood and live animal market, suggesting animal-to-person spread. Later, a growing number of patients reportedly did not have exposure to animal markets, indicating person-to-person spread. Chinese officials report that sustained person-to-person spread in the community is occurring in China.

Situation in the United States

Imported cases of 2019-nCoV infection in people have been detected in the U.S. No person-to-person spread has been detected with this virus at the time, and this virus is not currently spreading in the community in the United States.

Illness Severity

Both MERS and SARS have been known to cause severe illness in people. The complete clinical picture with regard to 2019-nCoV is still not fully clear. Reported illnesses have ranged from infected people with little to no symptoms to people being severely ill and dying.

Risk Assessment

Outbreaks of novel virus infections among people are always of public-health concern. The risk from these outbreaks depends on the characteristics of the virus, including whether and how well it spreads between people, the severity of the resulting illness, and the medical or other measures available to control the impact of the virus (for example, vaccine or treatment medications).

This is a serious public-health threat. The fact that this virus has caused severe illness and sustained person-to-person spread in China is concerning, but it is unclear how the situation in the United States will unfold at this time.

The risk to individuals is dependent on exposure. At this time, some people will have an increased risk of infection, for example, healthcare workers caring for 2019-nCoV patients and other close contacts. For the general American public, who are unlikely to be exposed to this virus, the immediate health risk from 2019-nCoV is considered low.

What to Expect

More cases are likely to be identified in the coming days, including more cases in the United States. Given what has occurred previously with MERS and SARS, it is likely that person-to-person spread will occur, including in the United States.

CDC Response

- The CDC is closely monitoring this situation and is working with the World Health Organization (WHO) and state and local public-health partners to respond to this emerging public-health threat.

- The goal of the ongoing U.S. public-health response is to contain this outbreak and prevent sustained spread of 2019-nCov in this country.
- The CDC established a 2019-nCoV Incident Management Structure on January 7, 2020. On January 21, 2020, the CDC activated its emergency response system to better provide ongoing support to the 2019-nCoV response.
- On January 27, 2020, the CDC issued updated travel guidance for China, recommending that travelers avoid all nonessential travel to all of the country.
- The CDC and customs and border protection (CBP) are continuing to conduct enhanced entry screening of passengers who have been in Wuhan within the past 14 days at 5 designated U.S. airports. Given travel out of Wuhan has been shut down, the number of passengers who meet this criteria is dwindling.
- Going forward, CBP officials will monitor for travelers with symptoms compatible with 2019-nCoV infection and a travel connection with China and will refer them to CDC staff for evaluation at all 20 U.S. quarantine stations.
- At the same time, ALL travelers from China will be given the CDC's travel Health Alert Notice (HAN), educating those travelers about what to do if they get sick with certain symptoms within 14 days after arriving in the United States.
- The CDC issued an updated interim HAN Advisory to inform state and local health departments and healthcare providers about this outbreak on January 17, 2020.
- The CDC has deployed multidisciplinary teams to Washington, Illinois, California, and Arizona to assist health departments with clinical management, contact tracing, and communications.
- The CDC has developed a real-time Reverse Transcription-Polymerase Chain Reaction (rRT-PCR) test that can diagnose 2019-nCoV in respiratory and serum samples from clinical specimens. On January 24, 2020, the CDC publicly posted the assay protocol for this test. Currently, testing for this virus must take place at the CDC, but in the coming days and weeks, the CDC will share these tests with domestic and international partners through the agency's International Reagent Resource (IRR).

- The CDC uploaded the entire genome of the virus from all 5 reported cases in the United States to GenBank.
- The CDC also is growing the virus in cell culture, which is necessary for further studies, including for additional genetic characterization.

Symptoms of 2019 Novel Coronavirus

For confirmed 2019-nCoV infections, reported illnesses have ranged from people being mildly sick to people being severely ill and dying. Symptoms can include:

- Fever
- Cough
- Shortness of breath

The CDC believes at this time that symptoms of 2019-nCoV may appear in as few as 2 days or as long as 14 after exposure. This is based on what has been seen previously as the incubation period of MERS viruses.

Transmission of 2019 Novel Coronavirus

Coronaviruses are a large family of viruses that are common in many different species of animals, including camels, cattle, cats, and bats. Rarely, animal coronaviruses can infect people and then spread between people such as with MERS and SARS.

When person-to-person spread has occurred with MERS and SARS, it is thought to have happened mainly via respiratory droplets produced when an infected person coughs or sneezes, similar to how influenza and other respiratory pathogens spread. Spread of SARS and MERS between people has generally occurred between close contacts.

It is important to note that how easily a virus spreads person-to-person can vary. Some viruses are highly contagious (like measles), while other viruses are less so. It is important to know this in order to better understand the risk associated with this virus. While the CDC considers this to be a very serious public-health threat, based on current information, the immediate health risk from 2019-nCoV to the general American public is considered low at this time.

Treatment of 2019 Novel Coronavirus

There is no specific antiviral treatment recommended for 2019-nCoV infection. People infected with 2019-nCoV should receive supportive care to help relieve symptoms. For severe cases, treatment should include care to support vital organ functions.

People who think they may have been exposed to 2019-nCoV should contact your healthcare provider immediately.

Prevention of Spreading 2019-nCoV in Homes and Communities

This interim guidance is based on what is currently known about 2019 novel coronavirus (2019-nCoV) and transmission of other viral respiratory infections. The CDC will update this interim guidance as needed and as additional information becomes available.

Coronaviruses are a large family of viruses, some causing illness in people and others that circulate among animals, including camels, cats and bats. Rarely, animal coronaviruses can evolve and infect people and then spread between people such as has been seen with MERS and SARS. The potential for human-to-human transmission of 2019-nCoV is unknown. The following interim guidance may help prevent this virus from spreading among people in homes and in communities.

This interim guidance is for:
- People confirmed to have 2019-nCoV infection, who do not need to be hospitalized and who can receive care at home
- People being evaluated by a healthcare provider for 2019-nCoV infection, who do not need to be hospitalized and who can receive care at home
- Caregivers and household members of a person confirmed to have, or being evaluated for, 2019-nCoV infection

- Other people who have had close contact with a person confirmed to have, or being evaluated for, 2019-nCoV infection

Prevention Steps for People Confirmed to Have or Being Evaluated for 2019-nCoV Infection Who Receive Care at Home

Your doctors and public-health staff will evaluate whether you can be cared for at home. If it is determined that you can be isolated at home, you will be monitored by staff from your local or state health department. You should follow the prevention steps below until a healthcare provider or local or state health department says you can return to your normal activities.

Stay Home except to Get Medical Care

You should restrict activities outside your home, except for getting medical care. Do not go to work, school, or public areas, and do not use public transportation or taxis.

Separate Yourself from Other People in Your Home

As much as possible, you should stay in a different room from other people in your home. Also, you should use a separate bathroom, if available.

Call Ahead before Visiting Your Doctor

Before your medical appointment, call the healthcare provider and tell them that you have, or are being evaluated for, 2019-nCoV infection. This will help the healthcare provider's office take steps to keep other people from getting infected.

Wear a Facemask

You should wear a facemask when you are in the same room with other people and when you visit a healthcare provider. If you cannot wear a facemask, the people who live with you should wear one while they are in the same room with you.

Cover Your Coughs and Sneezes

Cover your mouth and nose with a tissue when you cough or sneeze, or you can cough or sneeze into your sleeve. Throw used tissues in a lined trash can, and immediately wash your hands with soap and water for at least 20 seconds.

Wash Your Hands

Wash your hands often and thoroughly with soap and water for at least 20 seconds. You can use an alcohol-based hand sanitizer that contains at least 60 percent alcohol if soap and water are not available. Avoid touching your eyes, nose, and mouth with unwashed hands.

Avoid Sharing Household Items

You should not share dishes, drinking glasses, cups, eating utensils, towels, bedding, or other items with other people in your home. After using these items, you should wash them thoroughly with soap and water.

Monitor Your Symptoms

Seek prompt medical attention if your illness is worsening (e.g., you experience difficulty breathing). Before going to your medical appointment, call the healthcare provider and tell them that you have, or are being evaluated for, 2019-nCoV infection. This will help the healthcare provider's office take steps to keep other people from getting infected. Ask your healthcare provider to call the local or state health department.

Prevention Steps for Caregivers and Household Members

If you live with, or provide care at home for, a person confirmed to have, or being evaluated for, 2019-nCoV infection, you should:

- Make sure that you understand and can help the person follow the healthcare provider's instructions for medication and care. You should help the person with basic needs in the home and provide support for getting groceries, prescriptions, and other personal needs.
- Have only people in the home who are essential for providing care for the person.

- Other household members should stay in another home or place of residence. If this is not possible, they should stay in another room, or be separated from the person as much as possible. Use a separate bathroom, if available.
- Restrict visitors who do not have an essential need to be in the home.
- Keep elderly people and those who have compromised immune systems or chronic health conditions away from the person. This includes people with chronic heart, lung or kidney conditions, and diabetes.

- Make sure that shared spaces in the home have good air flow, such as by an air conditioner or an opened window, weather permitting.
- Wash your hands often and thoroughly with soap and water for at least 20 seconds. You can use an alcohol-based hand sanitizer that contains at least 60 percent alcohol if soap and water are not available. Avoid touching your eyes, nose, and mouth with unwashed hands.
- Wear a disposable facemask, gown, and gloves when you touch or have contact with the person's blood, body fluids and/or secretions, such as sweat, saliva, sputum, nasal mucus, vomit, urine, or diarrhea.
  - Throw out disposable facemasks, gowns, and gloves after using them. Do not reuse.
  - Wash your hands immediately after removing your facemask, gown, and gloves.
- Avoid sharing household items. You should not share dishes, drinking glasses, cups, eating utensils, towels, bedding, or other items with a person who is confirmed to have, or is being evaluated for, 2019-nCoV infection. After the person uses these items, you should wash them thoroughly (see "Wash laundry thoroughly" below).
- Clean all "high-touch" surfaces, such as counters, tabletops, doorknobs, bathroom fixtures, toilets, phones, keyboards, tablets, and bedside tables, every day. Also, clean any surfaces that may have blood, body fluids and/or secretions or excretions on them.

- Read the label of cleaning products and follow recommendations provided on product labels. Labels contain instructions for safe and effective use of the cleaning product, including precautions you should take when applying the product, such as wearing gloves or aprons and making sure you have good ventilation during use of the product.
- Use a diluted bleach solution or a household disinfectant with a label that says "EPA-approved." To make a bleach solution at home, add 1 tablespoon of bleach to 1 quart (4 cups) of water. For a larger supply, add ¼ cup of bleach to 1 gallon (16 cups) of water.
- Wash laundry thoroughly.
  - Immediately remove and wash clothes or bedding that have blood, body fluids and/or secretions or excretions on them.
  - Wear disposable gloves while handling soiled items. Wash your hands immediately after removing your gloves.
  - Read and follow directions on labels of laundry or clothing items and detergent. In general, wash and dry with the warmest temperatures recommended on the clothing label.
- Place all used disposable gloves, gowns, facemasks, and other contaminated items in a lined container before disposing of them with other household waste. Wash your hands immediately after handling these items.
- Monitor the person's symptoms. If they are getting sicker, call her or his medical provider and tell them that the person has, or is being evaluated for, 2019-nCoV infection. This will help the healthcare provider's office take steps to keep other people from getting infected. Ask the healthcare provider to call the local or state health department.
- Caregivers and household members who do not follow precautions when in close contact with a person who is confirmed to have, or is being evaluated for, 2019-nCoV infection, are considered "close contacts" and should monitor their health. Follow the prevention steps for close contacts below.
- Discuss any additional questions with you state or local health department.

Prevention Steps for Close Contacts

If you have had close contact with someone who is confirmed to have, or is being evaluated for, 2019-nCoV infection, you should:

- Monitor your health starting from the day you first had close contact with the person and continue for 14 days after you last had close contact with the person. Watch for these signs and symptoms:
  - Fever. Take your temperature twice a day.
  - Coughing
  - Shortness of breath or difficulty breathing
  - Other early symptoms to watch for are chills, body aches, sore throat, headache, diarrhea, nausea/vomiting, and runny nose.
- **If you develop fever or any of these symptoms, call your healthcare provider right away.**
- **Before** going to your medical appointment, be sure to tell your healthcare provider about your close contact with someone who is confirmed to have, or is being evaluated for, 2019-nCoV infection. This will help the healthcare provider's office take steps to keep other people from getting infected. Ask your healthcare provider to call the local or state health department.
- If you do not have any symptoms, you can continue with your daily activities, such as going to work, school, or other public areas.

Traveler's Guide
Traveling from China to the United States: Here Is What to Expect at the Airport

The CDC and U.S. Customs and Border Protection (CBP) are implementing enhanced health screenings to detect travelers with fever, cough, or difficulty breathing when entering the United States.

The screening procedures include:

- Travelers fill out a short questionnaire about their travel, any symptoms, and contact information.
- The CDC staff take the temperature of each traveler with a hand-held noncontact thermometer (thermometers that do not touch the skin)

and observe the traveler for cough or difficulty breathing. If sick travelers are identified, the CDC evaluates them further to determine whether they should be taken to a hospital for medical evaluation and to get care as needed.

- If the traveler does not have symptoms, the CDC staff will provide health information cards to take with them. The cards tell travelers what symptoms to look out for, and what to do if they develop symptoms within 14 days after leaving China.

This health assessment and request for persons to monitor their health is part of a layered approach to limiting the spread of disease. When used with other public-health measures, enhanced entry screening can strengthen the CDC efforts to protect the United States from 2019-nCoV and other diseases.

What Should I Do When I Arrive from China?

All travelers from China, including business travelers, people who visited friends and family, and humanitarian workers should take the following steps.

First, watch for any changes in your health for 14 days after leaving China. If you get a fever or develop a cough or difficulty breathing during this 14-day period, avoid contact with others. Call your doctor or healthcare provider to tell them about your symptoms and your recent travel. They will provide further instruction about steps to take before your medical visit to help reduce the risk that you will spread your illness to other people in the office or waiting room if that is what has made you sick. Do not travel while you are sick.

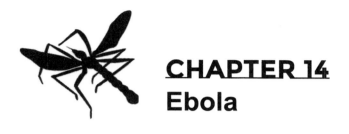

CHAPTER 14
Ebola

Chapter Contents

History of Ebola Virus Disease

This section includes text excerpted from "History of Ebola Virus Disease," Centers for Disease Control and Prevention (CDC), September 18, 2018.

The Emergence of Ebola in Humans

Ebola virus disease (EVD), one of the deadliest viral diseases, was discovered in 1976 when two consecutive outbreaks of fatal hemorrhagic fever occurred in different parts of Central Africa. The first outbreak occurred in the Democratic Republic of Congo (formerly Zaire) in a village near the Ebola River, which gave the virus its name. The second outbreak occurred in what is now South Sudan, approximately 500 miles (850 km) away.

Initially, public-health officials assumed these outbreaks were a single event associated with an infected person who traveled between the two locations. However, scientists later discovered that the two outbreaks were caused by two genetically distinct viruses: *Zaire ebolavirus* and *Sudan ebolavirus*. After this discovery, scientists concluded that the virus came from two different sources and spread independently to people in each of the affected areas.

Viral and epidemiologic data suggest that the Ebola virus existed long before these recorded outbreaks occurred. Factors such as population growth, encroachment into forested areas, and direct interaction with wildlife (such as bushmeat consumption) may have contributed to the spread of the Ebola virus.

Identifying a Host

Following the discovery of the virus, scientists studied thousands of animals, insects, and plants in search of its source (called "reservoir" among virologists, or people who study viruses). Gorillas, chimpanzees, and other mammals may be implicated when the first cases of an EVD outbreak in people occur. However, they—just as people—are "dead-end" hosts, meaning the organism dies following the infection and does not survive and spread the virus to other animals. Similar to other viruses of its kind, it is possible that the reservoir host animal of the Ebola virus does not experience acute illness despite the virus being present in its organs, tissues, and blood. Thus, the virus is likely maintained in the environment by spreading from host to host or through intermediate hosts or vectors.

African fruit bats are likely involved in the spread of the Ebola virus and may even be the source animal (reservoir host). Scientists continue to search for conclusive evidence of the bat's role in the transmission of Ebola. The most recent Ebola virus to be detected, the *Bombali virus*, was identified in samples from bats collected in Sierra Leone.

Since its discovery in 1976, the majority of cases and outbreaks of EVD have occurred in Africa. The Ebola outbreak between 2014 to 2016 in West Africa began in a rural area of southeastern Guinea, spread to urban areas and across borders within weeks, and became a global pandemic within months.

Understanding Pathways of Transmission

The use of contaminated needles and syringes during the earliest outbreaks enabled transmission and amplification of the Ebola virus. During the first outbreak in Zaire (now Democratic Republic of Congo (DRC)), nurses in the Yambuku mission hospital reportedly used 5 syringes for 300 to 600 patients a day. Close contact with infected blood, reuse of contaminated needles, and improper nursing techniques were the source for much of the human-to-human transmission during early Ebola outbreaks.

In 1989, *Reston ebolavirus* was discovered in research monkeys imported from the Philippines into the United States. Later, scientists confirmed that the virus spread throughout the monkey population through droplets in the air (aerosolized transmission) in the facility. However, such air-borne transmission is not proven to be a significant factor in human outbreaks of Ebola. The discovery of the Reston virus in these monkeys from the Philippines revealed that Ebola was no longer confined to African settings, but was present in Asia as well.

By the 1994 Cote d'Ivoire outbreak, scientists and public-health officials had a better understanding of how Ebola virus spreads and progress was made to reduce transmission through the use of face masks, gloves and gowns for healthcare personnel. In addition, the use of disposable equipment, such as needles, was introduced.

During the 1995 Kikwit, Zaire (now DRC) outbreak, the international public-health community played a strong role, as it is now widely agreed that containment and control of the Ebola virus were paramount in ending outbreaks. The local community was educated in how the disease spreads; the hospital was properly staffed and stocked with necessary equipment; and healthcare personnel were trained in disease reporting, patient-case identification, and methods for reducing transmission in the healthcare setting.

During the 2014 to 2015 Ebola outbreak in West Africa, healthcare workers represented only 3.9 percent of all confirmed and probable cases of EVD in Sierra Leone, Liberia, and Guinea combined. In comparison, healthcare workers accounted for 25 percent of all infections during the 1995 outbreak in Kikwit. During the 2014 to 2015 West Africa outbreak, the majority of transmission events were between family members (74%). Direct contact with the bodies of those who died from EVD proved to be one of the most dangerous—and effective—methods of transmission. Changes in behaviors related to mourning and burial, along with the adoption of safe burial practices, were critical in controlling that epidemic.

Section 14.2
Understanding Ebola

This section includes text excerpted from "Ebola (Ebola Virus Disease)," Centers for Disease Control and Prevention (CDC), November 5, 2019.

What Is Ebola Virus Disease?

Ebola virus disease (EVD) is a deadly disease with occasional outbreaks that occur primarily on the African continent. EVD most commonly affects people and nonhuman primates (such as monkeys, gorillas, and chimpanzees). It is caused by an infection with a group of viruses within the genus Ebolavirus:

- Ebola virus (species *Zaire ebolavirus*)
- Sudan virus (species *Sudan ebolavirus*)
- Taï Forest virus (species *Taï Forest ebolavirus*, formerly *Côte d'Ivoire ebolavirus*)
- Bundibugyo virus (species *Bundibugyo ebolavirus*)
- Reston virus (species *Reston ebolavirus*)
- Bombali virus (species *Bombali ebolavirus*)

Of these, only four (Ebola, Sudan, Taï Forest, and Bundibugyo viruses) are known to cause disease in people. Reston virus is known to cause disease in nonhuman primates and pigs, but not in people. It is unknown if the *Bombali virus*, which was recently identified in bats, causes disease in either animals or people.

Scientists do not know where the Ebola virus comes from. However, based on the nature of similar viruses, they believe the virus is animal-borne, with bats or nonhuman primates with bats or nonhuman primates (chimpanzees, apes, monkeys, etc.) being the most likely source. Infected animals carrying the virus can transmit it to other animals, such as apes, monkeys, duikers, and humans.

Ebola survivors may experience side effects after their recoveries, such as tiredness, muscle aches, eye, and vision problems and stomach pain.

Signs and Symptoms of Ebola Virus Disease

Symptoms may appear anywhere from 2 to 21 days after contact with the virus, with an average of 8 to 10 days. The course of the illness typically progresses from "dry" symptoms initially (such as fever, aches and pains, and fatigue), and then progresses to "wet" symptoms (such as diarrhea and vomiting) as the person becomes sicker.

Primary signs and symptoms of Ebola often include some or several of the following:

- Fever
- Aches and pains, such as severe headache, muscle, and joint pain, and abdominal (stomach) pain
- Weakness and fatigue
- Gastrointestinal symptoms including diarrhea and vomiting
- Abdominal (stomach) pain
- Unexplained hemorrhaging, bleeding or bruising

Other symptoms may include red eyes, skin rash, and hiccups (late-stage).

Many common illnesses can have the same symptoms as EVD, including influenza (flu), malaria, or typhoid fever.

Diagnosis of Ebola Virus Disease

Diagnosing EVD shortly after infection can be difficult. Early symptoms of EVD, such as fever, headache, and weakness are not specific to Ebola virus infection and often are seen in patients with other more common diseases, such as malaria and typhoid fever.

To determine whether EVD is a possible diagnosis, there must be a combination of symptoms suggestive of EVD AND a possible exposure to EVD within 21 days before the onset of symptoms.

If a person shows signs of EVD and has had a possible exposure, she or he should be isolated (separated from other people) and public-health authorities notified. Blood samples from the patient should be collected and tested to confirm infection. Ebola virus can be detected in blood after the onset of symptoms. It may take up to three days after symptoms start for the virus to reach detectable levels.

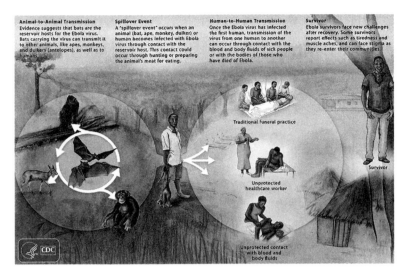

Figure 14.1. Ebola Virus Ecology and Transmission

Polymerase chain reaction (PCR) is one of the most commonly used diagnostic methods because of its ability to detect low levels of the Ebola virus. PCR methods can detect the presence of a few virus particles in small amounts of blood, but the ability to detect the virus increases as the number of virus increases during an active infection. When the virus is no longer present in great enough numbers in a patient's blood, PCR methods will no longer be effective. Other methods, based on the detection of antibodies an EVD case produces an infection, can then be used to confirm a patient's exposure and infection by the Ebola virus.

A positive laboratory test means that the Ebola infection is confirmed. Public-health authorities will conduct a public-health investigation, including identifying and monitoring all possibly exposed contacts.

Treatment of Ebola Virus Disease

Symptoms of EVD are treated as they appear. When used early, basic interventions can significantly improve the chances of survival. These include:

- Providing fluids and electrolytes (body salts) through infusion into the vein (intravenously)

You **CAN'T** get Ebola through **AIR**

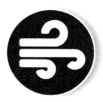

You **CAN'T** get Ebola through **WATER**

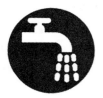

You **CAN'T** get Ebola through **FOOD** grown or legally purchased in the U.S.

Figure 14.2. Facts about Ebola in the United States
(Source: "Facts about Ebola in the U.S.," Centers for Disease Control and Prevention (CDC))

- Offering oxygen therapy to maintain oxygen status
- Using medication to support blood pressure, reduce vomiting and diarrhea, and to manage fever and pain
- Treating other infections, if they occur

Antiviral Drugs

There is currently no antiviral drug licensed by the U.S. Food and Drug Administration (FDA) to treat EVD in people.

During the 2018 eastern Democratic Republic of the Congo outbreak, 4 investigational treatments were initially available to treat patients with confirmed Ebola. For 2 of those treatments, called "Regeneron (REGN-EB3)" and "mAb114," overall survival was much higher. These two antiviral drugs currently remain in use for patients with confirmed Ebola.

Drugs that are being developed to treat EVD work by stopping the virus from making copies of itself.

Transmission of Ebola Virus Disease

Scientists think people are initially infected with the Ebola virus through contact with an infected animal, such as a fruit bat or nonhuman primate. This is called a "spillover event." After that, the virus spreads from person to person, potentially affecting a large number of people.

The virus spreads through direct contact (such as through broken skin or mucous membranes in the eyes, nose, or mouth) with:

- Blood or body fluids (urine, saliva, sweat, feces, vomit, breast milk, and semen) of a person who is sick with or has died from EVD.
- Objects (such as clothes, bedding, needles, and medical equipment) contaminated with body fluids from a person who is sick with or has died from EVD.
- Infected fruit bats or nonhuman primates (such as apes and monkeys).
- Semen from a man who recovered from EVD (through oral, vaginal, or anal sex). The virus can remain in certain body fluids (including semen) of a patient who has recovered from EVD, even if they no longer have symptoms of severe illness. There is no evidence that Ebola can be spread through sex or other contacts with vaginal fluids from a woman who has had Ebola.

When people become infected with Ebola, they do not start developing signs or symptoms right away. This period between exposure to illness and having symptoms is known as the "incubation period." A person can only spread Ebola to other people after they develop signs and symptoms of Ebola.

Additionally, the Ebola virus is not known to be transmitted through food. However, in certain parts of the world, the Ebola virus may spread through the handling and consumption of wild animal meat or hunted wild animals infected with Ebola. There is no evidence that mosquitoes or other insects can transmit Ebola virus.

Risk

Health workers who do not use proper infection control while caring for Ebola patients, and family and friends in close contact with Ebola patients, are at the highest risk of getting sick. Ebola can spread when people come into contact with infected blood or body fluids.

Ebola poses little risk to travelers or the general public who have not cared for or been in close contact (within three feet or one meter) with someone sick with Ebola.

Persistence of the Virus

The virus can remain in areas of the body that are immunologically privileged sites after acute infection. These are sites where viruses and pathogens, such as the Ebola virus, are shielded from the survivor's immune system, even after being cleared elsewhere in the body. These areas include the testes, interior of the eyes, placenta, and central nervous system (CNS), particularly the cerebrospinal fluid (CBF). Whether the virus is present in these body parts and for how long varies by the survivor. Scientists are now studying how long the virus stays in these body fluids among Ebola survivors.

During an Ebola outbreak, the virus can spread quickly within healthcare settings (such as clinics or hospitals). Clinicians and other healthcare personnel providing care should use dedicated, preferably disposable medical equipment. Proper cleaning and disposal of instruments such as needles and syringes are important. If instruments are not disposable, they must be sterilized before using it again.

Ebola virus can survive on dry surfaces, such as doorknobs, and countertops for several hours; in body fluids such as blood, the virus can survive up to several days at room temperature. Cleaning and disinfection should be performed using a hospital-grade disinfectant.

Prevention of Ebola Virus Disease

In the United States, EVD is a very rare disease that has only occurred because of cases that were acquired in other countries, eventually followed by person-to-person transmission. EVD is most common in parts of sub-Saharan Africa, with occasional outbreaks occurring in people. In these areas, the Ebola virus is believed to circulate at low rates in certain animal populations (enzootic). Occasionally people become sick with Ebola after coming into contact with these infected animals, which can then lead to Ebola outbreaks where the virus spreads between people.

When living in or traveling to a region where the Ebola virus is present, there are a number of ways to protect yourself and prevent the spread of EVD.

While in an area affected by Ebola, it is important to avoid the following:

- Contact with blood and body fluids (such as urine, feces, saliva, sweat, vomit, breast milk, semen, and vaginal fluids) of persons who are ill.
- Contact with semen from a man who has recovered from EVD, until testing verifies the virus is gone from the semen.
- Items that may have come in contact with an infected person's blood or body fluids (such as clothes, bedding, needles, and medical equipment).
- Funeral or burial rituals that require handling the body of someone who died from EVD.
- Contact with bats and nonhuman primates' blood, fluids, or raw meat prepared from these animals (bushmeat).
- Contact with the raw meat of an unknown source.

These same prevention methods apply when living in or traveling to an area affected by an Ebola outbreak. After returning from an area affected by Ebola, monitor your health for 21 days and seek medical care immediately if you develop symptoms of EVD.

Ebola Vaccine

There is currently no vaccine licensed by the U.S. Food and Drug Administration (FDA) to protect people from the Ebola virus. Several investigational vaccines for the prevention of Ebola virus infection are in development and are being evaluated in clinical trials.

An experimental vaccine, called "rVSV-ZEBOV," was found to be highly protective against the virus in a trial conducted by the World Health Organization (WHO) and other international partners in Guinea in 2015. Though still experimental, it was approved for use in the 2018 Ebola outbreak in the Democratic Republic of Congo (DRC) for emergency use. This vaccine has been shown to be safe and protective against the Zaire ebolavirus species of Ebola.

A second investigational vaccine will be introduced in 2019 in DRC under a research protocol. The second vaccine is a 2-dose regimen with an initial dose followed by a second "booster" dose 56 days later. The second vaccine is also designed to protect against Zaire ebolavirus species of Ebola.

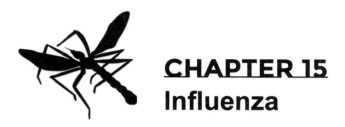

CHAPTER 15
Influenza

Chapter Contents

Influenza Pandemics of the 20th Century

This section includes text excerpted from "Influenza Pandemics of the 20th Century," Centers for Disease Control and Prevention (CDC), February 16, 2012. Reviewed January 2020.

Three worldwide (pandemic) influenza (flu) outbreaks occurred in the last century. Each differed from the others with respect to etiologic agents, epidemiology, and disease severity. They did not occur at regular intervals. In the case of the 2 that occurred within the era of modern virology (1957 and 1968), the hemagglutinin (HA) antigen of the causative viruses showed major changes from the corresponding antigens of immediately antecedent strains. The immediate antecedent to the virus of 1918 remains unknown, but that epidemic likely also reflected a major change in the antigens of the virus.

Brief Look Back at the 1918 Pandemic

The origin of this pandemic has always been disputed and may never be resolved. However, the observations of trained observers at that time are worth noting because they may bear on later genomic analysis of the resurrected 1918 virus nucleotide fragments and the abortive "swine flu" epidemic of 1976. In Richard Shope's Harvey lecture of 1936, he reviews evidence that in the late summer or early autumn of 1918, a disease not previously recognized in swine, and closely resembling influenza in humans, appeared in the American Middle West. Epidemiologic-epizootiologic evidence strongly suggested that the causative virus was moving from humans to swine rather than in the reverse direction. Similar observations were made on the other side of the world and reported in a little-known paper in the *National Medical Journal of China*. In the spring

157

of 1918, influenza in humans spread rapidly all over the world and was prevalent from Canton, China, to the most northern parts of Manchuria and from Shanghai to Sichuan. In October 1918, a disease diagnosed as influenza appeared in Russian and Chinese pigs in the area surrounding Harbin. Thus, epidemiologic evidence, fragmentary as it is, appears to favor the spread of the virus from humans to swine, in which it remained relatively unchanged until it was recovered more than a decade later by Shope in the first isolation of influenza virus from a mammalian species.

The virus of 1918 was undoubtedly uniquely virulent, although most patients experienced symptoms of typical influenza with a 3 to 5-day fever followed by complete recovery. Nevertheless, although diagnostic virology was not yet available, bacteriology was flourishing and many careful postmortem examinations of patients by academic bacteriologists and pathologists disclosed bacterial pathogens in the lungs. However, this was a time when bacterial superinfection in other virus diseases could lead to death; for example, measles in military recruits were often fatal. This is important in considering the question of "will there ever be another 1918?" To the degree that secondary bacterial infection may contribute to influenza death rates, it should at least be partially controllable by antimicrobial agents, as indeed was the case in 1957.

1957: Asian Influenza (H2N2)

After the influenza pandemic of 1918, influenza went back to its usual pattern of regional epidemics of lesser virulence in the 1930s, 1940s, and early 1950s. With the first isolation of a virus from humans in 1933, speculation began about the possible role of a similar virus in 1918. However, believing that this could have been the case was difficult until the pandemic of 1957. This was the first time the rapid global spread of a modern influenza virus was available for laboratory investigation. With the exception of persons >70 years of age, the public was confronted by a virus with which it had had no experience, and it was shown that the virus alone, without bacterial coinvaders, was lethal.

First Recognition of the Pandemic

In 1957, worldwide surveillance for influenza was less extensive than it is today. However, attentive investigators in Melbourne, London, and Washington, DC, soon had the virus in their laboratories after the initial recognition of a severe epidemic, followed by the publication in the *New York Times* of an article in 1957 describing an epidemic in Hong Kong that involved 250,000 people in a short period. Three weeks later, a virus was recovered from the outbreak and sent to the Walter Reed Army Institute for Research in Washington, DC, for study.

Nature of the Virus

The virus was quickly recognized as an influenza A virus by complement fixation tests. However, tests defining the HA antigen of the virus showed it to be unlike any previously found in humans. This was also true for the neuraminidase (NA) antigen. The definitive subtype of the Asian virus was later established as H2N2. The new virus had high sialidase/neuraminidase activity, and this activity was more stable than that of earlier strains. Different strains of the Asian virus also differed markedly with respect to sensitivity to either antibody neutralization or nonspecific inhibitors of hemagglutination. In animal studies, the new H2N2 viruses did not differ in their virulence characteristics from earlier influenza A subtypes. Viral isolates from the lungs of patients with fatal cases showed no discernible differences from those from throat-washing isolates of patients without pulmonary involvement within a small circumscribed hospital outbreak.

Primary Influenza Virus Pneumonia

Although secondary or concomitant bacterial infections of the lung were found to be a prominent feature of fatal cases in 1918 when a specific etiologic agent was sought, many cases of rapid death and lung consolidation or pulmonary edema occurred in which bacterial infection could not be demonstrated. As influenza persisted as an endemic disease with regional recurrences after the pandemic, lives continued to be occasionally claimed by bacterial pneumonia.

With the arrival of Asian influenza in 1957, the sheer number of cases associated with pandemics again brought the phenomenon of primary influenza virus pneumonia to the attention of physicians in teaching hospitals. In contrast to the observations in 1918, underlying chronic disease of the heart or lungs was found in most of these patients, although deaths of previously healthy persons were not uncommon. In the case of carefully studied patients at the New York Hospital, rheumatic heart disease (RHD) was the most common antecedent factor, and women in the third trimester of pregnancy were among those vulnerable.

Response to Vaccination in an Unprimed Population

The pandemic of 1957 provided the first opportunity to observe vaccination response in that large part of the population that had not previously been primed by novel HA and NA antigens not cross-reactive with earlier influenza A virus antigens. As summarized by world-renowned physician Gordon Meiklejohn at an international conference on Asian influenza held 3 years after the 1957 onslaught of H2N2, more vaccine was required to initiate a primary antibody response than with the earlier H1 vaccines (almost always observed in heterovariant primed subjects). In 1958, 1959, and 1960 (as recurrent infections occurred), mean initial antibody levels in the population increased (i.e., subjects were primed) and response to vaccination was more readily demonstrated. Divided doses given at intervals of <4 weeks were more beneficial than a single injection. Less benefit was derived from this strategy as the years passed. Intradermal administration of vaccine provided no special advantage over the conventional subcutaneous/ intramuscular route, even when the same small dose was given.

Nature of Endemic H2N2 Postpandemic Infection

The Asian influenza experience provided the first opportunity to study how the postpandemic infection and disease into an endemic phase subsided. In studies conducted in separate and disparate populations, the populations compared were Navajo school children and New York City medical students. In both groups, subclinical infections occurred each year during the three-year study period, and clinically manifested infections decreased in conjunction with an increasing level of H2N2-specific hemagglutination inhibition antibody.

A decreasing incidence of clinically manifested cases can be ascribed either to the increase in antibody levels in the community or to a change in the intrinsic virulence of the virus. Therefore, the nature of the disease during the endemic period is important to define. A study in 1960 of hospitalized patients with laboratory-confirmed infections demonstrated a spectrum of disease from uncomplicated 3-day illnesses to fatal pneumonia, all in the absence of discernible epidemic influenza in the community. Asian (H2N2) virus was destined for short survival in the human population and disappeared only 11 years after its arrival. It was supplanted by Hong Kong (H3N2) subtype.

1968: Hong Kong Influenza (H3N2)

As in 1957, a new influenza pandemic arose in Southeast Asia and acquired the sobriquet Hong Kong influenza on the basis of the site of its emergence to western attention. Once again, the daily press sounded the alarm with a brief report of a large Hong Kong epidemic in the *Times of London*. A decade after the 1957 pandemic, epidemiologic communication with mainland China was even less efficient than it had been earlier.

As this epidemic progressed, initially throughout Asia, important differences in the pattern of illness and death were noted. In Japan, epidemics were small, scattered, and desultory until the end of 1968. Most striking was the high illness and death rates in the United States following the introduction of the virus on the West Coast. This experience stood in contrast with the experience in western Europe, including the United Kingdom, in which increased illness occurred in the absence of increased death rates in 1968–1969 and increased death rates were not seen until the following year of the pandemic.

Since the Hong Kong virus differed from its antecedent Asian virus by its HA antigen but had retained the same (N2) NA antigen, researchers speculated that its more sporadic and variable impact in different regions of the world were mediated by differences in prior N2 immunity (16 to 19). Therefore, the 1968 pandemic has been aptly characterized as "smoldering."

Further evidence for the capacity of previous N2 experience to moderate the challenge of the Hong Kong virus was provided by Meiklejohn and colleague Theodore C. Eickhoff, and Meiklejohn, who showed that vaccination of Air Force cadets with an H2N2 adjuvant vaccine reduced subsequent influenza from verified H3N2 virus infection by 54 percent.

The amelioration of H3N2 virus infection by NA immunity alone is all the more remarkable because of the capacity of the virus to kill, as occurred in 1918 and 1957, although a broader spectrum of disease severity was apparent in 1968 than in 1957. Although not necessarily an indication of virulence, cross-species transmission of the virus was observed. 37 years later, the H3N2 subtype still reigns as the major and most troublesome influenza A virus in humans.

Section 15.2
Facts about Influenza

This section includes text excerpted from "Key Facts about Influenza (Flu)," Centers for Disease Control and Prevention (CDC), September 13, 2019.

What Is Influenza?

Influenza (flu) is a contagious respiratory illness caused by influenza viruses that infect the nose, throat, and sometimes the lungs. It can cause mild to severe illness, and at times can lead to death. The best way to prevent the flu is by getting a flu vaccine each year.

Influenza Symptoms

The flu can cause mild to severe illness, and at times can lead to death. The flu is different from a cold. The flu usually comes on suddenly. People who have the flu often feel some or all of these symptoms:

- Fever or feeling feverish/chills
- Cough
- Sore throat
- Runny or stuffy nose
- Muscle or body aches
- Headaches
- Fatigue (tiredness)

Some people may have vomiting and diarrhea, though this is more common in children than adults.

It is important to note that not everyone with flu will have a fever.

How Influenza Spreads

Most experts believe that flu viruses spread mainly by tiny droplets made when people with flu cough, sneeze or talk. These droplets can land in the mouths or noses of people who are nearby. Less often, a person might get the flu by touching a surface or object that has flu virus on it and then touching their own mouth, nose or possibly their eyes.

How Many People Get Sick with Influenza Every Year?

A 2018, the Centers for Disease Control and Prevention (CDC) study published in *Clinical Infectious Diseases* (*CID*) looked at the percentage of the United States population who were sickened by the flu using 2 different methods and compared the findings. Both methods had similar findings, which suggested that on average, about 8 percent of the United States population gets sick from the flu each season, with a range of between 3 and 11 percent, depending on the season.

Who Is Most Likely to Be Infected with Influenza?

The same *CID* study icon found that children are most likely to get sick from the flu and that people 65 and older are least likely to get sick from influenza. Median incidence values (or attack rate) by age group were 9.3 percent for children 0 to 17 years, 8.8 percent for adults 18 to 64 years, and 3.9 percent for adults 65 years and older. This means that children younger than 18 are more than twice as likely to develop asymptomatic flu infection than adults 65 and older.

How Is Seasonal Incidence of Influenza Estimated?

Influenza virus infection is so common that the number of people infected each season can only be estimated. These statistical estimations are based on the CDC-measured flu hospitalization rates that are adjusted to produce an estimate of the total number of influenza infections in the United States for a given flu season.

The estimates for the number of infections are then divided by the census population to estimate the seasonal incidence (or attack rate) of influenza.

Does Seasonal Incidence of Influenza Change Depend on the Severity of Flu Season?

Yes. The proportion of people who get sick from the flu varies. A paper published in *CID* found that between 3 percent and 11 percent of the United States population gets infected and develops flu symptoms each year. The 3 percent estimate is from the 2011 to 2012 season, which was an H1N1-predominant season classified as being of low severity. The estimated incidence of flu illness during two seasons was around 11 percent; 2012 to 2013 was an H3N2-predominant season classified as being of moderate severity, while 2014 to 2015 was an H3N2 predominant season classified as being of high severity.

Period of Contagiousness

You may be able to spread the flu to someone else before you know you are sick, as well as while you are sick.

- People with flu are most contagious in the initial three to four days after their illness begins.

- Some otherwise healthy adults may be able to infect others beginning one day before symptoms develop and up to five to seven days after becoming sick.
- Some people, especially young children and people with weakened immune systems might be able to infect others for an even longer time.

The Onset of Influenza Symptoms

The time from when a person is exposed and infected with flu to when symptoms begin is about two days but can range from about one to four days.

Complications of the Flu

Complications of the flu can include bacterial pneumonia, ear infections, sinus infections and worsening of chronic medical conditions, such as congestive heart failure, asthma, or diabetes.

People at High Risk from Influenza

Anyone can get the flu (even healthy people), and serious problems related to the flu can happen at any age, but some people are at high risk of developing serious flu-related complications if they get sick. This includes people 65 years and older, people of any age with certain chronic medical conditions (such as asthma, diabetes, or heart disease), pregnant women, and children younger than 5 years.

Preventing Seasonal Flu

The first and most important step in preventing the flu is to get a flu vaccine each year. The flu vaccine has been shown to reduce flu-related illnesses and the risk of serious flu complications that can result in hospitalization or even death. The CDC also recommends everyday preventive actions (such as staying away from people who are sick, covering coughs and sneezes and frequent handwashing) to help slow the spread of germs that cause respiratory (nose, throat, and lungs) illnesses, such as flu.

Diagnosing Influenza

It is very difficult to distinguish the flu from other viral or bacterial respiratory illnesses based on symptoms alone. There are tests available to diagnose the flu.

Treating Influenza

There are influenza antiviral drugs that can be used to treat the flu.

Section 15.3

Seasonal Flu versus Pandemic Flu

This section includes text excerpted from "Seasonal Flu versus Pandemic Flu Infographic," Centers for Disease Control and Prevention (CDC), June 26, 2018.

Influenza is one of the world's greatest infectious disease challenges. But did you know that the seasonal flu and pandemic flu are not the same?

What Is Seasonal Flu?

Influenza (flu) is a contagious respiratory illness caused by flu A and B viruses that infect the human respiratory tract. Annual flu epidemics occur among people worldwide.

What Is Pandemic Flu?

A flu pandemic is a global outbreak of the new flu A virus in people that is very different from current and recently circulating seasonal flu A viruses.

How Often Do Seasonal Flu Epidemics Occur?

Epidemics of seasonal flu happens every year. Fall and winter is the time for the flu in the United States.

How Often Do Flu Pandemics Occur?

Flu pandemics happen rarely. Four flu pandemics have happened in the past 100 years, but experts agree another one is inevitable.

How Do Seasonal Flu Viruses Spread?

Flu viruses are thought to spread mainly from person to person through droplets made when someone with the flu coughs, sneezes, or talks near a person (within six feet).

How Do Pandemic Flu Viruses Spread?

Pandemic flu viruses would spread in the same way as seasonal flu, but a pandemic virus will likely infect more people because few people have immunity to the pandemic flu virus.

Is There a Vaccine for Seasonal Flu?

Seasonal flu vaccines are made each year to vaccinate people against seasonal flu. Everyone six months and older should get a flu vaccine every year. For most people, only one dose of vaccine is needed.

Is There a Vaccine for Pandemic Flu?

Although the U.S. government maintains a limited stockpile of some prepandemic flu vaccines, a vaccine may not be widely available in the early stages of a pandemic. Two doses of pandemic flu vaccine will likely be needed.

Are There Medications to Treat Seasonal Flu?

Prescription medications called "antiviral drugs" can treat seasonal flu. During a severe flu season, there can be spot shortages of these drugs.

Are There Medications to Treat Pandemic Flu?

Flu antiviral medications may be used to treat pandemic flu if the virus is susceptible to these drugs. While a limited amount of flu antiviral drugs are stockpiled for use during a pandemic, supplies may not be enough to meet demand during a pandemic.

Who Is at Risk for Complications from Seasonal Flu?

Young children, people 65 years and older, pregnant women, and people with certain long-term medical conditions are more likely to have serious flu complications.

Who Is at Risk for Complications from Pandemic Flu?

Because this is a new virus not previously circulating in humans, it is not possible to predict who would be most at risk of severe complications in a future pandemic. In some past pandemics, healthy young adults were at high risk of developing severe flu complications.

Section 15.4
How the Flu Virus Can Change: "Drift" and "Shift"

This section includes text excerpted from "How the Flu Virus Can Change: 'Drift' and 'Shift,'" Centers for Disease Control and Prevention (CDC), October 15, 2019.

Influenza viruses are constantly changing. They can change in two different ways: antigenic drift and antigenic shift.

Antigenic Drift

One-way influenza viruses change is called "antigenic drift." These are small changes (or mutations) in the genes of influenza viruses that can lead to changes in the surface proteins of the virus: HA (hemagglutinin) and NA (neuraminidase). The HA and NA surface proteins of influenza viruses are "antigens," which means they are recognized by the immune system and are capable of triggering an immune response, including the production of antibodies that can block infection. The changes associated with antigenic drift happen continually over time as the virus replicates. Most flu shots are designed to target an influenza virus' HA surface proteins/antigens. The nasal spray flu vaccine Live attenuated influenza vaccine (LAIV) targets both the HA and NA of an influenza virus.

The small changes that occur from antigenic drift usually produce viruses that are closely related to one another, which can be illustrated by their location close together on a phylogenetic tree. Influenza viruses that are closely related to each other usually have similar antigenic properties. This means that antibodies your immune system creates against one influenza virus will likely recognize and respond to antigenically similar influenza viruses (this is called "cross-protection").

However, the small changes associated with antigenic drift can accumulate over time and result in viruses that are antigenically different (further away on the phylogenetic tree). It is also possible for a single (or small) change in a particularly important location on the HA to result in antigenic drift. When antigenic drift occurs, the body's immune system may not recognize and prevent sickness caused by the newer influenza viruses. As a result, a person becomes susceptible to flu infection again, as antigenic drift has changed the virus enough that a person's existing antibodies would not recognize and neutralize the newer influenza viruses.

Antigenic drift is the main reason why people can get the flu more than one time, and it is also a primary reason why the flu vaccine composition must be reviewed and updated each year (as needed) to keep up with evolving influenza viruses.

Antigenic Shift

The other type of change is called "antigenic shift." Antigenic shift is an abrupt, major change in influenza A virus, resulting in new HA and/or new HA and NA proteins in influenza viruses that infect humans. The shift can result in a new influenza A subtype in humans. One-way shift can happen is when an influenza virus from an animal population gains the ability to infect humans. Such animal-origin viruses can contain an HA or HA/NA combination that is so different from the same subtype in humans that most people do not have immunity to the new (e.g., novel) virus. Such a "shift" occurred in the spring of 2009 when an H1N1 virus with genes from North American swine, Eurasian swine, humans and birds emerged to infect people and quickly spread, causing a pandemic. When the shift happens, most people have little or no immunity against the new virus.

While influenza viruses change all the time due to antigenic drift, antigenic shift happens less frequently. Influenza pandemics occur very rarely; there have been four pandemics in the past 100 years. Type A viruses undergo both antigenic drift and shift and are the only influenza viruses known to cause pandemics, while influenza type B viruses change only by the more gradual process of antigenic drift.

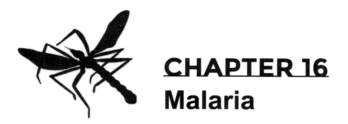

CHAPTER 16
Malaria

Chapter Contents

The Global Impact of Malaria

This section includes text excerpted from "Malaria,"
Centers for Disease Control and Prevention (CDC),
September 16, 2019.

Malaria is a mosquito-borne disease caused by a parasite. People with malaria often experience fever, chills, and flu-like illness. Left untreated, they may develop severe complications and die. Within the last decade, increasing numbers of partners and resources have rapidly increased malaria control efforts. This scale-up of interventions has saved 3.3 million lives globally and cut malaria mortality by 45 percent, leading to hopes and plans for elimination and ultimately eradication. In 2016, an estimated 216 million cases of malaria occurred worldwide and 445,000 people died, mostly children in the African Region.

About 1,700 cases of malaria are diagnosed in the United States each year. The vast majority of cases in the United States are in travelers and immigrants returning from countries where malaria transmission occurs, many from sub-Saharan Africa and South Asia.

Where malaria is found depends mainly on climatic factors, such as temperature, humidity, and rainfall. Malaria is transmitted in tropical and subtropical areas, where Anopheles mosquitoes can survive and multiply and malaria parasites can complete their growth cycle in the mosquitoes.

The highest transmission is found in Africa South of the Sahara and in parts of Oceania such as Papua New Guinea. In many temperate areas, such as western Europe and the United States, economic development and public-health measures have succeeded in eliminating malaria. However, most of these areas have Anopheles mosquitoes that can transmit malaria, and reintroduction of the disease is a constant risk.

While a number of companies and groups are working on developing a malaria vaccine, there is currently no effective vaccine on the market.

Malaria control is carried out through the recommended malaria treatment and prevention interventions. Prevention focuses on mosquito control (for example, through insecticides, water storage methods, and bed nets) and sometimes preventative antimalarial or fever treatment. Treatment of a patient with malaria depends on the country's national guidelines, which typically take into consideration the type (species) of the infecting parasite, the clinical status of the patient, any accompanying illness(es) or condition(s), pregnancy, drug allergies/other medications taken by the patient, and where the infection was acquired as well as the presence of antimalarial-drug resistance there.

Section 16.2
What Is Malaria?

This section includes text excerpted from "About Malaria—Frequently Asked Questions (FAQs)," Centers for Disease Control and Prevention (CDC), July 31, 2019.

Malaria is a serious and sometimes fatal disease caused by a parasite that commonly infects a certain type of mosquito which feeds on humans. People who get malaria are typically very sick with high fevers, shaking chills, and flu-like illness. Four kinds of malaria parasites infect humans: *Plasmodium falciparum*, *P. vivax*, *P. ovale*, and *P. malariae*. In addition, *P. knowlesi*, a type of malaria that naturally infects macaques in Southeast Asia, also infects humans, causing malaria that is transmitted from animal to human ("zoonotic" malaria). *P. falciparum* is the type of malaria that is most likely to result in severe infections and if not promptly treated, may lead to death. Although it can be a deadly disease, illness and death from malaria can usually be prevented.

About 1,700 cases of malaria are diagnosed in the United States each year. The vast majority of cases in the United States are in travelers and immigrants returning from parts of the world where malaria transmission occurs, including sub-Saharan Africa and South Asia.

Globally, the World Health Organization (WHO) estimates that in 2016, 216 million clinical cases of malaria occurred, and 445,000 people died of malaria, most of them children in Africa. Because malaria causes so much illness and death, the disease is a great drain on many national economies. Since many countries with malaria are already among the poorer nations, the disease maintains a vicious cycle of disease and poverty.

How People Get Malaria

Usually, people get malaria by being bitten by an infective female *Anopheles* mosquito. Only *Anopheles* mosquitoes can transmit malaria and they must have been infected through a previous blood meal taken from an infected person. When a mosquito bites an infected person, a small amount of blood is taken in which contains microscopic malaria parasites. About one week later, when the mosquito takes its next blood meal, these parasites mix with the mosquito's saliva and are injected into the person being bitten.

Because the malaria parasite is found in red blood cells (RBCs) of an infected person, malaria can also be transmitted through blood transfusion, organ transplant, or the shared use of needles or syringes contaminated with blood. Malaria may also be transmitted from a mother to her unborn infant before or during delivery ("congenital" malaria).

Malaria does not spread from one person to another, such as a cold or the flu, and it cannot be sexually transmitted. You cannot get malaria from casual contact with malaria-infected people, such as sitting next to someone who has malaria.

People at Risk of Getting Malaria

Anyone can get malaria. Most cases of malaria occur in people who live in countries with malaria transmission. People from countries with no malaria can become infected when they travel to countries with malaria or through a blood transfusion (although this is very rare). Also, an infected mother can transmit malaria to her infant before or during delivery.

Symptoms and Diagnosis of Malaria

Symptoms of malaria include fever and flu-like illness, including shaking chills, headache, muscle aches, and tiredness. Nausea, vomiting, and diarrhea may also occur. Malaria may cause anemia and jaundice (yellow coloring of the skin and eyes) because of the loss of red blood cells (RBCs). If not promptly treated, the infection can become severe and may cause kidney failure, seizures, mental confusion, coma, and death.

For most people, symptoms begin 10 days to 4 weeks after infection, although a person may feel ill as early as 7 days or as late as 1 year later. Two kinds of malaria, *P. vivax*, and *P. ovale* can occur again (relapsing malaria). In *P. vivax* and *P. ovale* infections, some parasites can remain dormant in the liver for several months up to about 4 years after a person is bitten by an infected mosquito. When these parasites come out of hibernation and begin invading red blood cells ("relapse"), the person will become sick.

Most people, at the beginning of the disease, have fever, sweats, chills, headaches, malaise, muscle aches, nausea, and vomiting. Malaria can very rapidly become a severe and life-threatening disease. The surest way for you and your healthcare provider to know whether you have malaria is to have a diagnostic test where a drop of your blood is examined under the microscope for the presence of malaria parasites. If you are sick and there is any suspicion of malaria (for example, if you have recently traveled to a country where malaria transmission occurs), the test should be performed without delay.

Preventing Malaria during Travel

Many effective antimalarial drugs are available. Your healthcare provider and you will decide on the best drug for you, if any, based on your travel plans, medical history, age, drug allergies, pregnancy status, and other factors.

To allow enough time for some of the drugs to become effective and for a pharmacy to prepare any special doses of medicine (especially doses for children and infants), you may need to visit your healthcare provider four to six weeks before travel. Other malaria medicines only need to be started the day before travel and so last-minute travelers can still benefit from a visit to their healthcare provider before traveling.

The drugs used to prevent malaria have been shown to be safe and well-tolerated for long term use.

Take Precautions

Anyone who goes to a country where malaria transmission occurs should take precautions against contracting malaria. During the time that you have spent in the United States, you have lost any malaria immunity that you might have had while living in your native country. Without frequent exposure to malaria parasites, your immune system has lost its ability to fight malaria. You are now as much at risk as someone who was born in the United States (a "nonimmune" person). Please consult with your healthcare provider or visit a travel clinic and get to know about precautions to take against malaria (preventive drugs and protection against mosquito bites) and against other diseases.

Buying Medications Abroad

Buying medications abroad has its risks. The drugs could be of poor quality because of the way they are produced. The drugs could contain contaminants or they could be counterfeit drugs, and therefore, may not provide you the protection you need against malaria. In addition, some medications that are sold overseas are not used anymore in the United States or were never sold here. These drugs may not be safe or their safety has never been evaluated.

It would be best to purchase all the medications that you need before you leave the United States. As a precaution, note the name of the medication(s) and the name of the manufacturer(s). That way, in case of accidental loss, you can replace the drug(s) abroad at a reliable vendor.

Vaccine for Malaria

Attempts at producing an effective malaria vaccine and vaccine clinical trials are ongoing. The malaria parasite is a complex organism with a complicated life cycle. The parasite has the ability to evade your immune system by constantly changing its surface, so developing a vaccine against these varying surfaces is very difficult. In addition, scientists do not yet totally understand the complex immune responses that protect humans against malaria. However, many scientists all over the world are working on developing an effective vaccine. Because other methods of fighting malaria, including drugs, insecticides, and insecticide-treated bed nets, have not succeeded in eliminating the disease, the search for a vaccine is considered to be one of the most important research projects in public health.

Other Preventive Measures

You and your family can most effectively prevent malaria by taking all three of these important measures:

- Taking antimalarial medication to kill the parasites and prevent becoming ill
- Keeping mosquitoes from biting you, especially at night
- Sleeping under insecticide-treated bed nets, using insect repellent, and wearing long-sleeved clothing if out of doors at night.

Treating Malaria

The disease should be treated early in its course before it becomes serious and life-threatening. Several good antimalarial drugs are available and should be taken early on. The most important step is to go see a doctor if you are sick and are presently in, or have recently been in an area with malaria so that the disease is diagnosed and treated right away.

Malaria can be cured with prescription drugs. The type of drugs and length of treatment depends on the type of malaria, where the person was infected, their age, whether they are pregnant, and how sick they are at the start of treatment.

If the right drugs are used, people who have malaria can be cured and all the malaria parasites can be cleared from their bodies. However, the disease can continue if it is not treated or if it is treated with the wrong drug. Some drugs are not effective because the parasite is resistant to them. Some people with malaria may be treated with the right drug, but at the wrong dose or for too short a period of time.

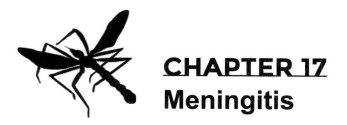

CHAPTER 17
Meningitis

What Is Meningitis?

Infections and other disorders affecting the brain and spinal cord can activate the immune system, which leads to inflammation. These diseases, and the resulting inflammation, can produce a wide range of symptoms, including fever, headache, seizures, and changes in behavior or confusion. In extreme cases, these can cause brain damage, stroke, or even death.

Inflammation of the meninges, the membranes that surround the brain and spinal cord, is called "meningitis."

What Causes Meningitis

Infectious causes of meningitis include bacteria, viruses, fungi, and parasites. For some individuals, environmental exposure (such as a parasite), recent travel, or immunocompromised state (such as human immunodeficiency virus (HIV), diabetes, steroids, chemotherapy treatment) are important risk factors. There are also noninfectious causes, such as autoimmune/rheumatological diseases and certain medications.

- **Bacterial meningitis** is a rare but potentially fatal disease. Several types of bacteria can cause an upper respiratory-tract infection (URTI) and then travel through the bloodstream to the brain.

This chapter includes text excerpted from "Meningitis and Encephalitis Fact Sheet," Centers for Disease Control and Prevention (CDC), August 13, 2019.

The disease can also occur when certain bacteria invade the meninges directly. Bacterial meningitis can cause stroke, hearing loss, and permanent brain damage.

- **Pneumococcal meningitis** is the most common form of meningitis and is the most serious form of bacterial meningitis. Some 6,000 cases of Pneumococcal meningitis are reported in the United States each year. The disease is caused by the bacterium *Streptococcus pneumoniae*, which also causes pneumonia, blood poisoning (septicemia), and ear and sinus infections. At particular risk are children under two years of age and adults with a weakened immune system. People who have had pneumococcal meningitis often suffer neurological damage ranging from deafness to severe brain damage. Immunizations are available for certain strains of the pneumococcal bacteria.

- **Meningococcal meningitis** is caused by the bacterium *Neisseria meningitides*. Each year in the United States about 2,600 people get this highly contagious disease. High-risk groups include infants under the age of 1 year, people with suppressed immune systems, travelers to foreign countries where the disease is endemic, and college students (freshmen in particular), military recruits, and others who reside in dormitories. Between 10 and 15 percent of cases are fatal, with another 10 to 15 percent causing brain damage and other serious side effects. If meningococcal meningitis is diagnosed, people in close contact with an infected individual should be given preventative antibiotics.

- ***Haemophilus influenzae* meningitis** was at one time the most common form of bacterial meningitis. Fortunately, the *Haemophilus influenzae* b vaccine has greatly reduced the number of cases in the United States. Those most at risk of getting this disease are children in child-care settings and children who do not have access to the vaccine.

Other forms of bacterial meningitis include Listeria monocytogenes meningitis (in which certain foods such as unpasteurized dairy or deli meats are sometimes implicated); *Escherichia coli* meningitis, which is most common in elderly adults and newborns and may be transmitted to a baby through the birth canal; and Mycobacterium tuberculosis (MTB) meningitis, a rare disease that occurs when the bacterium that causes tuberculosis attacks the meninges.

Viral, or aseptic, meningitis is usually caused by enteroviruses—common viruses that enter the body through the mouth and travel to the brain and surrounding tissues where they multiply. Enteroviruses are present in mucus, saliva, and feces, and can be transmitted through direct contact with an infected person or an infected object or surface. Other viruses that cause meningitis include varicella zoster (the virus that causes chickenpox and can appear decades later as shingles), influenza, mumps, HIV, and herpes simplex type 2 (HSV-2) (genital herpes).

Fungal infections can affect the brain. The most common form of fungal meningitis is caused by the fungus *cryptococcus neoformans* (found mainly in dirt and bird droppings). Cryptococcal meningitis mostly occurs in immunocompromised individuals such as those with acquired immunodeficiency syndrome (AIDS) but can also occur in healthy people. Some of these cases can be slow to develop and smolder for weeks. Although treatable, fungal meningitis often recurs in nearly half of affected persons.

Parasitic causes include cysticercosis (a tapeworm infection in the brain), which is common in other parts of the world, as well as cerebral malaria.

There are rare cases of amoebic meningitis, sometimes related to freshwater swimming, which can be rapidly fatal.

Who Is at Risk for Meningitis?

Anyone—from infants to older adults—can get meningitis. People with weakened immune systems, including those persons with HIV or those taking immunosuppressant drugs, are at increased risk.

How Is Meningitis Transmitted?

Some forms of bacterial meningitis are contagious and can be spread through contact with saliva, nasal discharge, feces, or respiratory and throat secretions (often spread through kissing, coughing, or sharing drinking glasses, eating utensils, or such personal items as toothbrushes, lipstick, or cigarettes). For example, people sharing a household, at a daycare center, or in a classroom with an infected person can become infected. College students living in dormitories—in particular, college freshmen—have a higher risk of contracting meningococcal meningitis than college students overall. Children who have not been given routine vaccines are at increased risk of developing certain types of bacterial meningitis.

Because these diseases can occur suddenly and progress rapidly, anyone who is suspected of having either meningitis should immediately contact a doctor or go to the hospital.

What Are the Signs and Symptoms of Meningitis?

The hallmark signs of meningitis include some or all of the following: sudden fever, severe headache, nausea or vomiting, double vision, drowsiness, sensitivity to bright light, and a stiff neck.

Meningitis often appears with flu-like symptoms that develop over one to two days. Distinctive rashes are typically seen in some forms of the disease. Meningococcal meningitis may be associated with kidney and adrenal gland failure and shock.

Important signs of meningitis to watch for in an infant include fever, lethargy, not waking for feedings, vomiting, body stiffness, unexplained/unusual irritability, and a full or bulging fontanel (soft spot on the top of the head).

How Is Meningitis Diagnosed?

Following a physical exam and medical history to review activities of the past several days or weeks (such as recent exposure to insects, ticks or animals, any contact with ill persons, or recent travel; preexisting medical conditions and medications), the doctor may order various diagnostic tests to confirm the presence of infection or inflammation. Early diagnosis is vital, as symptoms can appear suddenly and escalate to brain damage, hearing and/or speech loss, blindness, or even death.

Diagnostic tests include:

- A neurological examination involves a series of physical examination tests designed to assess motor and sensory function, nerve function, hearing and speech, vision, coordination and balance, mental status, and changes in mood or behavior.
- Laboratory screening of blood, urine, and body secretions can help detect and identify brain and/or spinal cord infection and determine the presence of antibodies and foreign proteins. Such tests can also rule out metabolic conditions that may have similar symptoms.
- Analysis of the cerebrospinal fluid (CSF) that surrounds and protects the brain and spinal cord can detect infections in the brain and/or spinal cord, acute and chronic inflammation, and other diseases. A small amount of CSF is removed by a special needle that is inserted into the lower back and the fluid is tested to detect the presence of bacteria, blood, and viruses. The testing can also measure glucose levels (a low glucose level can be seen in bacterial or fungal meningitis) and white blood cells (WBCs) (elevated white blood cell counts are a sign of inflammation), as well as protein and antibody levels.

Brain imaging can reveal signs of brain inflammation, internal bleeding or hemorrhage, or other brain abnormalities. Two painless, noninvasive imaging procedures are routinely used to diagnose meningitis.

- Computed tomography, also known as a "CT scan," combines x-rays and computer technology to produce rapid, clear, two-dimensional images of organs, bones, and tissues. Occasionally a contrast dye is injected into the bloodstream to highlight the different tissues in the brain and to detect signs of inflammation of the meninges.
- Magnetic resonance imaging (MRI) uses computer-generated radio waves and a strong magnet to produce detailed images of body structures, including tissues, organs, bones, and nerves. An MRI can help identify brain and spinal cord inflammation, infection, tumors, and other conditions. A contrast dye may be injected prior to the test to reveal more detail.

Additionally, electroencephalography, or EEG, can identify abnormal brain waves by monitoring electrical activity in the brain noninvasively through the skull. Among its many functions, EEG is used to help diagnose patterns that may suggest specific viral infections such as herpes virus and to detect seizures that do not show any clinical symptoms but may contribute to an altered level of consciousness in critically ill individuals.

How Is Meningitis Treated?

People who are suspected of having meningitis should receive immediate, aggressive medical treatment. Both diseases can progress quickly and have the potential to cause severe, irreversible neurological damage.

Early treatment of bacterial meningitis involves antibiotics that can cross the blood-brain barrier (a lining of cells that keeps harmful microorganisms and chemicals from entering the brain). Appropriate antibiotic treatment for most types of meningitis can greatly reduce the risk of dying from the disease. Anticonvulsants to prevent seizures and corticosteroids to reduce brain inflammation may be prescribed.

Infected sinuses may need to be drained. Corticosteroids such as prednisone may be ordered to relieve brain pressure and swelling and to prevent hearing loss that is common in *Haemophilus influenza* meningitis. Lyme disease is treated with antibiotics.

Antibiotics, developed to kill bacteria, are not effective against viruses. Fortunately, viral meningitis is rarely life-threatening and no specific treatment is needed. Fungal meningitis is treated with intravenous antifungal medications.

Can Meningitis Be Prevented?

People should avoid sharing food, utensils, glasses, and other objects with someone who may be exposed to or have the infection. People should wash their hands often with soap and rinse under running water.

Effective vaccines are available to prevent *Haemophilus influenza*, pneumococcal and meningococcal meningitis.

People who live, work, or go to school with someone who has been diagnosed with bacterial meningitis may be asked to take antibiotics for a few days as a preventive measure.

To lessen the risk of being bitten by an infected mosquito or other arthropod, people should limit outdoor activities at night, wear long-sleeved clothing when outdoors, use insect repellents that are most effective for that particular region of the country, and rid lawn and outdoor areas of free-standing pools of water, in which mosquitoes breed. Repellants should not be overapplied, particularly on young children and especially infants, as chemicals, such as DEET may be absorbed through the skin.

What Is the Prognosis for Meningitis?

The outcome generally depends on the particular infectious agent involved, the severity of the illness, and how quickly treatment is given. In most cases, people with very mild meningitis can make a full recovery, although the process may be slow.

Individuals who experience only headaches, fever, and stiff neck may recover in 2 to 4 weeks. Individuals with bacterial meningitis typically show some relief 48 to 72 hours following initial treatment but are more likely to experience complications caused by the disease. In more serious cases, these diseases can cause hearing and/or speech loss, blindness, permanent brain and nerve damage, behavioral changes, cognitive disabilities, lack of muscle control, seizures, and memory loss. These individuals may need long-term therapy, medication, and supportive care.

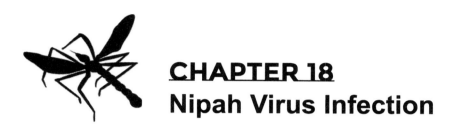

CHAPTER 18
Nipah Virus Infection

Nipah virus (NiV) is a member of the family *Paramyxoviridae*, genus *Henipavirus*. NiV was initially isolated and identified in 1999 during an outbreak of encephalitis and respiratory illness among pig farmers and people with close contact with pigs in Malaysia and Singapore. Its name originated from Sungai Nipah, a village in the Malaysian Peninsula where pig farmers became ill with encephalitis.

In the 1999 outbreak, NiV caused relatively mild disease in pigs, but nearly 300 human cases with over 100 deaths were reported. In order to stop the outbreak, more than a million pigs were euthanized, causing tremendous trade loss for Malaysia. Since this outbreak, no subsequent cases (in neither swine nor human) have been reported in either Malaysia or Singapore.

In 2001, NiV was again identified as the causative agent in an outbreak of human disease occurring in Bangladesh. Genetic sequencing confirmed this virus as NiV, but a strain different from the one identified in 1999. In the same year, another outbreak was identified retrospectively in Siliguri, India with reports of person-to-person transmission in hospital settings

This chapter contains text excerpted from the following sources: Text in this chapter begins with excerpts from "Nipah Virus (NiV)," Centers for Disease Control and Prevention (CDC), March 20, 2014. Reviewed January 2020; Text beginning with the heading "How Do People Get Nipah Virus Infection?" is excerpted from "Frequently Asked Questions: Nipah Virus," Centers for Disease Control and Prevention (CDC), May 30, 2018.

(nosocomial transmission). Unlike the Malaysian NiV outbreak, outbreaks occur almost annually in Bangladesh and have been reported several times in India.

How Do People Get Nipah Virus Infection?

People can get NiV infection from contact with the excrement or droppings of infected fruit bats, pigs, or other people infected with NiV. People can also get infected with NiV when they consume raw date palm sap (a drink found in parts of Asia) that is contaminated with bat droppings.

Do Animals Get Sick from Nipah Virus?

The main reservoir or carrier, an animal of NiV is a species of fruit bat found in Southeast Asia. Fruit bats do not get sick from NiV. However, they can pass the virus to other animals such as pigs, which can get sick. These animals can then pass the virus along to people.

How Can People Spread Nipah Virus to Each Other?

Nipah virus is spread from person to person through contact with infectious body fluids from another person such as nasal or respiratory droplets, urine, or blood.

How Can People Protect Themselves from Getting Nipah Virus Infection?

People can protect themselves from getting NiV infection by limiting their contact with fruit bats and sick pigs in affected areas of Southeast Asia, and by not drinking raw date palm sap. People should also avoid direct contact with body fluids from infected patients by wearing appropriate personal protective equipment such as gloves, gown, and facemask, and practicing good hand hygiene.

What Are the Symptoms of Nipah Virus Infection?

Typically, people become ill between 5 and 14 days after they are infected. Initial symptoms can include fever, headache, nausea and vomiting, shortness of breath, and may worsen to include drowsiness, confusion, and coma. Death can occur in as many as 80 percent of cases.

What Is the Treatment for Nipah Virus Infection?

At this time, the only treatment for NiV infection is supportive care. There are no antivirals or other medicines that have been found to conclusively treat NiV infection in people.

Is There a Vaccine for Nipah Virus Infection?

There is currently no vaccine available for NiV infection.

CHAPTER 19
Smallpox

Thousands of years ago, the variola virus (smallpox virus) emerged and began causing illness and deaths in human populations, with smallpox outbreaks occurring from time to time. Smallpox is a serious infectious disease caused by the variola virus. People who had smallpox had a fever and a distinctive, progressive skin rash. Most people with smallpox recover, but about 3 out of every 10 people with the disease died. Many smallpox survivors have permanent scars over large areas of their bodies, especially their faces. Some are left blind.

Thanks to the success of vaccination, smallpox was eradicated, and no cases of naturally occurring smallpox have happened since 1977. The last natural outbreak of smallpox in the United States occurred in 1949.

Transmission of Smallpox

Before smallpox was eradicated, it was mainly spread by direct and fairly prolonged face-to-face contact between people. Smallpox patients became contagious once the first sores appeared in their mouth and throat (early rash stage). They spread the virus when they coughed or sneezed and droplets from their nose or mouth spread to other people. They remained contagious until their last smallpox scab fell off.

This chapter includes text excerpted from "Smallpox," Centers for Disease Control and Prevention (CDC), July 12, 2017.

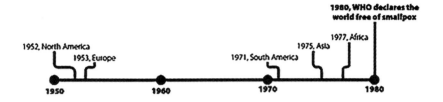

Figure 19.1. Smallpox Global Eradication—Timeline *(Source: "Global Smallpox Eradication," Centers for Disease Control and Prevention (CDC))*

These scabs and the fluid found in the patient's sores also contained the variola virus. The virus can spread through these materials or through the objects contaminated by them, such as bedding or clothing. People who cared for smallpox patients and washed their bedding or clothing had to wear gloves and take care to not get infected.

Rarely, smallpox has spread through the air in enclosed settings, such as a building (airborne route).

Smallpox can be spread by humans only. Scientists have no evidence that smallpox can be spread by insects or animals.

Signs and Symptoms of Smallpox

A person with smallpox goes through several stages as the disease progresses. Each stage has its own signs and symptoms.

Incubation Period

The incubation period is the length of time the virus is in a person's body before they look or feel sick. During this period, a person usually has no symptoms and may feel fine. This stage can last anywhere from 7 to 19 days (although the average length is 10 to 14 days) and is not contagious at this point in time.

Initial Symptoms

This stage lasts anywhere from two to four days. Smallpox may be contagious during this phase but is most contagious during the next two stages (early rash and pustular rash and scabs).

The first symptoms include:
- High fever
- Head and body aches
- Sometimes vomiting

At this time, people are usually too sick to carry on their normal activities.

Early Rash

This stage lasts about four days. At this time, the person is most contagious.

A rash starts as small red spots on the tongue and in the mouth. These spots change into sores that break open and spread large amounts of the virus into the mouth and throat. The person continues to have a fever.

Once the sores in the mouth start breaking down, a rash appears on the skin, starting on the face and spreading to the arms and legs, and then to the hands and feet. Usually, it spreads to all parts of the body within 24 hours. As this rash appears, the fever begins to decline, and the person may start to feel better.

By the fourth day, the skin sores fill with a thick, opaque fluid and often have a dent in the center. Once the skin sores fill with fluid, the fever may rise again and remain high until scabs form over the bumps.

Pustular Rash and Scabs

This stage lasts about 10 days and remains to be contagious. The sores become pustules (sharply raised, usually round and firm to the touch, such as peas under the skin). After about 5 days, the pustules begin to form a crust and then scab. By the end of the second week, after the rash appears, most of the sores have scabbed over.

Scabs for Off

This stage lasts about six days. Four weeks after the rash appears, all scabs should have fallen off. Once all the scabs have fallen off, the person is no longer contagious.

No Scabs

The person is no longer contagious. Four weeks after the rash appears, all scabs should have fallen off. Once all the scabs have fallen off, the person is no longer contagious.

Prevention and Treatment of Smallpox

There is a vaccine to protect people from smallpox. If there were a smallpox outbreak, health officials would use the smallpox vaccine to control it. While some antiviral drugs may help treat it or prevent the smallpox disease from getting worse, there is no treatment for it that has been proven effective in people sick with the disease.

Smallpox Vaccine

Smallpox can be prevented by the smallpox vaccine.

If you get the vaccine:
- Before contact with the virus, the vaccine can protect you from getting sick.
- Within three days of being exposed to the virus, the vaccine might protect you from getting the disease. If you still get the disease, you might get much less sick than an unvaccinated person would.
- Within four to seven days of being exposed to the virus, the vaccine likely gives you some protection from the disease. If you still get the disease, you might not get as sick as an unvaccinated person would.

Once you have developed the smallpox rash, the vaccine will not protect you.

The smallpox vaccine is not available to the general public because smallpox has been eradicated, and the virus no longer exists in nature. However, there is enough smallpox vaccine to vaccinate every person in the United States if a smallpox outbreak were to occur.

Antiviral Drugs

In July 2018, the U.S. Food and Drug Administration (FDA) approved tecovirimat (TPOXX) for the treatment of smallpox. Because these drugs were not tested in people sick with smallpox, it is not known if a person with smallpox would benefit from treatment with them. However, their use may be considered if there ever is an outbreak of smallpox.

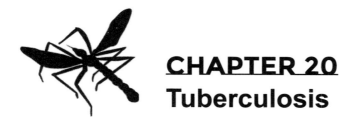

CHAPTER 20
Tuberculosis

The Global Impact of Tuberculosis

Tuberculosis (TB) is caused by a bacterium called "*Mycobacterium tuberculosis*." It usually attacks the lungs, but it can also attack other parts of the body such as the kidney, spine, and brain. Not everyone infected with TB bacteria becomes sick. As a result, two TB-related conditions exist latent TB infection (LTBI) and TB disease. If not treated properly, TB disease can be fatal.

In 2018, 1.7 billion people were infected by TB bacteria—roughly 23 percent of the world's population. TB is the leading infectious disease killer in the world, claiming 1.5 million lives each year. Of the 10 million individuals who became ill with TB in 2018, approximately three million were "missed" by health systems and do not get the care they need, allowing the disease to continue to be transmitted.

Resistance to anti-TB drugs can occur when these drugs are misused or mismanaged. Examples include when patients do not complete their full course of treatment; when healthcare providers prescribe the wrong treatment, the wrong dose, or length of time for taking the drugs; when

This chapter contains text excerpted from the following sources: Text under the heading "The Global Impact of Tuberculosis" is excerpted from "Global Health—Newsroom—Tuberculosis," Centers for Disease Control and Prevention (CDC), November 7, 2019: Text beginning with the heading "How Tuberculosis Spreads" is excerpted from "Basic TB Facts—How TB Spreads," Centers for Disease Control and Prevention (CDC), December 31, 2018.

the supply of drugs is not always available; or when the drugs are of poor quality.

Multidrug-resistant tuberculosis (MDR-TB) is TB resistant to two of the most important drugs used to treat TB: Isoniazid (INH) and Rifampin (RIF).

Extensively drug-resistant TB (XDR-TB) is a rare type of MDR-TB that is resistant to isoniazid and rifampin, plus any fluoroquinolone and at least one of three injectable second-line drugs (i.e., amikacin, kanamycin, or capreomycin). Because XDR-TB is resistant to the most potent TB drugs, patients are left with treatment options that are much less effective.

Extensively drug-resistant TB is of special concern for persons with HIV infection or other conditions that can weaken the immune system. These persons are more likely to develop TB disease once they are infected, and also have a higher risk of death once they develop TB.

Because the reach of TB is so broad, to effectively and fully address MDR-TB in the United States, MDR-TB must be addressed globally in the places hardest hit. TB anywhere is TB everywhere—it spreads from person to person and does not respect borders. Recent models show that unless efforts are scaled up to address this growing threat, the number of people dying from drug-resistant TB will nearly double every five years.

How Tuberculosis Spreads

Tuberculosis bacteria are spread through the air from one person to another. The TB bacteria are put into the air when a person with TB disease of the lungs or throat coughs, speaks or sings. People nearby may breathe in these bacteria and become infected.

Tuberculosis is NOT spread by:
- Shaking someone's hand
- Sharing food or drink
- Touching bed linens or toilet seats
- Sharing toothbrushes
- Kissing

When a person breathes in TB bacteria, the bacteria can settle in the lungs and begin to grow. From there, they can move through the blood to other parts of the body, such as the kidney, spine, and brain.

Tuberculosis disease in the lungs or throat can be infectious. This means that the bacteria can be spread to other people. TB in other parts of the body, such as the kidney or spine, is usually not infectious.

People with TB disease are most likely to spread it to people they spend time with every day. This includes family members, friends, and coworkers or schoolmates.

Signs and Symptoms of Tuberculosis

Symptoms of TB disease depend on where in the body the TB bacteria are growing. TB bacteria usually grow in the lungs (pulmonary TB). TB disease in the lungs may cause symptoms, such as:

- A bad cough that lasts three weeks or longer
- Pain in the chest
- Coughing up blood or sputum (phlegm from deep inside the lungs)

Other symptoms of TB disease are:

- Weakness or fatigue
- Weight loss
- No appetite
- Chills
- Fever
- Sweating at night

Symptoms of TB disease in other parts of the body depend on the area affected.

People who have latent TB infection do not feel sick, do not have any symptoms, and cannot spread TB to others.

Diagnosis of Tuberculosis

There are two kinds of tests that are used to detect TB bacteria in the body: the TB skin test (TST) and TB blood tests. A positive TB skin test or TB blood test only tells that a person has been infected with TB bacteria. It does not tell whether the person has latent TB infection or has progressed to TB disease. Other tests, such as a chest x-ray and a sample of sputum, are needed to see whether the person has TB disease. If a person is found to be infected with TB bacteria, other tests are needed to see if the person has latent TB infection or TB disease.

Tuberculosis Skin Test

The TB skin test is also called the "Mantoux tuberculin skin test." A TB skin test requires two visits to a healthcare provider.

On the first visit the test is placed; on the second visit, the healthcare provider reads the test.

The TB skin test is performed by injecting a small amount of fluid (called "tuberculin") into the skin on the lower part of the arm.

A person given the tuberculin skin test must return within 48 to 72 hours to have a trained healthcare worker look for a reaction on the arm.

The result depends on the size of the raised, hard area or swelling.

What the Test Results Mean

- **Positive skin test.** This means the person's body was infected with TB bacteria. Additional tests are needed to determine if the person has latent TB infection or TB disease.
- **Negative skin test.** This means the person's body did not react to the test, and that latent TB infection or TB disease is not likely.

There is no problem with repeating a TB skin test. If repeated, the additional test should be placed in a different location on the body.

The TB skin test is the preferred TB test for children under the age of five.

Tuberculosis Blood Test

Tuberculosis blood tests are also called "interferon-gamma release assays" or "IGRAs." Two TB blood tests are approved by the U.S. Food and Drug Administration (FDA) and are available in the United States: the QuantiFERON®—TB Gold In-Tube test (QFT-GIT) and the T-SPOT®. TB test (T-Spot).

A healthcare provider will draw a patient's blood and send it to a laboratory for analysis and results.

What the Test Results Mean

- **Positive TB blood test.** This means that the person has been infected with TB bacteria. Additional tests are needed to determine if the person has latent TB infection or TB disease.
- **Negative TB blood test.** This means that the person's blood did not react to the test and that latent TB infection or TB disease is not likely.

Tuberculosis blood tests are the preferred TB test for:
- People who have received the TB vaccine bacille Calmette–Guérin (BCG).
- People who have a difficult time returning for a second appointment to look for a reaction to the TST.

Who Should Be Tested?

Certain people should be tested for TB infection because they are at higher risk of being infected with TB bacteria, including:
- People who have spent time with someone who has TB disease
- People from a country where TB disease is common (most countries in Latin America, the Caribbean, Africa, Asia, eastern Europe, and Russia)
- People who live or work in high-risk settings (for example correctional facilities, long-term care facilities or nursing homes, and homeless shelters)
- Healthcare workers who care for patients at increased risk for TB disease
- Infants, children, and adolescents exposed to adults who are at increased risk for latent TB infection or TB disease

Many people who have latent TB infection never develop TB disease. But, some people who have latent TB infection are more likely to develop TB disease than others. Those at high risk for developing TB disease include:
- People with human immunodeficiency virus (HIV) infection
- People who became infected with TB bacteria in the last two years
- Babies and young children

- People who inject illegal drugs
- People who are sick with other diseases that weaken the immune system
- Elderly people
- People who were not treated correctly for TB in the past

Tuberculosis tests are generally not needed for people with a low risk of infection with TB bacteria.

Testing in bacille Calmette-Guerin-Vaccinated Persons

Many people born outside of the United States have been given a vaccine called "BCG."

People who were previously vaccinated with BCG may receive a TB skin test to test for TB infection. Vaccination with BCG may cause a false positive reaction to a TB skin test. A positive reaction to a TB skin test may be due to the BCG vaccine itself or due to infection with TB bacteria.

Tuberculosis blood tests (IGRAs), unlike the TB skin test, are not affected by prior BCG vaccination and are not expected to give a false-positive result in people who have received BCG. TB blood tests are the preferred method of TB testing for people who have received the BCG vaccine.

Treatment of Tuberculosis

When TB bacteria become active (multiplying in the body) and the immune system cannot stop the bacteria from growing, this is called "TB disease." TB disease will make a person sick. People with TB disease may spread the bacteria to people with whom they spend many hours.

It is very important that people who have TB disease are treated, finish the medicine, and take the drugs exactly as prescribed. If they stop taking the drugs too soon, they can become sick again; if they do not take the drugs correctly, the TB bacteria that are still alive may become resistant to those drugs. TB that is resistant to drugs is harder and more expensive to treat.

Tuberculosis disease can be treated by taking several drugs for 6 to 9 months. There are 10 drugs approved by the U.S. Food and Drug Administration (FDA) for treating TB. Of the approved drugs, the first-line anti-TB agents that form the core of treatment regimens are:

- Isoniazid
- Rifampin
- Ethambutol
- Pyrazinamide

Treatment Completion

Treatment completion is determined by the number of doses ingested over a given period of time.

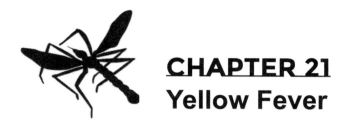

CHAPTER 21
Yellow Fever

The Global Impact of Yellow Fever

Yellow fever virus (YFV) is estimated to cause 200,000 cases of disease and 30,000 deaths each year, with 90 percent occurring in Africa. 20 to 50 percent of infected persons who develop severe disease die.

Yellow fever virus is transmitted to people primarily through the bite of infected *Aedes* or *Haemagogus* mosquitoes. People infected with yellow fever virus are infectious to mosquitoes shortly before the onset of fever and up to five days after onset. Outbreaks of yellow fever, which often occur when the disease is introduced to densely populated urban areas, can have disruptive effects on economies and healthcare systems.

Where Does the Yellow Fever Virus Occur?

Yellow fever virus is found in tropical and subtropical areas in South America and Africa. YFV is a very rare cause of illness in United States travelers to these areas.

This chapter contains text excerpted from the following sources: Text under the heading "The Global Impact of Yellow Fever" is excerpted from "Yellow Fever," Centers for Disease Control and Prevention (CDC), September 14, 2018: Text beginning with the heading "Where Does the Yellow Fever Virus Occur?" is excerpted from "Frequently Asked Questions," Centers for Disease Control and Prevention (CDC), January 15, 2019.

How Soon Do People Get Sick after Being Bitten by an Infected Mosquito?

The incubation period (time from infection to illness) is usually three to six days.

What Are the Symptoms of Yellow Fever?

Initial symptoms of yellow fever include sudden onset of fever, chills, severe headache, back pain, general body aches, nausea and vomiting, fatigue, and weakness. Most people improve after these initial symptoms. However, roughly 15 percent of people will have a brief period of hours to a day without symptoms and will then develop a more severe form of yellow fever disease. In severe cases, a person may develop a high fever, jaundice (a condition that involves yellow discoloration of the skin and the whites of the eyes), bleeding (especially from the gastrointestinal (GI) tract), and eventually shock and failure of many organs. Roughly 20 to 50 percent of people who develop the severe illness may die.

How Is Yellow Fever Diagnosed?

Diagnosis is usually based on blood tests that look for viruses or antibodies that a person's immune system makes against the viral infection.

What Is the Treatment for Yellow Fever?

No specific treatments have been found to help patients with yellow fever. If possible, patients with yellow fever should be hospitalized for the treatment of their symptoms and closely observed by healthcare workers. Rest, fluids, and use of pain medications and fever-reducing medications may relieve symptoms of fever and ache. Certain medications should be avoided, such as aspirin or other nonsteroidal anti-inflammatory drugs (NSAIDs) (such as ibuprofen and naproxen), because these may increase the risk of bleeding.

What Should You Do If You Think a Family Member Might Have Yellow Fever?

If you or anyone in your household has symptoms that are causing you concern, consult a healthcare provider promptly for proper diagnosis.

How Can People Reduce the Chance of Getting Infected with Yellow Fever Virus?

Yellow fever can be prevented by vaccination. The vaccine is a live but attenuated (less potent) strain of the virus. Travelers should also take action to prevent mosquito bites when in areas of Africa or South America with YFV transmission.

- **Use insect repellent.** When you go outdoors, use a U.S. Environmental Protection Agency (EPA)-registered insect repellents, such as those containing DEET, picaridin, IR3535, or oil of lemon eucalyptus on exposed skin. Even a short time outdoors can be long enough to get a mosquito bite.

- **Wear proper clothing to reduce mosquito bites.** When weather permits, wear long-sleeves, long pants and socks when outdoors. Mosquitoes may bite through thin clothing, so spraying clothes with repellent containing permethrin or another EPA-registered repellent will give extra protection. Clothing pretreated with permethrin is commercially available. Mosquito repellents containing permethrin are not approved for application directly to the skin.

- **Be aware of peak mosquito hours.** The peak biting times for many mosquito species is dusk to dawn. However, *Aedes aegypti*, one of the mosquitoes that transmit yellow fever virus, feeds during the daytime. Take extra care to use repellent and protective clothing during the daytime as well as during the evening and early morning. Staying in accommodations with screened or air-conditioned rooms, particularly during peak biting times, will also reduce the risk of mosquito bites.

Frequently Asked Questions about the Yellow Fever Vaccine

I Just Received the Yellow Fever Vaccine. Do I Need to Avoid Contact with My Immunocompromised Family Member?

No. There is no evidence that people who receive yellow fever vaccine shed the vaccine virus. Therefore, there is no need to avoid people, including those whose immune systems do not work well.

Who Should Get Yellow Fever Vaccine?

Yellow fever vaccine is recommended for people age nine months or older who are traveling to or living in areas at risk for yellow fever virus transmission in South America and Africa. Proof of yellow fever vaccine may be required for entry into certain countries.

Who Should Not Get Yellow Fever Vaccine?

Infants younger than six months of age should not get the vaccine. In addition, anyone with a severe allergy to any part of the vaccine, including eggs, chicken proteins, or gelatin should not get the vaccine. Anyone who has had a severe reaction to a previous dose of yellow fever vaccine should not be vaccinated again.

If you have any of the following conditions, your healthcare provider can help you decide whether you can safely receive the vaccine:

- Human immunodeficiency virus (HIV), acquired immunodeficiency syndrome (AIDS), or other diseases that affect the immune system
- Weakened immune system as a result of cancer or other medical conditions, transplant, or drug treatment (such as steroids, chemotherapy, or others that affect immune function)
- Thymus disorder
- Adults 60 years of age and older
- Infants 6 to 8 months of age
- Pregnant women and nursing mothers

How Long Does Yellow Fever Vaccination Last?

For most people, one dose of the vaccine provides long-lasting protection. Certain people may benefit from another dose of the vaccine either because they have problems with their immune system or they are in higher-risk settings.

Will I Have to Go to a Special Clinic to Get a Yellow Fever Vaccination?

Yes. Yellow fever vaccine is regulated by the International Health Regulations (IHRs), so only authorized providers can administer the vaccine. Most providers of the yellow fever vaccine can also give you other vaccines or medicines for travel.

Is Yellow Fever Vaccine Recommended for People 60 Years and Older Who Will Be Traveling to Areas with Risk for Yellow Fever?

People aged ≥60 years may be at increased risk for serious adverse events (serious disease or, very rarely, death) following vaccination, compared with younger persons. This is particularly true if they are receiving their first yellow fever vaccination. Travelers aged ≥60 years should discuss with their healthcare provider the risks and benefits of the vaccine given their travel plans. In addition to considering the vaccine, travelers to endemic areas should protect themselves from yellow fever and other vector-borne diseases. Preventive measures include wearing clothes with long sleeves and long pants and using an effective insect repellent, such as those with DEET, picaridin, IR3535, or oil of lemon eucalyptus.

What Are the Side Effects of Yellow Fever Vaccination?

Reactions to the yellow fever vaccine are generally mild. They can include mild headaches, muscle aches, and low-grade fevers. There have been reports of extremely rare but serious events following yellow fever vaccination.

I Think I Got Sick from the Vaccine, What Should I Do?

Consult with your healthcare provider. Ask your healthcare provider to report your case to the Vaccine Adverse Events Reporting System (VAERS) if she or he thinks the vaccine has made you sick.

Does the Yellow Fever Vaccine Contain Thimerosal?

No, the U.S. Food and Drug Administration (FDA)-approved yellow fever vaccine does not contain thimerosal.

How Long Should a Woman Wait to Conceive after Receiving a Yellow Fever Vaccination?

Yellow fever vaccination has not been known to cause any birth defects when given to pregnant women. Yellow fever vaccine has been given to many pregnant women without any apparent adverse effects on the fetus. However, since the yellow fever vaccine is a live virus vaccine, it poses a theoretical risk. While a two-week delay between yellow fever vaccination and conception is probably adequate, a one-month delay has been advocated as a more conservative approach. If a woman is inadvertently or of necessity vaccinated during pregnancy, she is unlikely to have any problems from the vaccine and her baby is very likely to be born healthy.

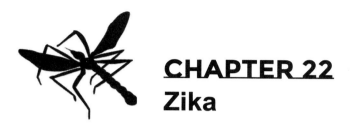

CHAPTER 22
Zika

Zika virus disease is caused by the Zika virus, which is spread to people primarily through the bite of an infected mosquito. The illness is usually mild with symptoms lasting up to a week, and many people do not have symptoms or will have only mild symptoms. However, Zika virus infection during pregnancy can cause a serious birth defect called "microcephaly" and other severe brain defects.

Symptoms of Zika

Many people infected with the Zika virus would not have symptoms or will only have mild symptoms. The most common symptoms of Zika are:

- Fever
- Rash
- Headache
- Joint pain
- Conjunctivitis (red eyes)
- Muscle pain

How Long Symptoms Last

Zika is usually mild with symptoms lasting for several days to a week. People usually do not get sick enough to go to the hospital, and they very

This chapter includes text excerpted from "Zika Virus," Centers for Disease Control and Prevention (CDC), May 20, 2019.

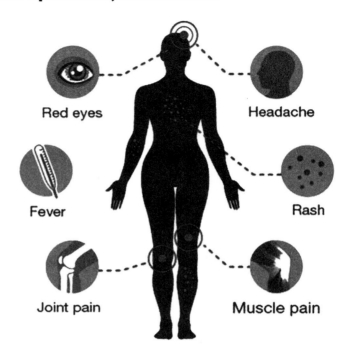

Figure 22.1. Common Symptoms of Zika

rarely die of Zika. For this reason, many people might not realize they have been infected. Symptoms of Zika are similar to other viruses spread through mosquito bites, such as dengue and chikungunya.

How Soon You Should Be Tested

Zika virus usually remains in the blood of an infected person for about a week. See your doctor or other healthcare providers if you develop symptoms and you live in or have recently traveled to an area with risk of Zika. Your doctor or other healthcare providers may order blood or urine tests to help determine if you have Zika. Once a person has been infected, she or he is likely to be protected from future infections.

When to See a Doctor or Healthcare Provider

See your doctor or other healthcare providers if you have symptoms described above and have visited an area with risk of Zika. This is especially important if you are pregnant. Be sure to tell your doctor or other healthcare providers where you traveled.

If You Think You Have Zika

- See your doctor or other healthcare providers for a diagnosis.
- Learn what you can do for treatment.
- Learn how you can protect others if you have Zika.

Zika Transmission

Zika virus is transmitted to people primarily through the bite of an infected *Aedes species* mosquito (*Ae. aegypti* and *Ae. albopictus*). These are the same mosquitoes that spread dengue and chikungunya viruses.

- These mosquitoes typically lay eggs in or near standing water in things, such as buckets, bowls, animal dishes, flower pots, and vases. They prefer to bite people and live indoors and outdoors near people.
- Mosquitoes that spread chikungunya, dengue, and Zika bite during the day and night.
- A mosquito gets infected with a virus when it bites an infected person during the period of time when the virus can be found in the person's blood, typically only through the first week of infection.
- Infected mosquitoes can then spread the virus to other people through bites.

From Mother to Child

- A pregnant woman can pass the Zika virus to her fetus during pregnancy. Zika is a cause of microcephaly and other severe fetal brain defects. The full range of other potential health problems that Zika virus infection during pregnancy may cause.
- A pregnant woman already infected with the Zika virus can pass the virus to her fetus during the pregnancy or around the time of birth.
- Zika virus has been found in breast milk. Possible Zika virus infections have been identified in breastfeeding babies, but Zika virus transmission through breast milk has not been confirmed. Additionally, we do not

yet know the long-term effects of the Zika virus on young infants infected after birth. Because current evidence suggests that the benefits of breastfeeding outweigh the risk of the Zika virus spreading through breast milk, the CDC continues to encourage mothers to breastfeed, even if they were infected or lived in or traveled to an area with risk of Zika. The CDC continues to study the Zika virus and the ways it can spread and will update recommendations as new information becomes available.

Through Sex

- Zika can be passed through sex from a person who has Zika to her or his partners. Zika can be passed through sex, even if the infected person does not have symptoms at the time. Learn how to protect yourself during sex.
  - It can be passed from a person with Zika before their symptoms start, while they have symptoms, and after their symptoms end.
  - Though not well documented, the virus may also be passed by a person who carries the virus but never develops symptoms.
- Studies are underway to find out how long Zika stays in the semen and vaginal fluids of people who have Zika, and how long it can be passed to sex partners. Zika can remain in semen longer than in other body fluids, including vaginal fluids, urine, and blood.

Through Blood Transfusion

- To date, there have not been any confirmed blood transfusion transmission cases in the United States.
- There have been multiple reports of possible blood transfusion transmission cases in Brazil.
- During the French Polynesian outbreak, 2.8 percent of blood donors tested positive for Zika and in previous outbreaks, the virus has been found in blood donors.

Through Laboratory and Healthcare Setting Exposure

- There are reports of laboratory-acquired Zika virus infections, although the route of transmission was not clearly established in all cases.

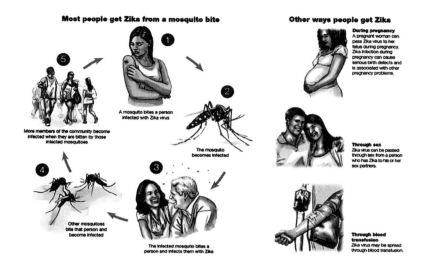

Figure 22.2. How Zika Spreads *(Source: "Zika Transmission," Centers for Disease Control and Prevention (CDC))*

- To date, no cases of Zika virus transmission in healthcare settings have been identified in the United States. Recommendations are available for healthcare providers to help prevent exposure to the Zika virus in healthcare settings.

Risks
- Anyone who lives in or travels to an area with risk of Zika and has not already been infected with the Zika virus can get it from mosquito bites. Once a person has been infected, she or he is likely to be protected from future infections.

Testing of Zika
How Zika Is Diagnosed
- To diagnose Zika, a doctor or other healthcare provider will ask about any recent travel and any signs and symptoms.
- They may order blood or urine tests to help determine if you have Zika.

Remember to ask for your Zika test results even if you are feeling better.

Only Some People Need Zika Testing

Following the Zika virus outbreaks in 2016, the number of Zika cases reported from most parts of the world declined and is now very low. Therefore, very few people need Zika testing.

Testing is recommended if you have symptoms of Zika and have traveled to a country with a current Zika outbreak (red areas).

Note: There are no countries or U.S. territories currently reporting an outbreak of Zika.

- Testing should take place as soon as possible, while you still have symptoms.
- Testing may include a molecular test that looks for the presence of the virus in the body or serological testing which looks for antibodies your body makes to fight infection.
- If you have questions talk to your healthcare provider.

Testing is recommended if you are a pregnant woman with symptoms of Zika and have traveled to an area with risk of Zika (purple areas) outside of the United States and its territories.

- Testing should take place as soon as possible, while you still have symptoms.
- Testing will be done using a molecular test that looks for the presence of the virus in the body.
- Serological testing is not recommended since antibodies against Zika persist for years and cross-react with other similar viruses, including dengue. For this reason, a positive lab result often cannot definitively tell you if you have a current or past infection or whether it is a Zika or dengue infection.
- If you have questions talk to your healthcare provider.

Testing is no longer routinely recommended if you are a pregnant woman with no symptoms of Zika but may be considered if you traveled to an area with a risk of Zika (purple areas).

- Upon your return from travel, testing should take place as soon as possible.
- Testing will be done using a molecular test that looks for the presence of the virus in the body.
- Serological testing is not recommended since antibodies against Zika persist for years and cross-react with other similar viruses, including dengue. For this reason, a positive lab result often cannot definitively tell you if you have a current or past infection or whether it is a Zika or dengue infection.
- If you have questions talk to your healthcare provider.

You should be tested for Zika if you are pregnant, traveled to an area with risk of Zika (purple areas) and your doctor sees Zika-associated abnormalities on an ultrasound or you deliver a baby with birth defects that may be related to Zika.

- Testing may include a molecular test that looks for the presence of the virus in the body or serological testing which looks for antibodies your body makes to fight infection.
- If you have questions talk to your healthcare provider.

Preconception Zika testing is NOT recommended.

If You Have Tested Positive for Zika
- If you are pregnant, you can pass Zika to your fetus.
- You can pass Zika to your sex partner(s).
- You can pass Zika to mosquitoes, which can bite you, get infected with the Zika virus, and spread the virus to other people.

Sexual Transmission and Testing
- A blood or urine test can help determine if you have Zika from the sexual transmission; however, testing blood, semen, vaginal fluids, or urine is not recommended to determine how likely a person is to pass the Zika virus through sex.

Treatment of Zika

There is no specific medicine or vaccine for the Zika virus.

- Treat the symptoms
- Get plenty of rest
- Drink fluids to prevent dehydration
- Take medicine, such as acetaminophen (Tylenol®) to reduce fever and pain.
- Do not take aspirin and other nonsteroidal anti-inflammatory drugs (NSAIDs) until dengue can be ruled out to reduce the risk of bleeding.
- If you are taking medicine for another medical condition, talk to your healthcare provider before taking additional medication.

If You Think You May Have or Had Zika

Tell your doctor or healthcare provider and take these steps to protect others.

If You Are Caring for a Person with Zika

Take steps to protect yourself from exposure to the person's blood and body fluids (urine, stool, vomit). If you are pregnant, you can care for someone with Zika if you follow these steps.

- Do not touch blood or body fluids or surfaces with these fluids on them with exposed skin.
- Wash hands with soap and water immediately after providing care.
- Immediately remove and wash clothes if they get blood or body fluids on them. Use laundry detergent and water temperature specified on the garment label. Using bleach is not necessary.
- Clean the sick person's environment daily using household cleaners according to label instructions.
- Immediately clean surfaces that have blood or other body fluids on them using household cleaners and disinfectants according to label instructions.

If you visit a family member or friend with Zika in a hospital, you should avoid contact with the person's blood and body fluids and surfaces with these fluids on them. Helping the person sit up or walk should not expose you. Make sure to wash your hands before and after touching the person.

Protect Yourself and Others
Use the Tips below to Protect Yourself and Others from Zika

Following the tips listed below, will help to protect you, your partner, your family, your friends, and your community from Zika. The more steps you take, the more protected you are. If you are caring for a family member or friend with Zika, take steps to protect yourself from exposure to the person's blood and body fluids.

Prevent Mosquito Bites
- Zika virus is spread to people mainly through the bite of an infected mosquito.
- Mosquitoes that spread Zika and other viruses bite during the day and night.
- The best way to prevent Zika is to protect yourself from mosquito bites.

Plan for Travel
- Outbreaks of Zika have occurred in different countries and territories.
- Zika virus will continue to infect people. It is difficult to know when and where the Zika virus will occur in the future.

Protect Yourself during Sex
- Zika can be passed through sex from a person who has Zika to her or his sex partners.
- It can remain in semen longer than in other body fluids, including vaginal fluids, urine, and blood.

If You Have Zika, Protect Others
- During the first week of infection, the Zika virus can be found in the blood and passed from an infected person to another mosquito through

mosquito bites. An infected mosquito can then spread the virus to other people.

- Zika can be passed through sex from a person who has Zika to her or his partners. Sex includes vaginal, anal and oral sex and the sharing of sex toys.

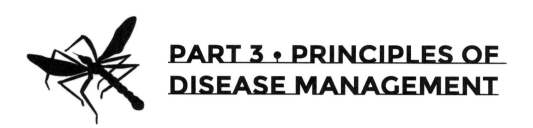

PART 3 • PRINCIPLES OF DISEASE MANAGEMENT

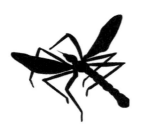

CHAPTER 23
Preventing Avoidable Epidemics

Chapter Contents

Immunization and Infectious Disease

This section includes text excerpted from "Immunization and Infectious Diseases," Office of Disease Prevention and Health Promotion (ODPHP), U.S. Department of Health and Human Services (HHS), March 15, 2010. Reviewed January 2020.

The increase in life expectancy during the 20th century is largely due to improvements in child survival. This increase is associated with reductions in infectious-disease mortality, due largely to immunization. However, infectious diseases remain a major cause of illness, disability, and death. Immunization recommendations in the United States target 17 vaccine-preventable diseases across the lifespan. Awareness of disease and completing prevention and treatment courses remain essential components for reducing infectious disease transmission.

Why Are Immunization and Infectious Diseases Important?

People in the United States continue to get diseases that are vaccine-preventable. Viral hepatitis, influenza, and tuberculosis (TB) remain among the leading causes of illness and death in the United States and account for substantial spending on the related consequences of infection.

The infectious disease public-health infrastructure, which carries out disease surveillance at the federal, state, and local levels, is an essential tool in the fight against newly emerging and re-emerging infectious diseases. Other important defenses against infectious diseases include:

- Proper use of vaccines
- Antibiotics
- Screening and testing guidelines
- Scientific improvements in the diagnosis of infectious disease-related health concerns

Understanding Immunization and Infectious Diseases

Immunization

Vaccines are among the most cost-effective clinical preventive services and are a core component of any preventive services package. Childhood immunization programs provide a very high return on investment. For example, for each birth cohort vaccinated with the routine immunization schedule (this includes DTap, Td, Hib, Polio, MMR, hepatitis B, and varicella vaccines), society:

- Saves 33,000 lives
- Prevents 14 million cases of the disease
- Reduces direct healthcare costs by $9.9 billion
- Saves $33.4 billion in indirect costs

Despite progress, approximately 42,000 adults and 300 children in the United States die each year from vaccine-preventable diseases*. Communities with pockets of unvaccinated and under-vaccinated populations are at increased risk for outbreaks of vaccine-preventable diseases. In 2008, imported measles resulted in 140 reported cases— nearly a 3-fold increase over the previous year. The emergence of new or replacement strains of the vaccine-preventable disease can result in a significant increase in serious illnesses and death.

This includes influenza, but does not include deaths due to 2009 H1N1.

Surveillance

The Nation's public-health goals focus on reducing illness, hospitalization, and death from vaccine-preventable diseases and other infectious diseases; expanding surveillance is crucial to those ends. Further efforts to improve disease surveillance will allow for earlier detection of the emergence and spread of diseases. Increased surveillance will save lives by allowing the maximum time possible for public-health responses, including vaccine production and the development of evidence-based recommendations on disease prevention and control. Surveillance enables rapid information sharing and facilitates the timely identification of people in need of immediate treatment. Increasing laboratory capacity is essential for these efforts.

Respiratory Diseases

Acute respiratory infections (ARI), including pneumonia and influenza, are the 8th leading cause of death in the United States, accounting for 56,000 deaths annually. Pneumonia mortality in children fell by 97 percent in the last century, but respiratory infectious diseases continue to be leading causes of pediatric hospitalization and outpatient visits in the United States. On average, influenza leads to more than 200,000 hospitalizations and 36,000 deaths each year. The 2009 H1N1 influenza pandemic caused an estimated 270,000 hospitalizations and 12,270 deaths (1,270 of which were of people younger than age 18) between April 2009 and March 2010.

Hepatitis and Tuberculosis

Viral hepatitis and TB can be prevented, yet healthcare systems often do not make the best use of their available resources to support prevention efforts. Because the United States healthcare system focuses on the treatment of illnesses, rather than health promotion, patients do not always receive information about prevention and healthy lifestyles. This includes advancing effective and evidence-based viral hepatitis and TB prevention priorities and interventions.

Emerging Issues in Immunization and Infectious Diseases

In the coming years, the United States will continue to face new and emerging issues in the area of immunization and infectious diseases. The public-health infrastructure must be capable of responding to emerging threats. State-of-the-art technology and highly-skilled professionals need to be in place to provide rapid response to the threat of epidemics. A coordinated strategy is necessary to understand, detect, control, and prevent infectious diseases. Below are some specific emerging issues.

- Providing culturally appropriate preventive healthcare is an immediate responsibility that will grow over the decade. As the demographics of the population continues to shift, public health and healthcare systems will need to expand their capacity to protect the growing needs of a diverse and aging population.
- New infectious agents and diseases continue to be detected. Infectious diseases must be looked at in a global context due to increasing:
  - International travel and trade
  - Migration
  - Importation of foods and agricultural practices
  - Threats of bioterrorism
- Inappropriate use of antibiotics and environmental changes multiply the potential for worldwide epidemics of all types of infectious diseases.

Infectious diseases are critical public health, humanitarian, and security concern; coordinated efforts will protect people across the nation and around the world.

Section 23.2
Understanding How Vaccines Work

This section includes text excerpted from "Understanding How Vaccines Work," Centers for Disease Control and Prevention (CDC), July 2018.

Vaccines prevent diseases that can be dangerous, or even deadly. Vaccines greatly reduce the risk of infection by working with the body's natural defenses to safely develop immunity to disease. This section explains how the body fights infection and how vaccines work to protect people by producing immunity.

The Immune System—the Body's Defense against Infection

To understand how vaccines work, it helps to first look at how the body fights illness. When germs, such as bacteria or viruses, invade the body, they attack and multiply. This invasion, called an "infection," is what causes illness. The immune system uses several tools to fight infection. Blood contains red blood cells (RBCs) for carrying oxygen to tissues and organs, and white or immune cells for fighting infection. These white blood cells (WBCs) consist primarily of macrophages, B-lymphocytes and T-lymphocytes:

- **Macrophages** are WBCs that swallow up and digest germs, plus dead or dying cells. The macrophages leave behind parts of the invading germs called "antigens." The body identifies antigens as dangerous and stimulates antibodies to attack them.
- **B-lymphocytes** are defensive WBCs. They produce antibodies that attack the antigens left behind by the macrophages.
- **T-lymphocytes** are another type of defensive WBC. They attack cells in the body that have already been infected.

The first time the body encounters a germ, it can take several days to make and use all the germ-fighting tools needed to get over the infection. After the infection, the immune system remembers what it learned about how to protect the body against disease.

The body keeps a few T-lymphocytes, called "memory cells," that go into action quickly if the body encounters the same germ again. When the familiar antigens are detected, B-lymphocytes produce antibodies to attack them.

How Vaccines Work

Vaccines help develop immunity by imitating an infection. This type of infection, however, almost never causes illness, but it does cause the immune system to produce T-lymphocytes and antibodies. Sometimes, after getting a vaccine, imitation infection can cause minor symptoms, such as fever. Such minor symptoms are normal and should be expected as the body builds immunity.

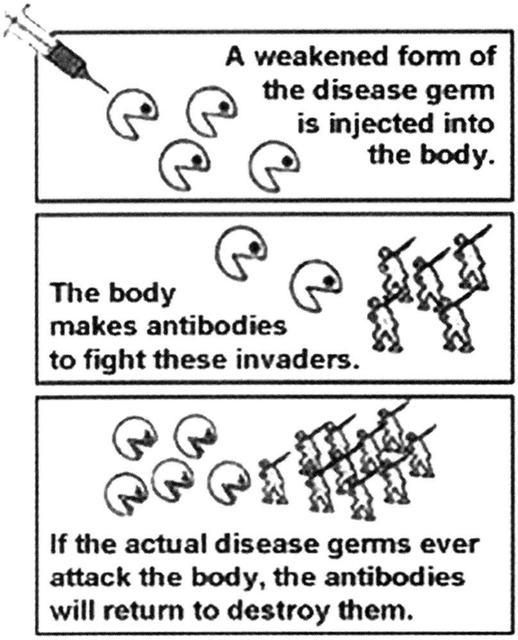

Figure 23.1. How Vaccines Work
(Source: "Why Are Childhood Vaccines So Important?" Centers for Disease Control and Prevention (CDC))

Once the imitation infection goes away, the body is left with a supply of "memory" T-lymphocytes, as well as B-lymphocytes that will remember how to fight that disease in the future. However, it typically takes a few weeks for the body to produce T-lymphocytes and B-lymphocytes after vaccination. Therefore, it is possible that a person infected with a disease just before or just after vaccination could develop symptoms and get a disease because the vaccine has not had enough time to provide protection.

Types of Vaccines

Scientists take many approaches to develop vaccines. These approaches are based on information about the infections (caused by viruses or bacteria) the vaccine will prevent, such as how germs infect cells and how the immune system responds to it. Practical considerations, such as regions of the world where the vaccine would be used, are also important because the strain of a virus and environmental conditions, such as temperature and risk of exposure, maybe different across the globe. The vaccine delivery options available may also differ geographically. Nowadays, there are five main types of vaccines that infants and young children commonly receive in the United States:

- **Live, attenuated vaccines** fight viruses and bacteria. These vaccines contain a version of the living virus or bacteria that have been weakened so that it does not cause serious disease in people with healthy immune systems. Because live, attenuated vaccines are the closest thing to a natural infection, they are good teachers for the immune system. Examples of living, attenuated vaccines include measles, mumps, and rubella vaccine (MMR) and varicella (chickenpox) vaccine. Even though they are very effective, not everyone can receive these vaccines. Children with weakened immune systems—for example, those who are undergoing chemotherapy—can not get live vaccines.

- **Inactivated vaccines** also fight viruses and bacteria. These vaccines are made by inactivating, or killing, the germ during the process of making the vaccine. The Inactivated polio vaccine is an example of this type of vaccine. Inactivated vaccines produce immune responses in different ways than live, attenuated vaccines. Often, multiple doses are necessary to build up and/or maintain immunity.

- **Toxoid vaccines** prevent diseases caused by bacteria that produce toxins (poisons) in the body. In the process of making these vaccines, the toxins are weakened so they cannot cause illness. Weakened toxins are called "toxoids." When the immune system receives a vaccine containing a toxoid, it learns how to fight off the natural toxin. The DTaP vaccine contains diphtheria and tetanus toxoids.

- **Subunit vaccines** include only parts of the virus or bacteria, or subunits, instead of the entire germ. Because these vaccines contain only the essential antigens and not all the other molecules that make up the germ, side effects are less common. Pertussis (whooping cough) component of the DTaP vaccine is an example of a subunit vaccine.

- **Conjugate vaccines** fight a different type of bacteria. These bacteria have antigens with an outer coating of sugar-like substances called "polysaccharides." This type of coating disguises the antigen, making it hard for a young child's immature immune system to recognize it and respond to it. Conjugate vaccines are effective for these types of bacteria because they connect (or conjugate) the polysaccharides to antigens that the immune system responds to very well. This linkage helps the immature immune system react to the coating and develop an immune response. An example of this type of vaccine is the *Haemophilus influenzae* type B (Hib) vaccine.

Vaccines Require More than One Dose

There are four reasons that babies—and even teens or adults—who receive a vaccine for the first time may need more than one dose:

- For some vaccines (primarily inactivated vaccines), the first dose does not provide as much immunity as possible. So, more than one dose is needed to build more complete immunity. The vaccine that protects against the bacteria Hib, which causes meningitis, is a good example.
- For some vaccines, after a while, immunity begins to wear off. At that point, a "booster" dose is needed to bring immunity levels back up. This booster dose usually occurs several years after the initial series of vaccine doses is given. For example, in the case of the DTaP vaccine, which protects against diphtheria, tetanus, and pertussis, the initial series of four shots that children receive as part of their infant immunizations helps build immunity. But, a booster dose is needed at 4 years through 6 years old. Another booster against these diseases is needed at 11 years or 12 years of age. This booster for older children—and teens and adults, too—is called "Tdap."
- For some vaccines (primarily live vaccines), studies have shown that more than one dose is needed for everyone to develop the best immune response. For example, after one dose of the MMR vaccine, some people may not develop enough antibodies to fight off infection. The second dose helps make sure that almost everyone is protected.
- Finally, in the case of flu vaccines, adults and children (6 months and older) need to get a dose every year. Children 6 months through 8 years old who have never gotten a flu vaccine in the past or have only gotten one dose in past years need two doses the first year they

are vaccinated. Then, an annual flu vaccine is needed because the flu viruses causing disease may be different from season to season. Every year, flu vaccines are made to protect against the viruses that research suggests will be most common. Also, the immunity a child gets from a flu vaccination wears off over time. Getting a flu vaccine every year helps keep a child protected, even if the vaccine viruses do not change from one season to the next.

The Bottom Line

Some people believe that naturally acquired immunity—immunity from having the disease itself—is better than the immunity provided by vaccines. However, natural infections can cause severe complications and be deadly. This is true even for diseases that many people consider mild, such as chickenpox. It is impossible to predict who will get serious infections that may lead to hospitalization.

Vaccines, such as any medication, can cause side effects. The most common side effects are mild. However, many vaccine-preventable disease symptoms can be serious, or even deadly. Although many of these diseases are rare in this country, they do circulate around the world and can be brought into the United States putting unvaccinated children at risk. Even with advances in healthcare, the diseases that vaccines prevent can still be very serious—and vaccination is the best way to prevent them.

Section 23.3

What Would Happen If We Stopped Vaccinations?

This section includes text excerpted from "What Would Happen If We Stopped Vaccinations?" Centers for Disease Control and Prevention (CDC), June 29, 2018.

Before the middle of the last century, diseases, such as whooping cough, polio, measles, *Haemophilus influenzae,* and rubella struck hundreds of thousands of infants, children and adults in the United States. Thousands died every year from them. As vaccines were developed and became widely used, rates of these diseases declined until today most of them are nearly gone from our country.

Nearly everyone in the United States got measles before there was a vaccine, and hundreds died from it each year. Nowadays, most doctors have never seen a case of measles.

More than 15,000 Americans died from diphtheria in 1921, before there was a vaccine. Only two cases of diphtheria have been reported to the Centers for Disease Control and Prevention (CDC) between 2004 and 2014.

An epidemic of rubella (German measles) in 1964 to 65 infected 12½ million Americans, killed 2,000 babies, and caused 11,000 miscarriages. Since 2012, 15 cases of rubella were reported to the CDC.

Given successes such as these, it might seem reasonable to ask, "Why should we keep vaccinating against diseases that we will probably never see?" Here is why:

Vaccines Do Not Just Protect Yourself

Most vaccine-preventable diseases are spread from person to person. If one person in a community gets an infectious disease, he can spread it to others who are not immune. But a person who is immune to a disease because she

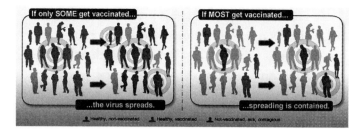

Figure 23.2. The Benefit of More People Getting Vaccinated

has been vaccinated cannot get that disease and cannot spread it to others. The more people who are vaccinated, the fewer opportunities a disease has to spread.

If one or two cases of the disease are introduced into a community where most people are not vaccinated, outbreaks will occur. In 2013, for example, several measles outbreaks occurred around the country, including large outbreaks in New York City and Texas—mainly among groups with low vaccination rates. If vaccination rates dropped to low levels nationally, diseases could become as common as they were before vaccines.

Diseases Have Not Disappeared

The United States has very low rates of vaccine-preventable diseases, but this is not true everywhere in the world. Only one disease—smallpox—has been totally erased from the planet. Polio is close to being eliminated but still exists in several countries. More than 350,000 cases of measles were reported from around the world in 2011, with outbreaks in the Pacific, Asia, Africa, and Europe. In that same year, 90 percent of measles cases in the United States were associated with cases imported from another country. Only the fact that most Americans are vaccinated against measles prevented these clusters of cases from becoming epidemics.

Disease rates are low in the United States. But, if people let themselves become vulnerable by not vaccinating, a case that could touch off an outbreak of some disease that is currently under control is just a plane ride away.

A Final Example: What Could Happen

It is a known fact that a disease that is apparently under control can suddenly return, because it has been happening in countries such as Japan, Australia, and Sweden. Here is an example from Japan: In 1974, about 80 percent of Japanese children were getting the pertussis (whooping cough) vaccine. That year there were only 393 cases of whooping cough in the entire country and not a single pertussis-related death. Then immunization rates began to drop until only about 10 percent of children were being vaccinated. In 1979, more than 13,000 people got whooping cough and 41 died. When routine vaccination was resumed, the disease numbers dropped again.

The chances of your child getting a case of measles or chickenpox or whooping cough might be quite low today. But, vaccinations are not just for protecting ourselves and are not just for today. They also protect the people around us (some of whom may be unable to get certain vaccines, or might have failed to respond to a vaccine, or might be susceptible for other reasons). And they also protect your children's children and their children by keeping diseases that you have almost defeated from making a comeback. What would happen if you stopped vaccinations? You could soon find yourselves battling epidemics of diseases you thought you had conquered decades ago.

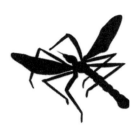

CHAPTER 24
Antimicrobial Drug Resistance and Emerging Infectious Disease

Chapter Contents

Section 24.1

History of Antibiotics and Resistance

This section includes text excerpted from "About Antibiotic Resistance," Centers for Disease Control and Prevention (CDC), November 4, 2019.

Antibiotic resistance happens when germs, such as bacteria and fungi develop the ability to defeat the drugs designed to kill them. That means the germs are not killed and continue to grow.

Infections caused by antibiotic-resistant germs are difficult and sometimes impossible, to treat. In most cases, antibiotic-resistant infections require extended hospital stays, additional follow-up doctor visits, and costly and toxic alternatives.

Antibiotic resistance does not mean the body is becoming resistant to antibiotics; it is that bacteria have become resistant to the antibiotics designed to kill them.

Antibiotic Resistance Threatens Everyone

Antibiotic resistance has the potential to affect people at any stage of life, as well as the healthcare, veterinary, and agricultural industries, making it one of the world's most urgent public-health problems.

Each year in the United States at least 2.8 million people are infected with antibiotic-resistant bacteria, and more than 35,000 people die as a result.

No one can completely avoid the risk of resistant infections, but some people are at greater risk than others (for example, people with chronic illnesses). If antibiotics lose their effectiveness, then the ability to treat infections and control public-health threats is lost.

Many medical advances are dependent on the ability to fight infections using antibiotics, including joint replacements, organ transplants, cancer therapy, and treatment of chronic diseases, such as diabetes, asthma, and rheumatoid arthritis (RA).

Brief History of Resistance and Antibiotics

Penicillin, the first commercialized antibiotic, was discovered in 1928 by Alexander Fleming. Ever since there has been discovery and acknowledgment of resistance alongside the discovery of new antibiotics. In fact, germs will always look for ways to survive and resist new drugs. More and more, germs are sharing their resistance with one another, making it harder for us to keep up.

Where Antibiotic Resistance Spreads
A Complex Web: Everything Is Connected

Antibiotic-resistant germs can quickly spread across settings, including communities, the food supply, healthcare facilities, the environment (e.g., soil, water), and around the world. Antibiotic resistance is a One Health problem — the health of people is connected to the health of animals and the environment (soil, water).

It can affect the progress in healthcare, food production, and life expectancy. Antibiotic resistance is not only a U.S. problem — it is a global crisis. New forms of resistance emerge and can spread with remarkable speed between continents through people, goods, and animals.

Healthcare Facilities

Antibiotic-resistant germs, including new and emerging resistance, can spread within and between healthcare facilities. These germs can cause infections in patients, called "healthcare-associated infections," and can spread to the community or environment.

Community

Germs, including antibiotic-resistant germs, live and spread within the community and sometimes make people sick.

Environment

Human activity can introduce antibiotics and antibiotic-resistant germs into the environment, but it remains unclear how to spread in the environment impacts human and animal health.

Table 24.1. Select Germs Showing Resistance over Time

Antibiotic Approved or Released	Year Released	Resistant Germ Identified	Year Identified
Penicillin	1943	Penicillin-resistant *Streptococcus pneumoniae*	1967
		Penicillinase-producing *Neisseria gonorrhoeae*	1976
Vancomycin	1958	Plasmid-mediated vancomycin-resistant *Enterococcus faecium*	1988
		Vancomycin-resistant *Staphylococcus aureus*	2002
Amphotericin B	1959	Amphotericin B-resistant *Candida auris*	2016
Methicillin	1960	Methicillin-resistant *Staphylococcus aureus*	1960
Extended-spectrum cephalosporins	1980 (Cefotaxime)	Extended-spectrum beta-lactamase-producing *Escherichia coli*	1983
Azithromycin	1980	Azithromycin-resistant *Neisseria gonorrhoeae*	2011
Imipenem	1985	*Klebsiella pneumoniae* carbapenemase (KPC)-producing *Klebsiella pneumoniae*	1996
Ciprofloxacin	1987	Ciprofloxacin-resistant *Neisseria gonorrhoeae*	2007
Fluconazole	1990 (FDA approved)	Fluconazole-resistant *Candida*	1988
Caspofungin	2001	Caspofungin-resistant *Candida*	2004
Daptomycin	2003	Daptomycin-resistant methicillin-resistant *Staphylococcus aureus*	2004
Ceftazidime-avibactam	2015	Ceftazidime-avibactam-resistant KPC-producing *Klebsiella pneumoniae*	2015

Food, Farms, and Animals

Animals, such as people, carry germs in their gut, including antibiotic-resistant germs. The United States food supply is among the safest in the world, but these germs can get into the food supply and make people sick.

Section 24.2

Influenza Antiviral Drug Resistance

This section includes text excerpted from "Influenza Antiviral Drug Resistance," Centers for Disease Control and Prevention (CDC), February 20, 2019.

What Are Reduced Susceptibility and Antiviral Resistance?

When an antiviral drug is fully effective against a virus, the virus is said to be susceptible to that antiviral drug. Influenza viruses are constantly changing, and can sometimes change in ways that might make antiviral drugs work less well or not work at all against these viruses. When an influenza virus changes in the active site where an antiviral drug works, that virus shows reduced susceptibility to that antiviral drug. Reduced susceptibility can be a sign of potential antiviral drug resistance. Antiviral drugs may not work as well in viruses with reduced susceptibility. Influenza viruses can show reduced susceptibility to one or more influenza antiviral drugs.

In the United States, there are four U.S. Food and Drug Administration (FDA)-approved antiviral drugs recommended by the Centers for Disease Control and Prevention (CDC) this season. Three are neuraminidase inhibitor antiviral drugs: oseltamivir (available as a generic version or under the trade name Tamiflu®) for oral administration, zanamivir (trade name Relenza®) for oral inhalation using an inhaler device, and peramivir (trade name Rapivab®) for intravenous administration. The fourth is a cap-dependent endonuclease (CEN) inhibitor, baloxavir marboxil (trade name Xofluza®) for oral administration, approved for use in the United States during the 2018 to 2019 season by the FDA in October of 2018.

There is another class of influenza antiviral drugs (amantadine and rimantadine) called the "adamantanes" (which have activity against only influenza A viruses) that are not recommended for use in the United States at this time because of widespread antiviral resistance in circulating influenza A viruses.

How Widespread Are Reduced Susceptibility and Antiviral Resistance in the United States?

In the United States, the majority of the circulating influenza viruses have been fully susceptible to the neuraminidase inhibitor antiviral medications and to baloxavir. On the other hand, many flu A viruses are resistant to the adamantane drugs which is why they are not recommended for use at this time.

How Does Reduced Susceptibility and Antiviral Resistance Happen?

Influenza viruses are constantly changing; they can change from one season to the next and can even change within the course of one flu season. As a flu virus replicates (i.e., make copies of itself), the genetic makeup may change in a way that results in the virus becoming less susceptible to one or more of the antiviral drugs used to treat or prevent influenza. Influenza viruses can become less susceptible to antiviral drugs spontaneously or emerge during the course of antiviral treatment. Viruses that are less susceptible or resistant vary in their ability to transmit to other people.

How Are Reduced Susceptibility and Antiviral Resistance Detected?

The CDC routinely tests flu viruses collected through domestic and global surveillance to see if they have indications of reduced susceptibility to any of the FDA-approved flu antiviral drugs, as this can suggest the potential for antiviral resistance. This data informs public-health policy recommendations about the use of flu antiviral medications.

Detection of reduced susceptibility and antiviral resistance involves several laboratory tests, including specific functional assays and molecular techniques (sequencing and pyrosequencing) to look for genetic changes that are associated with reduced antiviral susceptibility.

How Has the CDC Prepared to Test for Reduced Susceptibility and Antiviral Resistance to the New Flu Antiviral Baloxavir?

The CDC's Influenza Division has taken specific laboratory actions to incorporate the new antiviral drug baloxavir into routine virologic surveillance. This includes the creation and validation of new assays to determine baloxavir susceptibility, and the training of laboratorians to conduct baloxavir susceptibility testing.

Seasonal influenza A and B viruses in humans, as well as several influenza A viruses that circulate in animals, were tested to establish baseline susceptibility to baloxavir. In addition, the susceptibility of other distantly related influenza viruses to baloxavir was tested. The CDC also is collaborating with the Association of Public Health Laboratories (APHL) and the Wadsworth Center New York State Department of Health (NYSDOH), a National Influenza Reference Center (NIRC), to establish laboratory-testing capacity for baloxavir susceptibility. The CDC has trained staff within these partner organizations to use the CDC's new method for assessing baloxavir susceptibility.

What Is Oseltamivir Resistance and What Causes It?

Flu viruses are constantly changing. Changes that occur in circulating flu viruses typically involve the structures of the viruses' two primary surface proteins: neuraminidase (NA) and hemagglutinin (HA).

Oseltamivir is the most commonly prescribed of the recommended antiviral drugs in the United States that is used to treat flu illness. Oseltamivir is known as an "NA inhibitor" because this antiviral drug binds to NA proteins of the flu virus and inhibits the enzymatic activity of these proteins. By inhibiting NA activity, oseltamivir prevents flu viruses from spreading from infected cells to other healthy cells.

If the NA proteins of the flu virus change, oseltamivir can lose its ability to bind to and inhibit the function of the virus's NA proteins. This results in "oseltamivir resistance" (nonsusceptibility). A particular genetic change known as the "H275Y" mutation is the only known mutation to confer oseltamivir resistance in 2009 H1N1 flu viruses. The H275Y mutation makes oseltamivir ineffective in treating illnesses with that flu virus by preventing oseltamivir from inhibiting NA activity, which then allows the virus to spread to healthy cells. The H275Y mutation also reduces the effectiveness of peramivir to treat influenza virus infections with this mutation.

How Does the CDC Improve Monitoring of Influenza Viruses for Reduced Susceptibility and Antiviral Resistance?

The CDC continually improves the ability to rapidly detect influenza viruses with antiviral reduced susceptibility and antiviral resistance through improvements in laboratory methods; increasing the number of surveillance sites domestically and globally, and increasing the number of laboratories that can test for reduced susceptibility and antiviral resistance. Enhanced surveillance efforts have provided the CDC with the capability to detect resistant viruses more quickly, and enabled the CDC to monitor for changing trends over time.

How Did Influenza Antiviral Susceptibility Patterns Change during the Previous (2017 to 2018) Influenza Season?

Antiviral susceptibility patterns changed very little in 2017 to 2018 compared with the previous season (2016 to 2017). During the 2016 to

2017 season, no oseltamivir resistance was found. During the 2017 to 2018 influenza season, only a small number of viruses were resistant to oseltamivir. Most of the influenza viruses tested during 2017 to 2018 continued to be susceptible to the antiviral drugs recommended for influenza by the CDC and the Advisory Committee on Immunization Practices (ACIP) (oseltamivir, zanamivir, and peramivir). Resistance to the adamantane class of antiviral drugs among A/H3N2 and A/H1N1 viruses remained widespread (influenza B viruses are not susceptible to adamantane drugs).

Specifically, for the 2017 to 2018 season:

- The CDC tested 1,147 influenza A(H1N1)pdm09, 2,354 influenza A (H3N2), and 1,118 influenza B viruses for reduced susceptibility and resistance to antiviral medications (i.e., oseltamivir, zanamivir, or peramivir).
- While the majority of the tested viruses showed susceptibility to antiviral drugs, 11 (1.0%) A(H1N1)pdm09 viruses were resistant to both oseltamivir and peramivir but were sensitive to zanamivir.
- As indicated by these results, oseltamivir, zanamivir, and peramivir remained recommended antiviral treatment options for flu illness during the 2017 to 2018 flu season.
- High levels of resistance to the adamantanes (amantadine and rimantadine) persisted among circulating influenza A viruses, and adamantanes are also not effective against influenza B viruses — adamantane drugs were not recommended for use against influenza at this time.

The CDC conducts ongoing surveillance and testing of influenza viruses for antiviral reduced susceptibility and resistance among seasonal and novel influenza viruses, and guidance is updated as needed. Because there were no dramatic changes in antiviral susceptibility patterns during the 2017 to 2018 flu season, the guidance for the 2018 to 2019 flu season on the use of influenza antiviral drugs remains unchanged.

What Can People Do to Protect Themselves against Flu Viruses with Reduced Susceptibility and Antiviral Resistance?

Getting a yearly seasonal flu vaccination is the best way to reduce the risk of flu and its potentially serious complications. Flu vaccines protect against an influenza A(H1N1) virus, an influenza A(H3N2) virus, and one or two influenza B viruses (depending on the vaccine). The CDC recommends that everyone six months of age and older gets vaccinated each year. If you are in a group at high risk of serious flu-related complications and become ill with flu symptoms, call your doctor right away, you may benefit from early treatment with an influenza antiviral drug. If you are not at high risk, if possible, stay home from work, school, and errands when you are sick. This will help prevent you from spreading your illness to others.

What Implications Do Reduced Susceptibility and Antiviral Resistance Have for the United States Antiviral Stockpile That Was Created as Part of the United States Pandemic Plan?

Antiviral drugs are one component of a multifaceted approach to pandemic preparedness planning and response. The U.S. Strategic National Stockpile (SNS) contains supplies of three neuraminidase inhibitor (NAI) antiviral medications, including oseltamivir (for oral administration), zanamivir (for oral inhalation) and peramivir (for intravenous administration). These medications are to be used in the event that a novel influenza A virus, such as avian influenza A(H7N9) virus, gains the ability to spread easily among people in a sustained manner, and is susceptible to NAI antiviral drugs.

During the 2009 H1N1 pandemic, antiviral drugs were released from the SNS and used to treat the infection with the pandemic virus, now referred to as influenza A (H1N1) pdm09 virus. Antivirals in the SNS are for use during public-health emergencies in the United States, such as an influenza pandemic, but not for seasonal influenza epidemics. Since antiviral drug resistance can emerge in influenza viruses, including to the

NAI antivirals, new antivirals with mechanisms of action that are different than the NAIs are needed for the SNS.

Section 24.3
Antimicrobial Resistance— A Global Threat

This section includes text excerpted from "Antimicrobial Resistance—A Global Threat," Centers for Disease Control and Prevention (CDC), September 19, 2018.

Antibiotic resistance requires a collaborative approach across countries to detect, prevent, and respond to these threats. Global leaders are joining the Centers for Disease Control and Prevention's (CDC) Antimicrobial Resistance (AMR) Challenge by committing to action across healthcare, food, communities, and the environment (soil and water) to accelerate the fight.

Antibiotic resistance, when germs (i.e., bacteria, fungi) develop the ability to defeat the drugs designed to kill them, is a top threat to the public's health and a priority across the globe. In the United States alone, it causes more than 2 million infections and 23,000 deaths per year. Worldwide, antibiotic resistance threatens the progress in healthcare, food production, and ultimately life expectancy.

Antibiotic resistance has been found in all regions of the world. Modern travel of people, animals, and goods means antibiotic resistance can easily spread across borders and continents. Collaborative, coordinated efforts will help slow the development and spread of antibiotic resistance and protect people.

The Centers for Disease Control and Prevention Collaborates to Support Global Action

Through the CDC's Antibiotic Resistance (AR) Solutions Initiative, the agency collaborates with countries throughout the world to improve antibiotic use, track resistance, and implement infection prevention and control activities in healthcare settings, where antibiotic resistance can emerge and amplify the spread.

The CDC shares expertise and deploys experts to investigate and contain resistance outbreaks, and assists other countries as they:

- Implement infection prevention and control programs and antibiotic stewardship programs in healthcare settings
- Establish or strengthen national tracking systems to respond rapidly to outbreaks, identify emerging pathogens, and track trends
- Enhance laboratory capacity to detect and report resistance
- Develop and implement national action plans to address the threat of antibiotic resistance

Progress Made, but More Work Needed

Germs will inevitably find ways to resist antibiotics, which is why aggressive action is needed. In September 2018, the United States is launching the AMR Challenge at a United Nations' General Assembly side event to accelerate the fight against antibiotic resistance.

The AMR Challenge is a year-long effort for governments, private industries, and nongovernmental organizations worldwide to make formal commitments that further progress against antibiotic resistance. The AMR Challenge includes five commitment areas: tracking and data; infection prevention and control; antibiotic use; sanitation and environment; and vaccines, therapeutics, and diagnostics.

Antibiotic resistance has the potential to affect people at any stage of life, as well as the healthcare, veterinary, and agriculture industries. Everyone has a role to play in fighting antibiotic resistance.

Section 24.4

National Strategy for Combating Antibiotic-Resistant Bacteria

This section contains text excerpted from the following sources: Text in this section begins with excerpts from "U.S. National Strategy for Combating Antibiotic-Resistant Bacteria (National Strategy)," Centers for Disease Control and Prevention (CDC), September 10, 2018; Text under the heading "The United States Action to Combat Antibiotic Resistance" is excerpted from "U.S. Action to Combat Antibiotic Resistance," Centers for Disease Control and Prevention (CDC), November 4, 2019.

The National Strategy is a plan for the United States to work with domestic and international partners to reduce the national and international threat of antibiotic resistance.

The National Strategy was released alongside Executive Order 13676 and a report on combating antibiotic resistance by the President's Council of Advisors on Science and Technology (PCAST). These materials informed the United States National Action Plan for Combating Antibiotic-Resistant Bacteria, released in 2015.

All of us who depend on antibiotics must join in a common effort to detect, stop, and prevent the emergence and spread of resistant bacteria."

Guiding Principles

The National Strategy takes into account both the causes of antibiotic resistance and opportunities to combat the threat, including:

- Using antibiotics, including misuse and overuse, in healthcare and food production to accelerate the development of antibiotic resistance
- Detecting and responding to antibiotic resistance by adoption of a One Health approach to data collection, recognizing that the health of people is connected to the health and animals and the environment

- Implementing evidence-based infection control practices to prevent the spread of resistance
- Encouraging the development of more therapies and drugs to treat infections
- Identifying opportunities to use innovations and new technologies to develop next-generation tools to support human and animal health
- Recognizing that antibiotic resistance is a global health problem that requires international attention and collaboration

Main Goals

The National Strategy identified five main goals to guide collaborative action taken by the United States federal government:

- Slow the emergence of resistant bacteria and prevent the spread of resistant infections.
- Strengthen national One Health surveillance efforts to combat resistance.
- Advance development and use of rapid and innovative diagnostic tests for identification and characterization of resistant bacteria.
- Accelerate basic and applied research and development for new antibiotics, other therapeutics, and vaccines objectives.
- Improve international collaboration and capacities for antibiotic resistance prevention, surveillance, control, and antibiotic research and development.

National and International Partnerships

The National Strategy requires cooperation from the public and private sector in the United States including:

- Healthcare providers and leaders
- Veterinarians
- Agriculture industry leaders
- Manufacturers
- Universities
- Scientists and researchers

- Policymakers
- Patients

The National Strategy also calls for partnerships with international human and animal health organizations, including:
- Ministries of health, agriculture, and food safety
- World Health Organization (WHO)
- Transatlantic Taskforce on Antimicrobial Resistance (TATFAR)
- Global Health Security Agenda (GHSA)
- Food and Agriculture Organization (FAO) of the United Nations
- World Organization for Animal Health (OIE)

The United States Action to Combat Antibiotic Resistance

Antibiotic resistance is a national priority, and the U.S. government has taken ambitious steps to fight this threat. For example, it established a U.S. National Strategy for Combating Antibiotic-Resistant Bacteria (National Strategy) and an accompanying the U.S. National Action Plan for Combating Antibiotic-Resistant Bacteria (National Action Plan).

Federal agencies are working together to:
- Respond to new and ongoing public-health threats
- Strengthen detection of resistance
- Enhance efforts to slow the emergence and spread of resistance
- Improve antibiotic use and reporting
- Advance development of rapid diagnostics
- Enhance infection control measures
- Accelerate research on new antibiotics and antibiotic alternatives

Section 24.5

Combatting Antimicrobial Resistance Globally

This section includes text excerpted from "Combat Antimicrobial Resistance Globally," Centers for Disease Control and Prevention (CDC), November 5, 2019.

A Global Problem and Priority

Antimicrobial resistance has been found in all regions of the world. Modern travel of people, animals, and goods means antimicrobial resistance can easily spread across borders and continents.

Fighting this threat is a public-health priority. It requires a collaborative global approach across sectors to detect, prevent, and respond to these threats when they occur.

Global Strategies to Fight Resistance

Every country can take steps to slow antimicrobial resistance. Commit to setting goals across multiple sectors, including:

- Healthcare
- Food
- Communities (local and global)
- Environment (soil and water)

Create and implement a comprehensive plan with a One Health approach to achieve those goals, and track progress.

Every country plan can consider the following actions to prevent resistant infections and their spread:

- Implement infection prevention and control practices
- Improve antibiotic use, including ensuring access
- Implement data and tracking systems to track resistance, guide prevention strategies, and report results at the local and global level
- Improve lab capacity to identify resistant bacteria

In addition to these important actions, it is also critical to join the global effort to develop new drugs, diagnostics, vaccines, and therapeutics to treat infections.

The CDC Collaborates to Support Global Action

The CDC works with world leaders and experts to implement the United States National Action Plan for Combating Antimicrobial Resistant Bacteria. Through the CDC's Antibiotic Resistance Solutions Initiative, the agency supports activities in high burden countries throughout the world to improve antibiotic use, track resistance, and implement infection prevention and control activities.

The Global Health Security Agenda (GHSA), which elevates global health security as a national and global priority, also contributes to combating antimicrobial resistance through its "action package."

The CDC's Global Action

The CDC shares expertise and deploys scientists to investigate and contain resistance outbreaks, and assists other countries in:

- Contributing to the development and implementation of national action plans
- Implementing programs in healthcare settings to prevent the spread of resistance (infection prevention and control programs) and support the appropriate use of antimicrobials (antimicrobial stewardship programs)
- Enhancing laboratory capacity to detect and report resistance that has global health implications
- Establishing or strengthening national tracking systems to respond rapidly to outbreaks, identify emerging pathogens, and track trends
- Supporting a national network of travel clinics to better understand the spread of resistance across the United States to ultimately improve the health of international travelers

In addition, the CDC collaborates in global activities, including:

- Participating in and acts as the secretariat for the Transatlantic Taskforce on Antimicrobial Resistance (TATFAR), a collaborative effort between Canada, the European Union, Norway, and the United States to address antimicrobial resistance together
- Hosting a World Health Organization (WHO) Collaborating Center, part of the AMR Surveillance and Quality Assessment Collaborating Centres Network that support countries in building capacity to track antimicrobial resistance by strengthening international collaboration and improving coordination
- Supporting the World Health Organization (WHO) tracking platforms, including the Global AMR Surveillance System (GLASS), which provides a standardized approach to the collection, analysis, and sharing of global antimicrobial resistance data; ultimately, GLASS will alert countries worldwide when new resistance emerges

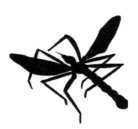

CHAPTER 25
Hospital-Based Infections

Chapter Contents

Section 25.1

Common Types of Healthcare-Associated Infections

This section includes text excerpted from "Types of Healthcare-Associated Infections," Centers for Disease Control and Prevention (CDC), March 26, 2014. Reviewed January 2020.

Modern healthcare employs many types of invasive devices and procedures to treat patients and to help them recover. Infections can be associated with the devices used in medical procedures, such as catheters or ventilators.

These healthcare-associated infections (HAIs) include central line-associated bloodstream infections, catheter-associated urinary tract infections (UTIs), and ventilator-associated pneumonia. Infections may also occur at surgery sites, known as "surgical site infections" (SSIs).

Central Line-Associated Bloodstream Infection

Central line-associated bloodstream infections (CLABSIs) result in thousands of deaths each year and billions of dollars in added costs to the U.S. healthcare system, yet these infections are preventable.

Catheter-Associated Urinary Tract Infections

A UTI is an infection involving any part of the urinary system, including urethra, bladder, ureters, and kidneys. UTIs are the most common type of healthcare-associated infections reported to the National Healthcare Safety Network (NHSN). Among UTIs acquired in the hospital, approximately 75 percent are associated with a urinary catheter, which is a tube inserted into the bladder through the urethra to drain urine. Between 15 to 25 percent of hospitalized patients receive urinary catheters during their hospital stay.

The most important risk factor for developing a catheter-associated UTI (CAUTI) is prolonged use of the urinary catheter. Therefore, catheters should only be used for appropriate indications and should be removed as soon as they are no longer needed.

Surgical Site Infection

A surgical site infection (SSI) is an infection that occurs after surgery in the part of the body where the surgery took place. SSIs can sometimes be superficial infections involving the skin only. Other SSIs are more serious and can involve tissues under the skin, organs, or implanted material. The CDC provides guidelines and tools to the healthcare community to help end SSIs and resources to help the public understand these infections and take measures to safeguard their own health when possible.

Ventilator-Associated Pneumonia

Ventilator-associated pneumonia is a lung infection that develops in a person who is on a ventilator. A ventilator is a machine that is used to help a patient breathe by giving oxygen through a tube placed in a patient's mouth or nose, or through a hole in the front of the neck. An infection may occur if germs enter through the tube and get into the patient's lungs.

Section 25.2

Data on Biggest Antimicrobial Resistance Threats

This section includes text excerpted from "Biggest Threats and Data," Centers for Disease Control and Prevention (CDC), November 14, 2019.

The Centers for Disease Control and Prevention's (CDC) Antibiotic Resistance Threats in the United States, 2019 report includes the latest national death and infection estimates that underscores the continued threat of antibiotic resistance in the United States.

According to the report, more than 2.8 million antibiotic-resistant infections occur in the U.S. each year, and more than 35,000 people die as a result. In addition, 223,900 cases of *Clostridioides difficile* occurred in 2017 and at least 12,800 people died.

Dedicated prevention and infection control efforts in the U.S. are working to reduce the number of infections and deaths caused by antibiotic-resistant germs, but the number of people facing antibiotic resistance is still too high. More action is needed to fully protect people.

The rising resistant infections in the community, which can put more people at risk, make spread more difficult to identify and contain, and threaten the progress made to protect patients in healthcare is a matter of concern.

The report lists 18 antibiotic-resistant bacteria and fungi into three categories based on the level of concern to human health—urgent, serious, and concerning—and highlights:
- Estimated infections and deaths since the 2013 report
- Aggressive actions are taken
- Gaps slowing progress

The report also includes a watch list with three threats, urgent threats, serious threats, and concerning threats, that have not spread resistance widely in the U.S. but could become common without a continued aggressive approach.

The urgent threat includes:

- Carbapenem-resistant *Acinetobacter*
- *Candida auris*
- Clostridioides difficile
- Carbapenem-resistant Enterobacteriaceae
- Drug-resistant *Neisseria gonorrhoeae*

Serious threats include:

- Drug-resistant *Campylobacter*
- Drug-resistant *Candida*
- ESBL-producing Enterobacteriaceae
- Vancomycin-resistant *Enterococci (VRE)*
- Multidrug-resistant *Pseudomonas aeruginosa*
- Drug-resistant nontyphoidal *Salmonella*
- Drug-resistant *Salmonella* serotype Typhi
- Drug-resistant *Shigella*
- Methicillin-resistant *Staphylococcus aureus (MRSA)*
- Drug-resistant *Streptococcus pneumoniae*
- Drug-resistant tuberculosis

Concerning threats include:

- Erythromycin-resistant Group A *Streptococcus*
- Clindamycin-resistant Group B *Streptococcus*

Section 25.3
Patient Safety Information

This section includes text excerpted from "Patient Safety: What You Can Do to Be a Safe Patient," Centers for Disease Control and Prevention (CDC), November 6, 2019.

You go to the hospital to get well, right? Of course, but did you know that you can get infections in the hospital while you are being treated for something else?

Time in the hospital can put you at risk for healthcare-associated infection (HAI), such as blood, surgical site, or urinary tract infection (UTI). Every day, patients get infections in healthcare facilities while they are being treated for something else. These infections can have devastating emotional, financial, and medical effects. Worst of all, they can be deadly.

Healthcare procedures can leave you vulnerable to germs that cause HAIs. These germs can be spread in healthcare settings from patient to patient on unclean hands of healthcare personnel or through the improper use or reuse of equipment. These infections are not limited to hospitals. For example, in the past 10 years alone, there have been more than 30 outbreaks of hepatitis B and hepatitis C in nonhospital-healthcare settings such as:

- Outpatient clinics
- Dialysis centers
- Long-term care facilities

Protect Yourself and Your Family from Harmful Germs That Can Cause Infections

Keep your hands clean. Regular hand-cleaning is one of the best ways to remove germs, avoid getting sick, and prevent spreading germs.

Take antibiotics only when your provider thinks you need them. Ask if your antibiotic is necessary. If you take antibiotics when you do not need them, you are only exposing yourself to unnecessary risk of side effects and potentially serious infections in the future. If you do need antibiotics, take them exactly as they are prescribed.

Watch for signs of infection and its complications, such as sepsis. Get care right away—do not delay.

- Tell your doctor if you think you have an infection, or if your infection is not getting better or is getting worse.

Watch out for life-threatening diarrhea caused by *C. difficile*. If you have been taking an antibiotic, tell your doctor if you have 3 or more diarrhea episodes in 24 hours.

Get vaccinated against the flu and other infections to avoid complications.

Be a Safe Patient in the Hospital

Tell your doctor if you have been hospitalized in another facility, have recently received healthcare outside of the United States, or have recently had an infection.

Ask your healthcare provider what they and the facility will do to protect you and your family from an antibiotic-resistant infection.

- If you have a catheter, ask daily your doctor when it can be removed.
- If you are having surgery, ask your doctor how they prevent infections. Also, ask how you can prepare for surgery to reduce your infection risk.

Keep your hands clean. Make sure everyone cleans their hands before touching you. Remind healthcare personnel and your visitors to clean their hands.

Let your doctors check you for resistant germs if needed. Hospitals need to screen patients if they are exposed, and this helps protect you and those around you.

Understand that if you have a resistant bacteria, healthcare providers may use gowns and gloves when caring for you.

Allow people to clean your room while you are in the hospital, even when it feels inconvenient for you.

- Environmental services workers are the people who clean patient rooms in the hospital, and they are important members of the healthcare team.
- Allowing them to clean and disinfect your room helps keep you safe by reducing your risk of developing an infection—do not say, "come back later."

Section 25.4

Containment Strategy for Healthcare-Associated Infections

This section includes text excerpted from "Containment Strategy Responding to Emerging AR Threats," Centers for Disease Control and Prevention (CDC), June 27, 2019.

When launched at the first sign of a problem, the Centers for Disease Control and Prevention's (CDC) Containment Strategy keeps new or rare forms of antibiotic resistance from spreading. Containment complements foundational CDC strategies, including improving antibiotic use and preventing infections, and builds on existing detection and response structure. The entire package is needed to address urgent threats such as *Candida Auris* and carbapenem-resistant *Enterobacteriaceae* (CRE) before they gain a foothold. Working together, public-health teams can defend the nation from new threats and help protect patients.

Containment Strategy

The Containment Strategy includes:

- Rapid identification
- Infection control assessments

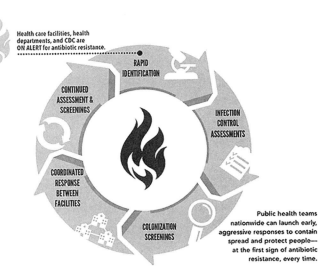

Figure 25.1. The Containment Strategy *(Source: "Containing Unusual Resistance,"* Centers for Disease Control and Prevention *(CDC))*

- Colonization screenings when needed
- A coordinated response between facilities
- Continue assessments and colonization screenings until spread is controlled

Containment Response Tiers

These three response tiers help health departments launch effective and tailored responses once a threat is confirmed by the laboratory:

- **Tier 1:** Genes and germs for which no treatment options exist or genes and germs which have never or only rarely been detected in the United States
- **Tier 2:** Genes and germs not commonly detected in a geographic area
- **Tier 3:** Genes and germs that are known threats in a geographic area but not endemic

Unusual Antibiotic Resistance Threats

There is a need for health departments to lead aggressive detection and response activities when new or rare genes and germs are identified. This includes threats such as germs resistant to all antibiotics, Vancomycin-resistant *Staphylococcus aureus* (VRSA), *Candida auris*, and certain types of "nightmare bacteria" such as CRE and carbapenem-resistant *Pseudomonas aeruginosa* (CRPA).

Antibiotic resistance threats vary by state. Health departments should make sure all healthcare facilities know what isolates (pure samples of a germ) to send for testing, and what state and local laboratory support is available.

Examples of unusual antibiotic resistance germs include those that:

- Are resistant to all or most antibiotics tested, making them hard to treat
- Are uncommon in a geographic area in the United States
- Have special genes that allow them to spread their resistance to other germs

What Can Be Done?

Germs are constantly developing resistance against new and older antibiotics. While antibiotic resistance threats vary nationwide, AR has been found in every state and new types of resistance are constantly developing and spreading. When resistance spreads, it accelerates the threat of untreatable infections.

Enhanced capacity nationwide that supports early, aggressive responses to every case of unusual resistance and vigilant prevention strategies can reduce the number of infections caused by these organisms.

The federal government is:

- Monitoring resistance and sounding the alarm when threats emerge. The CDC develops and provides new lab tests so health departments can quickly identify new threats.
- Improving identification through the CDC's AR Lab Network in all 50 states, 5 large cities, and Puerto Rico, including 7 regional labs and a national tuberculosis lab for specialty testing
- Supporting prevention experts and programs in every state, and providing data and recommendations for local prevention and response

- Testing innovative infection control and prevention strategies with healthcare and academic partners
- The CDC funds innovative research to support safe healthcare

State and local health departments and labs can:
- Make sure all healthcare facilities know what state and local lab support is available and what isolates (pure samples of a germ) to send for testing. Develop a plan to respond rapidly to unusual genes and germs when they first appear.
- Assess the quality and consistency of infection control in healthcare facilities across the state, especially in facilities with high-risk patients and long stays. Help improve practices.
- Coordinate with affected healthcare facilities, the AR Lab Network regional lab, and the CDC for every case of unusual resistance. Investigations should include onsite infection control assessments and colonization screenings for people who might have been exposed to unusual resistance. They could spread it to others. Continue both until spread is controlled.
- Provide timely lab results and recommendations to affected healthcare facilities and providers. If the patient came from or was transferred to another facility, alert that facility.

Healthcare facilities can:
- Plan for unusual resistance arriving at your facility.
- **Leadership.** Work with the health department to stop the spread of unusual resistance. Review and support infection control in the facility.
- **Clinical labs.** Know what isolates to send for testing. Establish protocols that immediately notify the health department, healthcare provider, and infection control staff of unusual resistance. Validate new tests to detect the latest threats. If needed, use isolates from ARIsolateBank.
- **Healthcare providers, epidemiologists, and infection control staff.**
  - Place patients with unusual resistance on contact precautions, assess and enhance infection control, and work with the health department to screen others.

- Communicate about patient status if transferred.
- Continue infection control assessments and colonization screenings until spread is controlled. Ask about any recent travel or healthcare at-risk patients.

Everyone can:

- Inform your healthcare provider if you recently received healthcare in another country or facility
- Talk to your healthcare provider about preventing infections, taking good care of chronic conditions and getting recommended vaccines
- Practice good hygiene, such as keeping hands clean with handwashing or alcohol-based hand rubs, and keep cuts clean until healed

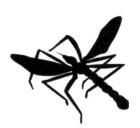

CHAPTER 26
Laboratory-Guided Detection of Disease Outbreaks

Chapter Contents

Culture-Independent Diagnostic Tests

This section includes text excerpted from "Culture-Independent Diagnostic Tests," Centers for Disease Control and Prevention (CDC), October 28, 2019.

What Are Culture-Independent Diagnostic Tests and How Do They Affect Food-Borne Illness?

The culture-independent diagnostic tests (CIDTs) are changing the way that clinical laboratories diagnose patients with food-borne illnesses. These tests can identify the general type of bacteria causing illness within hours, without having to culture, or grow bacteria in a laboratory. (The pure bacterial strain that grows is called an "isolate.") These tests allow doctors to rapidly determine the cause of a patient's illness. However, a shift toward CIDTs means that clinical laboratories may stop culturing, or producing bacterial isolates from patients with food-borne illnesses. For example, the percentage of *Campylobacter* diarrheal illnesses diagnosed only by CIDTs in FoodNet sites increased from 13 percent in 2012 to 2014 to 38 percent in 2018.

Without a bacterial isolate from the culturing process, public-health scientists cannot perform tests that determine an organism's strain or subtype (such as deoxyribonucleic acid (DNA) fingerprints), resistance pattern, or other characteristics. This information is needed to detect and prevent outbreaks, track antibiotic resistance, and monitor disease trends to know if prevention measures are working.

How Do Culture-Independent Diagnostic Tests Affect the Ability of Public-Health Officials to Detect and Prevent Outbreaks?

PulseNet, a laboratory network that connects food-borne illness cases to detect outbreaks, extracts important information from the bacteria that are found in samples from sick people. PulseNet needs bacterial isolates to determine the precise strains making people ill, using DNA fingerprinting methods, including a new precise method known as "whole-genome sequencing" (WGS).

Public-health officials look at PulseNet data for clusters of matching DNA fingerprints. If epidemiologists find that the cluster has a common source, it is called an "outbreak."

The CIDTs skip the step of producing an isolate and as a result, DNA fingerprints cannot be produced for PulseNet. Without DNA fingerprints from the bacteria, PulseNet will not be able to continue detecting clusters. Without PulseNet cluster detection, outbreaks may not even be recognized, contaminated products may remain on shelves and in pantries, more people may become sick, and valuable opportunities for improving the safety of food may be lost.

PulseNet prevents an estimated 270,000 illnesses every year and saves about $507 million every year in medical costs and lost work productivity.

How Do Culture-Independent Diagnostic Tests Affect the Ability to Track and Contain Antibiotic Resistance?

Public-health officials gather information about antibiotic resistance by analyzing bacterial isolates after they are grown in culture. If cultured bacterial isolates are not available to be analyzed, it will be impossible to know how resistant they are to antibiotics. This may affect how the illness is treated and make it difficult to monitor trends in resistance over time.

Monitoring antibiotic resistance sometimes results in regulatory action to protect the health, such as the ban of fluoroquinolone use in poultry after scientific data showed its use was causing an increase in antibiotic-resistant *Campylobacter*, which cause food-borne illnesses.

How Do Culture-Independent Diagnostic Tests Affect the Ability to Monitor Disease Trends?

The CIDTs may improve the ability to monitor certain types of disease trends, such as diseases caused by bacteria, viruses, or parasites for which practical tests were formerly not available.

It does not produce bacterial isolates that are needed to distinguish between strains and subtypes of bacteria. Therefore, public-health officials are not able to track important changes in rates of illnesses caused by specific types of bacteria. This also limits the ability to detect, investigate, and control multistate outbreaks.

Regulatory agencies and industries need information from outbreak investigations and disease trends to take action to make food safer.

Short- and Long-Term Solutions

The Centers for Disease Control and Prevention (CDC) is encouraging clinical laboratories to work with public-health laboratories to continue culturing and isolating the harmful bacteria from ill people with positive CIDTs. Patient specimens with a positive CIDT for Salmonella, Shiga toxin-producing *E. coli*, and *Shigella* should be cultured to isolate the bacterial strain. Selected laboratories should also do this for *Campylobacter*. It is considering ways to make follow-up cultures easier and cheaper for clinical laboratories. It is working closely with the Association of Public Health Laboratories (APHL), public-health officials, regulatory agencies, diagnostic laboratories, CIDT kit manufacturers, and clinicians to make sure that cultures are obtained in clinical labs when CIDTs are positive, or the positive specimen from the patient is provided to public health laboratories so they can culture it.

The CDC is encouraging companies that make CIDTs to design the tests in a way that keeps the bacteria alive so they can be cultured if the test is positive. It is adapting surveillance systems, such as the Foodborne Diseases Active Surveillance Network, or FoodNet, to include infections diagnosed only by CIDTs. It is working with partners to develop advanced testing methods that will not require bacterial isolates to provide the information needed by public-health officials. These tests may also provide additional information to healthcare providers about the germ's potential for antibiotic resistance or the likelihood of causing serious illness.

These innovations are in the early stages of development and could be years away from implementation. Researchers hope that the use of these methods will eventually eliminate the need for culturing bacterial isolates from most patients and speed up the process of detecting and solving outbreaks. Culture-derived bacterial isolates from patients will still be needed for a long time to identify emerging problems.

Section 26.2

Rapid Diagnostic Tests

This section includes text excerpted from "Rapid Diagnostic Tests: How They Work," Centers for Disease Control and Prevention (CDC), July 23, 2018.

Rapid diagnostic tests (RDTs) most often use a dipstick or cassette format and provide results in about 20 minutes. A blood specimen collected from the patient is applied to the sample pad on the test card along with certain reagents. Approved RDTs for use in the malaria-endemic world can detect 2 types of malaria antigens; one is specific for *P. falciparum* and the other is found in all 4 human species of malaria. After 15 to 20 minutes (depending on the test), the presence of specific bands in the test card window indicates whether the patient is infected with *P. falciparum* or one of the other 3 species of human malaria.

Rapid Diagnostic Tests Importance in Diagnosis and Treatment in the Malaria-Endemic World

Rapid diagnostic tests offer a useful alternative to microscopy in situations where a reliable microscopic diagnosis is not available—or is not available right away. This is the case in most of the malaria-endemic world.

Malaria RDTs are being widely used in malaria-endemic countries, but the use of an RDT does not completely eliminate the need for malaria microscopy. Because RDTs may not be able to detect some infections with lower numbers of malaria parasites in the patient's blood and the less common species of malaria, *P. ovale*, and *P. malariae*, in the malaria-endemic world:

- Patients with negative RDT results can be followed up by microscopy where available to confirm the result
- Patients with positive RDT results who are not responding to initial antimalarial treatment should be evaluated for other causes of their symptoms to determine whether the treatment was appropriate and to examine parasites in the blood by microscopy to determine the possibility of drug resistance

Other Considerations
Test Performance and Cost

For RDTs to be optimally useful, the tests must perform well. At this time, product testing has shown that some tests on the market perform much better than others. In addition, care must be taken during the transport and storage of RDTs. High temperatures and high humidity, in particular, can contribute to poor performance. The tests must also be affordable to national malaria programs. The costs of the tests have fallen in the last few years; even so, many malaria control programs find that procuring the large numbers of test kits needed to ensure the universal diagnosis is a considerable expense.

Health-Worker Training

New methodologies require training. Healthcare workers need training both in the new test methodology, as well as in using the results to treat patients. Available resources can limit the amount and quality of training available under real-world conditions.

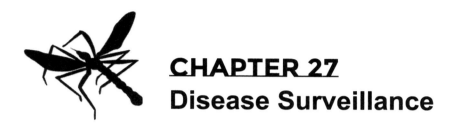

CHAPTER 27
Disease Surveillance

Chapter Contents

Section 27.1

Role of Surveillance in Disease Elimination Programs

This section includes text excerpted from "Surveillance Manual—Indicators," Centers for Disease Control and Prevention (CDC), November 17, 2017.

In routine disease control programs, traditional, passive-disease surveillance systems are usually adequate to meet program demands despite their limitations. In contrast, in disease elimination or eradication programs, routine surveillance activities are inadequate once the goal is near. In advanced disease elimination and eradication programs, every case counts. Without adequate surveillance, the elimination of vaccine-preventable diseases cannot be achieved and sustained. This section describes surveillance for diseases in various stages of prevention and control and discusses surveillance indicators that have been developed to evaluate the appropriateness, completeness, accuracy, and timeliness of surveillance systems. For the Nationally Notifiable Diseases Surveillance System (NNDSS), components include case reporting from the healthcare provider to public-health officials in a jurisdiction, the public-health case investigation, and case notification from jurisdiction to the Centers for Disease Control and Prevention (CDC).

Traditionally, communicable disease surveillance programs have relied on passive reporting, in which reports are received from physicians and other healthcare providers. For diseases and conditions for which laboratory confirmation is routinely obtained, laboratory-based reporting has virtually replaced traditional healthcare provider-based reporting in many jurisdictions, because case ascertainment is far more complete. However, even when supplemented by laboratory-based reports, reporting in traditional passive surveillance systems remains incomplete. Despite this limitation, these data remain useful because they are used primarily for monitoring trends in disease occurrence rather than for initiating public-health action in response to each individual case.

In disease elimination programs, the role of surveillance is different. To achieve a goal of zero cases of a disease, aggressive efforts must be made to identify factors that allow cases to continue to occur despite the low incidence of disease. The occurrence of these cases may indicate the need for new prevention strategies, but in order to track the impact of any such strategies, surveillance data are essential. In addition, timely notification is necessary so that public-health action can be taken to limit the spread of disease. This was illustrated during the global smallpox eradication program. The continued occurrence of cases of smallpox despite high vaccination coverage led to the development of a new strategy for smallpox eradication; i.e., a wide circle of contacts around each case-patient was identified and vaccinated, creating a wall of immunity around the remaining patients. These efforts led ultimately to the global eradication of smallpox. This goal could not have been achieved without recognition of the need for an additional strategy and without the ability to rapidly identify and respond to individual cases.

To achieve and maintain the eradication status of a specific disease within an area, it is necessary:

- To obstruct transmission until endemicity ceases
- To prevent or nullify the reestablishment of the disease from carriers, relapsing cases, or imported sources of infection

Accordingly, an adequate surveillance organization must be developed to identify and cope with these threats to the achievement of disease eradication.

Development of Surveillance Indicators

Because of the essential role of surveillance in disease elimination, methods to monitor its quality were developed in 1988 by the Pan American Health Organization (PAHO) as part of the polio eradication effort in the Western Hemisphere. Surveillance indicators included measures of surveillance infrastructure (e.g., the number of reporting units reporting on a weekly basis), timeliness of notification (e.g., the interval between case onset and notification), adequacy of case investigation (e.g., the proportion of cases with appropriately timed laboratory specimens obtained), and timeliness of laboratory testing. Although not generally done outside of evaluation projects in routine disease control programs, monitoring these attributes would undoubtedly provide useful information for any surveillance system. These attributes overlap with those recommended by the CDC for the evaluation of surveillance systems.

Indicators of Reporting Completeness

The unique requirements of surveillance in disease elimination programs led PAHO to also develop an indicator that allowed monitoring of the completeness of reporting. In disease elimination programs, it is critical to have some measure of the adequacy of case ascertainment as well as a measure of how well cases were investigated once they were reported as suspected cases. It is not sufficient to adequately investigate reported cases if most cases are never reported. More importantly, as disease incidence declines, it becomes increasingly difficult to interpret the absence of reported cases. How can you tell if zero means zero? Does it mean there were no cases, or does it mean no one looked?

The PAHO developed one successful strategy to address this problem during the polio eradication effort in Latin America. Surveillance was performed not for paralytic poliomyelitis but for a syndrome that includes both paralytic polio and other conditions, including Guillain-Barré Syndrome (GBS), among children younger than 15 years of age—that is, the surveillance system was organized to identify cases that were clinically consistent with polio (suspected cases), and then to track the cases as laboratory investigation was performed to either accept or rule out a diagnosis of polio due to wild poliovirus. If adequate laboratory testing was not obtained to definitively determine or rule out the diagnosis of polio, the case was classified as compatible and considered a failure of case investigation and surveillance. In the absence of polio, GBS and other conditions causing acute flaccid paralysis (AFP) in children occur at a fairly constant rate over time, thus the adequacy of ascertainment of suspected polio cases could be monitored by tracking the incidence of AFP among children younger than 15 years of age. In countries or regions reporting rates of AFP of 1 per 100,000 children younger than 15 years of age and without confirmed or compatible polio cases, one could be reasonably confident that the absence of reported polio cases, in fact, meant the absence of polio. In contrast, if AFP rates were less than 1 per 100,000 among children in this age group, the absence of cases might reflect inadequate surveillance rather than the absence of polio. Monitoring the rate of AFP reporting in Latin America was a critical component of PAHO's effort to monitor the adequacy of polio surveillance. By tracking this closely at the regional and national levels, investigators could identify and assist areas with inadequate surveillance and document resulting improvements.

Unfortunately, few other examples of vaccine-preventable diseases exist for which indicators analogous to the AFP rate are known. For example, no external standard for determining the completeness of measles surveillance exists that would be equivalent to the rate of AFP in the surveillance of polio.

While monitoring all cases of AFP is highly sensitive, it is not specific. Another part of the PAHO approach is essential—that is, classifying incompletely evaluated cases as "compatible." In a disease elimination program, the aim is to capture all the true cases by having a case definition that is very sensitive; nonetheless, it is also important to exclude noncases by adequate case investigation and laboratory testing. The PAHO strategy captured both these elements, enhancing the sensitivity and specificity of the surveillance system.

Surveillance Indicators in the United States

The purpose of vaccine-preventable disease surveillance indicators in the United States is to ensure the adequate performance of the essential components of surveillance and case investigation and to identify components of each that need improvement. Surveillance indicators for selected vaccine-preventable diseases were proposed by the CDC and approved by the Council of State and Territorial Epidemiologists (CSTE) in 1994. Since then, the indicators have continued to evolve to maximize their usefulness. The CDC currently monitors the following indicators on a regular basis.

Indicators for Measles Surveillance

- The proportion of confirmed cases reported to the National Notifiable Diseases Surveillance System (NNDSS) with complete information (clinical case definition, hospitalization, laboratory testing, vaccination history, date reported to the health department, transmission setting, outbreak-related, epidemiologic linkage, date of birth, and onset date)
- The interval between the date of symptom onset and date of public-health notification
- The proportion of confirmed cases that are laboratory confirmed
- The proportion of cases that have an imported source
- The proportion of cases for which at least one clinical specimen for virus isolation was submitted to the CDC
- The number of discarded measles-like illness (MLI) reports (discontinued January 2006)

Indicators for Mumps Surveillance

- The proportion of confirmed cases reported to the NNDSS with complete information (clinical case definition, hospitalization, laboratory testing, vaccination history, date reported to the health department, transmission setting, outbreak-related, epidemiologic linkage, date of birth, and onset date)
- The interval between the date of symptom onset and date of public-health notification
- The proportion of confirmed cases that are laboratory confirmed
- The proportion of cases that have an imported source

Indicators for Rubella Surveillance

- The proportion of confirmed cases reported to the NNDSS with complete information (clinical case definition, hospitalization, laboratory testing, vaccination history, date reported to the health department,

transmission setting, outbreak-related, epidemiologic linkage, date of birth, and onset date)
- The interval between the date of symptom onset and date of public-health notification
- The proportion of confirmed cases that are laboratory confirmed
- The proportion of cases that have an imported source
- The proportion of confirmed cases among women of child-bearing age with known pregnancy status

Indicators for Haemophilus Influenzae Type B Invasive Disease Surveillance

- The proportion of cases reported to the NNDSS with complete information (clinical case definition—species, specimen type; vaccination history; and serotype testing)
- The proportion of cases among children younger than five years of age with complete vaccination history
- The proportion of cases among children younger than five years of age in which an isolate was serotyped

Indicators for Pertussis Surveillance

- The proportion of cases reported to the NNDSS with complete information (clinical case definition, complications, antibiotic treatment, laboratory testing, vaccination history, and epidemiologic data (e.g., outbreak/epidemiological linkage))
- The interval between the date of symptom onset and date of public-health notification
- The proportion of cases meeting clinical case definition that are laboratory tested
- The proportion of case-patients with complete vaccination history

Indicators for Invasive Pneumococcal Disease Surveillance

- The proportion of cases reported to the NNDSS with complete information (clinical case definition, serotype, and vaccine history)

- The proportion of cases that are serotyped
- The proportion of case-patients with complete vaccination history

Indicators for Meningococcal Disease Surveillance

- The proportion of cases reported to the NNDSS with complete information (birthdate or age and event date)
- The proportion of cases that are reported as confirmed
- The proportion of cases with known outcome
- The proportion of confirmed cases with serogroup testing
- The proportion of case-patients with complete vaccination history

Indicators for Varicella Disease Surveillance

- The proportion of cases reported to the NNDSS with complete information on age, number of lesions, and hospitalization
- The proportion of cases that are reported as confirmed
- The proportion of confirmed cases with laboratory testing
- The proportion of cases with an outbreak linkage
- The proportion of case-patients with complete vaccination history

Additional Approaches and Future Directions

Although these indicators have been useful for identifying major problems with case investigation and reporting, given the small number of cases of most vaccine-preventable diseases now reported in the United States, a critical issue remaining is the sensitivity of the surveillance system, i.e., does the absence of cases from a particular jurisdiction indicate that there were, in fact, no cases?

One approach to improving the completeness of reporting is to implement active surveillance, that is, to make contact and solicit reports from all providers and institutions responsible for reporting on a regular basis. Active surveillance has been shown to increase reporting of measles, rubella, salmonellosis, and hepatitis in demonstration projects but is generally too expensive to perform routinely.

Active surveillance is supported by the following assumptions:

- Cases are occurring in the community.
- Case-patients seek medical attention or otherwise come to the attention of institutions subject to reporting requirements.
- The condition is recognized by the provider or institution.
- Cases are not reported because filling out reporting forms or calling the health department is too much trouble.
- If the administrative reporting burden for providers is reduced, cases will be reported.

For rare diseases (i.e., most vaccine-preventable diseases in the United States) these conditions are rarely met. Indeed, previous demonstrations of the usefulness of active surveillance have focused on diseases that were relatively common or at least endemic in the population under surveillance. In many communities and states, no cases of measles or rubella have occurred in years, and in the absence of a large, ongoing outbreak, participating in active surveillance for these conditions is unlikely to be of much interest to providers.

As part of the polio eradication effort in the Western Hemisphere, PAHO instituted a system of weekly negative reporting that allowed them to monitor the surveillance infrastructure (i.e., the number of clinics and other facilities that participated in the surveillance system). Each reporting unit was to include in the weekly notifiable diseases report not only cases of disease identified, but for AFP only, a negative report if no cases were identified that week (i.e., "no cases of acute flaccid paralysis"). It was implicitly assumed that any such cases would be recognized because the patient would seek medical care. This was an attempt to gain the benefits of active surveillance within a passive surveillance system without the investment of resources needed to conduct active surveillance. However, an evaluation in one country suggested that at the local level, negative reporting was not accompanied by efforts at case finding, and substantial training was needed to make negative reporting meaningful at the local level.

What approach can provide firm evidence that the absence of reported cases means the absence of disease in the population? Several methods may be useful: application of external standards, identification of imported cases, monitoring the level of reporting for suspected cases that are ruled out as cases by epidemiologic and laboratory investigation, monitoring diagnostic effort, and monitoring circulation of the organism.

Section 27.2
The National Notifiable Noninfectious Diseases Surveillance System

This section includes text excerpted from "About Notifiable Noninfectious Disease and Conditions Data," Centers for Disease Control and Prevention (CDC), August 2, 2017.

Public-health surveillance of noninfectious conditions and disease outbreaks at the local, state, and territorial levels protects the public's health by ensuring the proper identification of conditions and health hazards. With these data, local public-health officials monitor trends in these conditions, identify populations or geographic areas at high risk, plan prevention and control policies and other interventions, allocate resources effectively, coordinate activities, and assess the effectiveness of their efforts. Local, state, and territorial health departments also use these data to assist the federal government in meeting requirements under the international health regulations to identify, respond to, and share information about adverse-health events that might constitute a public-health emergency of international concern (PHEIC).

Completeness and Surveillance System Characteristics

Although the sources of data for national notifiable infectious diseases and for national notifiable noninfectious conditions and disease outbreaks are the same (i.e., local, state, and territorial jurisdictions' data on reportable conditions) and have the same general purpose (i.e., monitoring and responding to the condition to improve population health), there are a number of differences that should be considered when comparing findings across conditions and by time, location, and demographic characteristics. Under-reporting of noninfectious conditions and disease outbreaks to local and state health departments occurs, and the completeness of reporting, and therefore, of notifications to the Centers for Disease Control and Prevention (CDC), varies by condition. Moreover, variations in data collection methods also influence comparative observations across conditions and disease outbreaks. For example, case-based surveillance of acute pesticide-related illness or injury, elevated blood-lead levels, and cancer are focused on collecting information on cases that meet the criteria specified in national condition-specific case definitions and on collecting information about those persons' conditions. In contrast, surveillance of outbreaks of food-borne and water-borne illness seeks to identify clusters of sick persons with a common exposure (as opposed to persons with a specific disease). "Food-borne disease outbreaks" are defined as two or more cases of a similar illness resulting from the ingestion of food. "Water-borne disease outbreaks" are defined as two or more cases of a similar illness resulting from common exposure to water or water-associated chemicals. For these conditions, information is collected about the characteristics of the disease outbreaks, including data from epidemiologic and environmental investigations.

Even among conditions for which case-based surveillance methods are used, there is substantial variation in what a condition means. For example, for a condition, such as elevated blood-lead levels, surveillance uses laboratory findings to identify persons who have been exposed to a hazard but does not require a clinical diagnosis of lead poisoning. In contrast, for many other conditions, a diagnosis based on clinical and/or pathological criteria is needed to meet the case definition for a notification to the CDC.

The meaning of the date of the occurrence of the condition also varies among the conditions and across jurisdictions. For cancer, as for some infectious diseases, including tuberculosis (TB) and human immunodeficiency virus (HIV) infection diagnosis, the date of occurrence is assigned based on the date the condition is diagnosed. For silicosis, the date of occurrence represents the date of the initial report (e.g., the date of a hospital discharge report, clinician report, or a workers' compensation claim). For lead-screening test results, the date of occurrence is the date the sample was tested. For acute pesticide-related illness, it is the date of pesticide exposure, which is generally identical to the date of symptom onset since symptom onset is within seconds to hours of exposure. For disease outbreaks, the date of occurrence represents the date of illness onset of the first case in the outbreak.

The source and definitions of race and ethnicity also vary over time and among conditions. For example, information about race and ethnicity for lead exposure is based on self-report. Whereas for cancer incidence it is based on medical records, which might or might not be based on self-report, or from matching the names of persons with cancer with lists of surnames for different ethnic groups or with tribal registries. For silicosis, race and ethnicity are based on a self-report, report from next-of-kin, or from medical records. Race- and ethnicity-specific information among the conditions might also vary depending on the jurisdictions' systems for submitting notifications to the CDC and the need to protect private-health information. There are also variations across conditions in terms of which specific U.S. Census Bureau data sets were used to calculate rates of occurrence of the conditions.

Section 27.3
Investigating an Outbreak

This section includes text excerpted from "Conducting a Field Investigation," Centers for Disease Control and Prevention (CDC), December 13, 2018.

When a threat to the public's health occurs, epidemiologists are ready responders who investigate the problem so they can identify causes and risk factors, implement prevention and control measures, and communicate with everyone involved. Epidemiologic-field investigations are a core function of epidemiology and perhaps the most obvious way information is transformed into action to ensure public health and safety. This section describes the step-by-step process required in performing an epidemiologic-field investigation. This section describes a field investigation in the context of a public-health response to a presumed acute infectious-disease outbreak, although this approach also applies to other scenarios and problems.

Background Considerations

An "outbreak" is defined as the occurrence of more cases of disease than expected in a given area or among a specific group of people over a particular period of time. When there are clearly many more cases than usual that is distributed across a larger geographic area, the term "epidemic" can be used. An "outbreak" is a situation that usually needs a rapid public-health response. Notification of a suspected outbreak can come from different sources, including astute clinicians, laboratory scientists, public-health surveillance data, or the media.

After the decision is made to start an investigation, clearly defining the objective of the investigation is crucial. Field investigations of common outbreak scenarios have standard objectives and time-tested methods that can be implemented rapidly. For example, because transmission modes associated with food-borne and water-borne outbreaks are well-known (i.e., spread by contact with infected persons, animals, or contaminated food or water), epidemiologists have developed the National Hypothesis Generating Questionnaire (NHGQ), a standardized questionnaire to help develop hypotheses and collect information from ill persons regarding demographics and specific exposures. In contrast, at the time of initial recognition, many outbreaks have no obvious or known cause, which challenges the epidemiologist to establish a clear objective early—albeit one that is broad and can be revised as the investigation evolves—and to generate hypotheses.

Finally, a certain urgency to field investigations and pressure to find an answer quickly will always exist. For example, rapid surveys or other study designs used in outbreak investigations might lack the level of statistical power or proof of causality that often are possible in prospectively planned research studies. Likewise, delays caused by waiting for all laboratory samples to be tested can delay the determination of pathogens or modes of spread and, consequently, implementation of control measures. However, the goal is to be both timely and accurate. Because of these considerations, coordinating with all partners and establishing priorities early is key to a successful investigation.

The Investigation

Epidemiologists use a systematic multistep approach to field investigations. Although these steps are presented here in numeric order, they might be conducted out of order or concurrently to meet the demands of the investigation. For example, in certain circumstances, implementing a control measure soon after notification and confirmation of an outbreak might be possible and even advisable. Often, steps 2 and 3 are performed at the same time. These two steps highlight the need for increased collaboration (or teamwork) early in the investigation among public-health officials, laboratory personnel, clinicians, and other stakeholders.

Step 1. Prepare for Field Work

An important first step in any field investigation is addressing the operational aspects related to preparing for fieldwork. This preparation includes ensuring that all persons involved agree on the purpose of the investigation and that the required official approvals for the field investigation have been received. A formal invitation for assistance must be received from an authorized official; for example, when a state requests assistance from the Centers for Disease Control and Prevention (CDC) to conduct an investigation, the Governor or an appropriate public-health officer such as the state epidemiologist would be authorized to extend that invitation. In addition, the roles and responsibilities of those involved in the investigation must be delineated. For most investigations, laboratory testing will play a crucial role; thus, discussions with laboratory colleagues about types of testing and specimens need to occur before the field investigation begins. Concerns related to the safety of the field team (e.g., whether personal protective equipment will be needed) should also be considered during this first step. Ensuring that this early preparation for the field investigation is completed will prevent misunderstandings and other problems later.

Step 2. Confirm the Diagnosis

Confirming or verifying the diagnosis ensures, to the extent possible, that you are addressing the problem that was reported initially and rules out misdiagnosis and potential laboratory error. For example, in a communicable-disease outbreak, the real clustering of false infections—a consequence of misdiagnosis and laboratory error—can result in a pseudo epidemic. The term "pseudoepidemic" refers to a situation in which there is an observed increase in positive test results or the incidence of disease-related to something other than a true increase in disease. Diagnoses can be confirmed by implementing some or all of the following activities:

- Interviewing the affected persons
- Clinical examination of the affected persons by healthcare personnel when indicated and possible
- Reviewing medical records and other pertinent clinical information (e.g., radiography and other imaging studies)
- Confirming the results of laboratory testing; if the epidemiologist does not have the expertise to assess the adequacy, accuracy, or meaning of the laboratory findings, laboratory scientists and other personnel should be consulted

Although laboratory data might be the best and the only link between a putative cause and case, not every case requires laboratory confirmation before further action can be taken. A related step to confirming the diagnosis is the need to obtain specimens (e.g., microbiologic strains already isolated) before they have been discarded so that they are available for further analysis if new questions arise later in an investigation.

Step 3. Determine the Existence of an Outbreak

Determining the existence of an outbreak is a sometimes difficult step that should be completed before committing program resources to a full-scale investigation. This step also is necessary to rule out spurious problems (e.g., pseudoepidemics or reporting increases caused by surveillance artifacts). As noted previously, pseudoepidemics might result from real clustering of false infections (e.g., inadvertent contaminants of laboratory specimens) or artifactual clustering of real infections (e.g., increases in the number of reported cases because of changes in surveillance procedures introduced by the health department or implemented by a healthcare-delivery system.) Problems potentially associated with pseudoepidemics include risks related to unnecessary or inappropriate treatment and unnecessary diagnostic procedures.

To confirm the existence of an outbreak, the field investigation team must first compare the number of cases during the suspected outbreak period with the number of cases that would be expected during a nonoutbreak time frame by:

- Establishing a comparison timeframe in the suspected epidemic setting by considering, for example, whether it should be the period (e.g., hours, days, weeks, or months) immediately preceding the current problem or the corresponding period from the previous year
- Taking into account potential problems or limitations in determining comparison timeframes (e.g., lack of data, varying or lack of case definitions, incomplete reporting, and other reasons for inefficient surveillance)
- Calculating occurrence rates, when possible, between the period of the current problem and a comparator period

For certain problems, an outbreak can be rapidly confirmed through the use of existing surveillance data. For others, however, substantial time lags might occur before a judgment can be made about the existence of an outbreak

Step 4. Identify and Count Cases
The aim of this step is to identify or ascertain, as many cases as possible without including noncases. As a practical matter, this entails casting a broad net through the use of a classification scheme—the case definition—that maximizes sensitivity (i.e., correctly identifies persons who have cases

of the condition (true-positives)) and optimizes specificity (i.e., does not include persons who do not have cases of the condition (false-positives)).

The "case definition" is a statement consisting of three elements that together specify a person:

- With a condition consisting of (a) a set of symptoms (e.g., myalgia or headache) or (b) signs (e.g., elevated temperature, maculopapular rash, or rales) or (c) laboratory findings (e.g., leukocytosis or positive blood culture)
- With the condition occurring during a particular period, usually referred to as the "epidemic period"
- With the condition occurring after the person was in one or more specific settings (e.g., a hospital, school, place of work, or community or neighborhood, or among persons who participated in a gathering, such as a wedding or meeting

Although the case definition might be broad at the onset of an epidemiologic field investigation, it is a flexible classification scheme that is often revised and narrowed as the investigation progresses.

To minimize the likelihood of ascertainment bias (i.e., a systematic distortion in measurement due to the way in which data are collected), cases ideally are sought and counted through systematic searches of a multiplicity of potential sources to identify the maximum number or a representative sample of cases. Examples of sources include:

- Public-health agency surveillance data
- Medical system records from hospitals, laboratories, or ambulatory care settings
- Institutional setting records (e.g., school and workplace attendance records)
- Special surveys

Information about identified cases (e.g., coded patient identifiers, age, sex, race/ethnicity, date of illness onset or diagnosis, symptoms, signs, laboratory findings, or other relevant data) should be systematically recorded in a spreadsheet or through other means (e.g., a line listing or similar epidemiologic database) for subsequent analysis and for use in conducting further investigative studies (e.g., hypothesis testing). All staff involved in data collection and maintenance should be trained to use the forms and questionnaires (whether these be on paper or electronic) and to store the forms to protect personal information while facilitating rapid data analysis.

Depending on the nature, scope, and extent of the outbreak, consideration should be given to the need for additional active case finding and surveillance once sufficient information has been collected to support prevention and control efforts. Specifically, ongoing or intensified surveillance can be paramount in subsequent efforts to evaluate the effectiveness of control measures for curbing and terminating the epidemic.

Step 5. Tabulate and Orient the Data in Terms of Time, Place, and Person

This step involves translating and transforming data from the line listing into a basic epidemiologic description of the outbreak. This description characterizes the outbreak in terms of time, place, and person (referred to as "descriptive epidemiology"). Through a systematic review of data in the line listing, key actions typically involve:

- Drawing epidemic curves
- Constructing spot maps or other special spatial projections
- Comparing groups of persons

In addition, these key actions contribute to developing initial hypotheses for explaining the potential cause, source, and mode of spread of the outbreak's causative agent(s).

Time

Establishing the time of the outbreak or epidemic requires the following actions:

- Develop a chronologic framework by collecting information about and ordering key events identified during the creation of the line listing or through other inquiry, including:
  - Time of onset of illness (symptoms, signs, or laboratory test positivity) among affected persons

- Period of likely exposure to the causal agent(s) or risk factor(s)
- The time when treatments were administered or control measures were implemented
- Time of potentially related events or unusual exposures. This includes examples of epidemic curves displaying the types of information that can be analyzed to aid in conducting a field investigation.
- Develop an epidemic curve by graphing the number of cases on the y-axis in relation to units of time (e.g., hours, days, months) on the x-axis—note that time intervals conventionally should be less than (i.e., one-fourth to one-third) the known or suspected incubation period.
- Use the epidemic curve configuration to make preliminary inferences about the modes of spread (e.g., person-to-person, common-source, or continuing point source) of a suspected causative agent.
- If the agent is known, use knowledge of the incubation period to look retrospectively at the period of likely exposure among affected persons.
- If the agent is unknown, but a common event or exposure period is likely, consider potential causal agents on the basis of the possible incubation period.
- When indicated, construct epidemic curves relative to specific sites (e.g., workplace settings, hospital units, classrooms, or neighborhoods) or groups identified by other potential risk characteristics.

Place

Use information collected for the line listing and through other inquiry to orient cases in relation to locations, including:

- Place of residence
- Place of occupation
- Venues for recreational activity
- Activity sites (e.g., rooms or units in which persons were hospitalized; rooms visited during a convention or meeting; or seating or activity locations on transportation conveyances, such as planes or cruise ships)

Using information about the place, construct spot maps or other visual methods to depict locations of cases at the time of onset of illness or possible exposure to causal agents or factors, including:
- Within buildings
- City blocks or neighborhoods
- Geographic or geopolitical areas (e.g., cities, counties, states, or regions)

Person
Use information collected for the line listing to describe cases in relation to such factors as:
- Demographic characteristics (e.g., age, sex, and race/ethnicity), occupation, and diagnoses
- Features shared by affected persons

When possible and where indicated, obtain denominator data (e.g., total cookout attendees in a food-borne disease outbreak) to develop preliminary estimates of rates of illness in relation to demographic, exposure, and other characteristics.

Step 6. Consider Whether Control Measures Can Be Implemented Now
Control measures include two categories of interventions:
- Those that can be directed at the source(s) of most infectious and other disease-causing agents (e.g., treating infected persons and animals or isolating infected persons who are contagious)
- Those that can be directed at persons who are susceptible to such agents (administering postexposure prophylaxis, vaccinating in advance, or employing barrier techniques)

In concept, control measures are implemented only after the preceding and subsequent steps—including developing and testing hypotheses about the cause or mode of spread—have been implemented. In practice, however, decisions about control measures might be necessary at any step in the sequence, and preliminary-control measures can be instituted on the basis of limited initial information and then modified as needed as the investigation proceeds. Control measures should be considered again after more systematic studies are complete.

Step 7. Develop and Test Hypotheses

Hypotheses about the disease-causing agent, source or reservoir of the agent, transmission mode, and risk factors for disease can be developed based on information from multiple sources including:

- Expert subject-matter knowledge by field epidemiologists, laboratory colleagues, and others
- Descriptive epidemiologic findings resulting from analysis of the line listing of identified affected persons
- Information obtained from interviews of individuals or groups of affected persons by using structured questionnaires or open-ended questioning
- Anecdotes, impressions, and ideas from affected persons or others in the affected area
- Consideration of outlier cases (i.e., cases with onset occurring at the beginning or end of the outbreak period)

In certain instances, descriptive epidemiologic findings alone, or results of cross-sectional survey data or other studies will be sufficient for developing hypotheses. Often, however, analytic epidemiologic methods—especially cohort or case-control studies—will be needed for identifying possible risk and other causative factors and for testing the strength of the association of the factors with the disease. The process of hypothesis testing, therefore, can entail multiple iterations of hypothesis-generating and testing, serial studies, and collection, analysis, and management of considerable additional data.

Typically, statistically significant (e.g., small p-value) findings of associations alone do not constitute an adequate body of evidence to support conclusions about the validity of hypotheses and to implement interventions to terminate an outbreak. Instead, all key information and investigative findings should be viewed as a whole in relation to such standards as the Bradford Hill tenets of causation.

Step 8. Plan One or More Systematic Studies

At this stage of most epidemiologic-field investigations, the purposes of systematic or other studies might include improving the quality of information underlying the investigation's conclusions about the problem (e.g., improving the quality of numerators or denominators). Additional examples include refining the accuracy of the estimates of persons at risk and examining other germane concerns (e.g., expanding characterization of the causative agent and its epidemiology).

Step 9. Implement and Evaluate Control and Prevention Measures

The ultimate purpose of an epidemiologic field investigation is to implement scientifically rational and advisable control measures for preventing additional outbreak-associated morbidity or mortality. Control measures implemented in outbreaks will vary based on the causative agent; modes of spread; size and characteristics of the population at risk; setting; and other considerations, such as available resources, politics, and community concerns. Categories of control measures used for terminating outbreaks are described in step 6. Evaluating the impact of control measures is essential. Therefore, evaluation efforts should be implemented concurrently with control measures to assess their effectiveness in attenuating and ultimately terminating the outbreak. If not yet in place, active surveillance should be initiated to monitor for new cases and for evidence of the effect of the control measures and to guide decision-making about additional needs (e.g., further investigation, additional studies, or modifications to the control measures).

Regardless of the intervention, the ethical implications of any action must be considered. Because outbreak investigations typically involve the collection of private, personally identifiable information from individual persons, and often from their families, coworkers, or other acquaintances, epidemiologists should be familiar with applicable local, state, and federal laws regarding privacy protection.

Step 10. Communicate Findings

Field epidemiologists must be diligent and effective communicators throughout and after outbreak investigations. The information they provide helps keep the public and stakeholders accurately apprised during an outbreak, informs decisions about actions to halt the outbreak, and documents the investigation.

This step requires the following actions:

- Establish a communications plan at the onset of the investigation.
- Identify and designate a spokesperson or a consistent point of contact who will serve as the primary communicator for the investigative team. This will optimize the team's efficiency by concentrating on the communications role in one person who is accessible to the news media and others. This also minimizes the potential for confusion or misunderstanding by ensuring consistency in messaging throughout the investigation.
- Provide oral briefings and written communications, as might be indicated.
- Written reports can be customized for multiple purposes, including formally conveying recommendations, meeting institutional requirements for documentation, providing a record for future reference, and facilitating rapid dissemination of investigation findings to the requesting authority, stakeholders, scientific colleagues, and others.
- Before departing the field, the investigative team should provide a preliminary written report and oral briefing to the requesting authority and local stakeholders that document all activities; communicates the findings; and conveys recommendations. A final, more detailed, report might be provided later, especially if additional analyses and studies are planned.
- Brief reports published rapidly in public-health bulletins (e.g., *Morbidity and Mortality Weekly Report*) can help alert colleagues about the problem.

Summing Up

Although no steps should be skipped, they might be conducted concurrently or out of order depending on the circumstances of the investigation. Although descriptive epidemiologic findings are sufficient for supporting initiation of public-health action in certain investigations, more extensive inquiry, including analytic studies, often is required to provide a scientifically rational basis for interventions. Regardless of complexity, the list of steps that organize epidemiologic field investigations helps to ensure focus and thoroughness throughout the investigative response.

Section 27.4
Collecting Epidemiologic Data

This section includes text excerpted from "Collecting Data," Centers for Disease Control and Prevention (CDC), December 13, 2018.

Epidemiologic data are paramount to targeting and implementing evidence-based control measures to protect the public's health and safety. Nowhere is data more important than during a field-epidemiologic investigation to identify the cause of an urgent public-health problem that requires immediate intervention. Many of the steps to conducting a field investigation rely on identifying relevant existing data or collecting new data that address the key investigation objectives.

The challenge is not the lack of data but rather how to identify the most relevant data for meaningful results and how to combine data from various sources that might not be standardized or interoperable to enable analysis. Epidemiologists need to determine quickly whether existing data can be analyzed to inform the investigation or whether additional data need to be collected and how to do so most efficiently and expeditiously.

Epidemiologists working in applied public health have myriad potential data sources available to them. Multiple factors must be considered when identifying relevant data sources for conducting a field investigation. These include investigation objectives and scope, whether requisite data exist and can be accessed, to what extent data from different sources can be practically combined, methods for and feasibility of primary data collection, and resources (e.g., staff, funding) available.

Sources of data and approaches to data collection vary by topic. Although public-health departments have access to notifiable disease case data (primarily for communicable diseases) through mandatory reporting by providers and laboratories, data on chronic diseases and injuries might be available only through secondary sources, such as hospital discharge summaries. Existing data on health-risk behaviors might be available from population-based surveys, but these surveys generally are conducted only among a small proportion of the total population and are de-identified. Although some existing data sources (e.g., death certificates) cover many disease outcomes, others are more specific (e.g., reportable disease registries).

Accessing or collecting clean, valid, reliable, and timely data challenges most field-epidemiologic investigations. New data collected in the context of field investigations should be evaluated for attributes similar to those for surveillance data, such as quality, definitions, timeliness, completeness, simplicity, generalizability, validity, and reliability. Epidemiologists would do well to remember garbage in, garbage out (GIGO) when delineating their data collection plans.

Data Collection Activities

Collecting data during a field investigation requires the epidemiologist to conduct several activities. Although it is logical to believe that a field investigation of an urgent public-health problem should roll out sequentially—first identification of study objectives, followed by questionnaire development; data collection, analysis, and interpretation; and implementation of control measures—in reality, many of these activities must be conducted in parallel, with information gathered from one part of the investigation informing the approach to another part. Moreover, most, if not all, field investigations will be done by a larger team. The importance of developing a protocol, identifying the roles and responsibilities of team members, and documenting all activities and processes should not be underestimated.

Determine Decisions Regarding Control Measure Implementation

The epidemiologist must keep in mind that the primary purpose of a field investigation into an urgent public-health problem is to control the problem and prevent further illness. The range of public-health control measures is broad. Many of these control measures, such as recalling contaminated food products, closing business establishments, recommending antibiotic prophylaxis or vaccination, and requiring isolation of an infectious person, considerably burden individuals, businesses, or the community. Therefore, it is incumbent on the epidemiologists to determine upfront which decisions need to be made and what information is needed to support these decisions.

Define the Investigation's Objectives and Determine Data Needed

Determining whether an urgent public-health problem exists (i.e., an excess of observed cases of illness above what is expected) depends on knowing the expected background rate of endemic disease. The background rate generally is determined by accessing existing data sources, such as reportable disease registries or vital statistics. For foodborne outbreaks, most states and local jurisdictions publish data at least annually; however, for chronic diseases (e.g., cancer) or birth outcomes (e.g., microcephaly), expected baseline rates might have to be extrapolated by applying previously published rates to the population of concern. Although not specific, data from syndromic surveillance systems (e.g., from emergency departments) can be useful in determining background rates of prediagnostic signs or symptoms, such as fever, respiratory illness, or diarrhea.

After the epidemiologist has confirmed the existence of an urgent public-health problem, the next important task in a field investigation is to define the specific objectives and determine what data are necessary and sufficient to justify the control measures. Is the objective to identify a point source (e.g., a contaminated food item) of an outbreak to recall the product? Is the objective to identify specific behaviors that put people at increased risk (e.g., cross-contamination during food handling)? Is the objective to identify factors in the environment that might be causing disease (e.g., elevated lead levels in drinking water)?

Although engaging stakeholders, such as other public-health agencies, community partners, industry leaders, affected businesses, healthcare practitioners, customers, and regulatory agencies, early in an investigation is time-consuming, including them is essential. Discussing up front the purpose of the investigation and the data collection processes will prove invaluable in the long run when collaborators are needed during case finding, data collection, implementation of control measures, and communication with affected populations and the public.

Develop a Study Protocol

The ability to conduct an epidemiologic-field investigation efficiently and effectively depends on understanding the interconnectedness of its parts. Many investigation activities must be conducted in parallel and are interdependent and iterative, with the results informing edits or amendments. For example, the available resources will influence how complex data collection efforts can be; the timeline for an investigation of an infectious-disease outbreak needing urgent control measures might require a quick-and-dirty data collection process, whereas an investigation of a cancer cluster that has unfolded over several years may permit a more in-depth data collection and analysis. Therefore, writing a protocol before embarking on any data collection is paramount.

The urgency of most field investigations requires that the epidemiologist act quickly but thoughtfully. An important and potentially time-saving step is to review prior epidemiologic investigations of similar illnesses and, whenever possible, use or adapt existing protocols, including standard data collection approaches and case definitions. Doing so facilitates data exchange with other systems if the outbreak extends to other jurisdictions.

A field-investigation protocol does not have to be lengthy, but it must include the following:

- Investigation objectives
- Study design (e.g., cohort study, a case-control study)

- Study population, case definition, sample size, and selection
- Data collection procedures, variables to be collected, procedures to safeguard participants
- Data security, privacy, confidentiality, information technology controls
- Analysis plan
- Logistics, including budget, personnel, and timeline
- Legal considerations, including statutes, rules, and regulations

Identifying up front which software package(s) will be used for questionnaire development, data collection, data entry, and analysis also is useful. One such tool, Epi Info, was developed by the Centers for Disease Control and Prevention (CDC) and is a public-domain suite of interoperable software tools designed for public-health practitioners.

Considering all the different elements of an investigation from the beginning will minimize errors that potentially can lead to inconclusive results. Major sources of error that need to be considered during data collection include the following:

- Lack of generalizability because of selection bias, variable participation rates
- Information bias, such as measurement error, self-report bias, and interviewer bias
- Uncontrolled confounding or bias introduced in the association between exposure and outcome because of the third variable
- Small sample size, resulting in inadequate power to detect differences between groups

Identify Possible Data Sources

Keeping in mind the investigation objectives, the epidemiologist should evaluate whether existing data sources (e.g., vital statistics, notifiable disease registries, population surveys, healthcare records, environmental data) are useful for addressing the investigation objectives, whether these data are accurate and readily accessible for analysis, whether existing data systems are interoperable, and what additional data, if any, need to be collected de novo.

Mortality Statistics

Collecting mortality statistics and classifying the causes of death dates to the 1500s in London, when the *Bill of Mortality* was periodically published. During the 1800s, Dr. William Farr developed a disease classification system that ushered in the era of modern vital statistics. During the same period, Dr. John Snow, known as the "father of modern epidemiology," mapped deaths from cholera in London and determined the Broad Street Pump as the source of contaminated water. The story of removing the pump handle is the quintessential public-health intervention based on scientific data. Vital statistics remain an important source of data for understanding leading and unusual causes of death (e.g., childhood influenza-associated, viral hemorrhagic fever, variant Creutzfeldt-Jakob disease (CJD)), and their timeliness is improving thanks to the electronic death reporting system, which many states have implemented.

Notifiable Diseases Reporting

In the United States, the legal framework for reporting infectious diseases to public-health authorities for investigation and control dates to 1878, when Congress authorized the Public Health Service to collect reports of cholera, smallpox, plague, and yellow fever from consuls overseas to implement quarantine measures to prevent their introduction into the United States.

In 1951, the first conference of state epidemiologists determined which diseases should be nationally notifiable to the Public Health Service and later to the CDC. This process continues to-the-day; the Council of State and Territorial Epidemiologists determines which diseases and conditions are designated as nationally notifiable to the CDC, but each state and territory legally mandated reporting in its jurisdiction. Although the list comprises primarily-infectious diseases, in 1995, the first noninfectious condition—elevated blood lead levels—was added.

Laboratory Data

Data from laboratories are critical for investigating infectious-disease outbreaks. By law, most states require laboratories that identify causative agents of notifiable diseases to send case information electronically to state public-health agencies. In addition, most states require laboratories to send cultures to the public-health laboratory in their jurisdiction for confirmation, subtyping, and cataloging results in state and national databases. These data are invaluable for determining whether an apparent cluster of cases might be linked and require further investigation or caused by a random clustering of events. Genotyping data on specific infectious agents (e.g., *Salmonella* strains) produced by state public-health laboratories are loaded to the CDC's PulseNet database to enable identification of cases across jurisdictions that might have a common source

Ongoing Population Surveys

Ongoing population surveys are important for understanding the prevalence of health risk behaviors in the general population. The predominant survey conducted in all states is the Behavioral Risk Factor Surveillance System (BRFSS), a random-digit dialed household survey of noninstitutionalized U.S. adults. Other ongoing surveys include the Youth Risk Behavior Survey (YRBS), Pregnancy Risk Assessment Monitoring System (PRAMS), and the National Health and Nutrition Examination Survey (NHANES). Several states conduct population-based food preference surveys; such surveys are valuable in assessing the background rate of consumption of various food items and can help the field epidemiologist determine whether a food-borne outbreak in which many case-patients report eating a particular food item needs to be investigated further.

Environmental Exposure Data
Distribution of Vectors

Many emerging infectious diseases are zoonotic in origin, so related data are needed. For example, understanding the distribution of vectors for each infection and patterns of the diseases in animals is paramount. During the 2016 epidemic of Zika virus infection, understanding the ecological niche for the *Aedes* mosquito vector was important when investigating an increase in febrile-rash illnesses.

Environmental Contaminants

Illness resulting from exposure to environmental contaminants is another area of public-health importance requiring surveillance. For example, elevated childhood blood-lead levels are a reportable condition, prompting an investigation into possible environmental sources of lead. From 2014 to 2015, a sharp increase in the percentage of children with elevated blood-lead levels in Flint, Michigan, resulted from exposure to drinking water after the city introduced a more corrosive water source containing higher levels of lead.

Additional Existing Sources of Data

Additional existing data sources can help identify cases, determine background rates of human illness, or assess exposures to disease-causing agents (e.g., pathogenic bacteria, vectors, environmental toxins) in a field investigation. Examples of clinical data sources include medical record abstraction, hospital discharge data (e.g., for cases of hemolytic uremic syndrome), syndromic surveillance systems (e.g., for bloody diarrhea during a Shiga toxin-producing Escherichia coli outbreak), poison control center calls (e.g., exposure to white powder during anthrax-related events), and school and work absenteeism records (e.g., New York City school absenteeism in students traveling to Mexico at the beginning of the influenza A (H1N1) pandemic). Examples of data sources for assessing possible exposures include sales receipts (e.g., meals ordered online or food items purchased from a particular store) and law-enforcement data (e.g., drug seizures involving illicit fentanyl in conjunction with opioid-overdose deaths due to fentanyl).

Newer Sources of Data

Electronic health records (EHRs) appear to be a promising source of data for public-health surveillance and for assessing the prevalence of a disease or behavioral-risk factors in the population seeking healthcare. Furthermore, EHRs contain potentially useful data on healthcare use, treatment, and outcomes of a disease—elements not typically assessed by more traditional public-health data sources.

With the advent of personal computers in most households and smartphones in many pockets, epidemiologists are evaluating the utility of the Internet and social media as data sources for identifying outbreaks or case finding during outbreak investigations. Many of these data sources are promising in theory, and epidemiologists are busy evaluating their utility in outbreak detection and case identification. Examples of these data sources include Google hits for antidiarrheal or antipyretic medications to detect outbreaks of gastrointestinal illness or influenza and social media (e.g., Facebook, Twitter, blogs) to identify contacts of patients with sexually transmitted infections (STIs), restaurants where case-patients ate or products they ate before becoming sick, or levels of disease activity during influenza season. Online order forms or electronic grocery receipts may be useful in identifying the names of customers to contact to determine illness status.

Determine Data Collection Method

After evaluating whether existing data can address the study objectives, the field epidemiologist must determine whether additional data need to be collected and, if so, what and how. An important initial step in collecting data as part of a field investigation is determining the mode of data collection (e.g., self-administered, mailed, phone or in-person interview, online survey). The mode in part dictates the format, length, and style of the survey or questionnaire.

Factors to consider when deciding on data collection methods include the following:

- **The feasibility of reaching participants through different modes.** What type of contact information is available? Do participants have access to phones, mailing addresses, or computers?
- **Response rate.** Mailed and Internet surveys traditionally yield lower response rates than phone surveys; however, the response rate for phone surveys also has declined during the past decade.
- **The sensitivity of questions.** Certain sensitive topics (e.g., sexual behaviors) might be better for a self-administered survey than a phone survey.

- **Length and complexity of the survey.** For example, for a long survey or one with complex skip patterns, an interviewer-administered survey might be better than a self-administered one.
- **Control over completeness and order of questions.** Interviewer-administered surveys provide more control by the interviewer than self-administered ones.
- **Cost (e.g., interviewer time).** A mixed-mode of survey administration (e.g., a mailed survey with phone follow-up) might be less expensive to conduct than a phone-only survey, but it also increases study complexity.

Develop the Questionnaire or Survey Instrument

Before developing a survey instrument, review the investigation objectives (i.e., study questions) to identify the specific variables that need to be collected to answer the questions. Similar to developing a protocol, the most efficient and effective means for developing a survey instrument might be to identify an existing survey questionnaire or template that can be adapted for current use. Pay special attention to ensuring that survey instruments can be used across multiple sites in the event that the outbreak involves multiple jurisdictions.

Information and variables to include in a survey instrument are:

- Unique identifier for each record
- Date questionnaire is completed
- A description of the purpose of the investigation for participants
- Participant demographics
- Outcome measures
- Measures of exposure
- Possible confounders and effect modifiers
- Information about who participants should contact with questions

If the survey is interviewer-administered, it should include fields for the interviewer's name and interview date. A cover sheet with attempts to contact, code status of the interview (e.g., completed), and notes can be helpful.

In writing survey questions, borrow from other instruments that have worked well (e.g., that are demonstrated to be reliable and accurate) whenever possible. Write questions that are clear and use vocabulary understandable to the study population and that contain only one concept.

Three basic types of questions are:

- **Close-ended questions.** These questions ask participants to choose from predetermined response categories. An "other (specify)—" field can capture any other responses. They are quick for participants to respond to and easy to analyze.
- **Open-ended questions.** These questions enable participants to answer in their own words and can provide rich information about new topics or context to close-ended questions; however, responses to these questions can be time-consuming to code and analyze.
- **Precoded, open-ended questions.** These questions can be used on interviewer-administered surveys. They enable participants to answer unprompted, but the interviewer selects from precoded response categories.

Close-ended questions usually are used for outbreak investigations. They can have various response categories (e.g., nominal, numeric, Likert scales). Consider including "don't know" and "refused" response categories. Ideally, code response categories in advance and on the instrument to facilitate data entry and analysis (e.g., yes = 1, no = 0). Close-ended questions could include cascading questions, which can be an efficient way to get more detailed information as one filters down through a hierarchy of questions (e.g., first you ask the participant's state of residence, then a menu of that state's counties drops down).

In compiling questions, consider the flow, needed skip patterns, and order (e.g., placing more sensitive questions toward the end). For self-administered surveys, the format needs to be friendly, well-spaced, and easy to follow, with clear instructions and definitions.

Content experts should review the draft questionnaire. The epidemiologist should pilot the questionnaire with a few colleagues and members of the study population and edit as necessary. This will save time in the long run; many epidemiologists have learned the hard way that a survey question was not clear or was asking about more than one concept, or that the menu of answers was missing a key response category.

Calculate the Sample Size and Select the Sample

Good sample selection can help improve the generalizability of results and ensure sufficient numbers of study participants. Information about determining whom to select is covered in study design discussions, but the sample size is worth briefly mentioning here. If the study comprises the entire study population, it is a census; a subset of the study population is a sample. A sample can be selected through probability sampling or nonprobability sampling (e.g., purposive sampling or a convenience sample). Probability sampling is a better choice for statistical tests and statistical inferences. For probability sampling procedures other than a simple random sample (e.g., stratified or cluster sampling), consult with a survey sampling expert.

How large a sample to select depends on resources, study timeline (generally the larger the sample, the more expensive and time-consuming), the analyses to be conducted, and the effect size you want to detect. For example, to detect a difference in proportions between two groups using a chi-square test, consider how much of a difference needs to be detected to be meaningful.

Review Legal Authority, Rules, and Policies Governing Data Collection

Generally, government public-health agencies have the authority to access healthcare system data (with justification). The Health Insurance Portability and Accountability Act (HIPAA) of 1996 has a specific language allowing for the use of personal-health information by government agencies to perform public-health activities.

Nonetheless, accessing data sources that are not specifically collected and maintained by public-health authorities can be challenging. Many outside parties are not familiar with the legal authority that public-health agencies have to investigate and control diseases and exposures that affect the public's health and safety. The field epidemiologist may find it useful to consult her or his agency's attorney for legal counsel regarding data collection during a specific public-health event.

Other scenarios that challenge epidemiologists trying to access external data include concern by healthcare systems that requests for data on hospitalizations, clinic visits, or emergency department visits breach privacy of protected health information; concern by school officials that access to information about children during an outbreak associated with a school activity violates provisions of the Family Educational Rights and Privacy Act (FERPA); and concerns by businesses that case-patients in an outbreak associated with a particular food item or establishment might pursue legal action or lawsuits. Legal counsel can help address these concerns.

Collect the Data

Having a written data collection section as part of the overall study protocol is essential. As with survey development, borrowing from previous data collection protocols can be helpful. This protocol can include the following:

- An introductory letter to participants
- Introductory script for interviewers
- Instructions for recruiting and enrolling participants in the survey, including obtaining consent for participation. Although field epidemiologic investigations of an urgent public-health problem are legally considered to be public-health practice and not research, including elements of informed consent might be useful to ensure that participants are aware of their rights, participation is voluntary, and the confidentiality of their health information will be protected.
- Instructions on conducting the interviews, especially if there are multiple interviewers, include the importance of reading the questions verbatim, term definitions, the pace of the interview, answers to frequently asked questions, and ways to handle urgent situations
- Instructions related to the protection of participants (e.g., maintaining confidentiality, data security)

Train staff collecting data on the protocol, reviewing instructions carefully and modifying as needed. Involve interviewers in pilot testing the survey instrument and provide feedback. Have a plan for quality checks during questionnaire administration (if the survey is not computer-based). Review the first several completed surveys to check the completeness of fields, inconsistencies in responses, and how well skip patterns work. In addition, debrief interviewers about issues they might have encountered (e.g., if participants cannot understand certain questions, those questions might need rewording).

Similarly, data entry must have quality checks. When starting data entry, check several records against the completed survey instrument for accuracy and consider double data entry of a sample of surveys to check for errors.

The subsequent section discusses the details of the data analysis. However, it is important to consider conducting some preliminary data analysis even before data collection is complete. Understanding how participants are interpreting and answering questions can enable corrections to the wording before it is too late. Many an epidemiologist has bemoaned a misinterpreted question, confusing survey formatting, or a missing confounding variable resulting in study questions without meaningful results.

Issues and Challenges with Data Collection

The important attributes of a public-health surveillance system can and should be applied to data collected in response to an urgent event. Infield investigations, tradeoffs exist between these attributes; for example, a more timely collection of data might lead to lower quality data, fewer resources might mean less complete data, and retrospective analysis of preexisting data might be more cost-effective, although prospective data collection from case-patients might enable more targeted questions about specific exposures.

The media can play an important and sometimes conflicting role during an outbreak. The media can be useful in alerting the public to an outbreak and assisting with additional case finding. In contrast, if the public believes an outbreak resulted from eating a specific food item or eating at a specific restaurant, that belief can preclude the field epidemiologist's ability to obtain accurate data after a press release has been issued because it might cause self-report bias among study participants. In addition, with the current calls for government transparency and accountability, field epidemiologists might be reluctant to release information too early, thereby risking additional exposures to the suspected source.

Changes in technology also challenge data collection. Such changes range from laboratories moving to nonculture diagnostic methods for isolating infectious pathogens, which decreases the epidemiologist's ability to link cases spread out in space and time, to the increasing use of social media to communicate, which limits response rates from time-honored methods of data collection, such as landline telephones. Conversely, many new sources of data are opportunities made possible by the expanded use of computer technology by individuals, businesses, and health systems. It is incumbent upon field epidemiologists to adapt to these changes to be able to investigate and control urgent public-health threats.

Summing Up

Responding to urgent public-health issues expeditiously requires balancing the speed of response with the need for accurate data and information to support the implementation of control measures. Adapting preexisting protocols and questionnaires will facilitate timely response and consistency across jurisdictions. In most epidemiologic studies the activities are not done linearly and sequentially; rather, the steps frequently are conducted in parallel and are iterative, with the results informing edits or amendments. The analyses and results are only as good as the quality of the data collected.

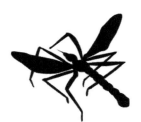

CHAPTER 28
Role of Technology and Surveillance Systems in Public-Health Response

Public-health surveillance has benefitted from and has often pioneered, informatics analyses and solutions. However, the field of informatics also serves other facets of public health including emergency response, environmental health, nursing, and administration. "Public-health informatics" has been defined as the systematic application of information and computer science and technology to public-health practice, research, and learning. It is an interdisciplinary profession that applies mathematics, engineering, information science, and related social sciences (e.g., decision analysis) to important public-health problems and processes. Public-health informatics is a subdomain of the larger field known as "biomedical or health informatics." Health informatics is not synonymous with the term "health information technology" (health IT). Although the concept of health IT encompasses the use of technology in the field of healthcare, one can think of health informatics as defining the science, how and why behind health IT. For example, health IT professionals should be able to resolve infrastructure problems with a network connection, whereas trained public-health informaticians should be able to support public-health decisions by facilitating the availability of timely, relevant, and high-quality information. In other words, they should always be able to provide advice on methods

This chapter includes text excerpted from "The Role of Public Health Informatics in Enhancing Public Health Surveillance," Centers for Disease Control and Prevention (CDC), July 27, 2012. Reviewed January 2020.

for achieving a public-health goal faster, better, or at a lower cost by leveraging computer science, information science, or technology.

This chapter proposes a vision for informatics in enhancing public-health surveillance, identifies challenges and opportunities, and suggests approaches to attain the vision. This topic was identified by the Centers for Disease Control and Prevention (CDC) leadership as one of six major concerns that must be addressed by the public-health community to advance public-health surveillance in the 21st century. This chapter is intended to continue the conversations with the public-health community for a shared vision for public-health surveillance in the 21st century.

The work of public-health informatics can be divided into three categories. First the study and description of complex systems (e.g., models of disease transmission or public-health nursing workflow). Second is the identification of opportunities to improve the efficiency and effectiveness of public health systems through innovative data collection or use of information. The third is the implementation and maintenance of processes and systems to achieve such improvements.

The informatics perspective can provide insights and opportunities to improve each of the seven ongoing elements of any public health surveillance system. Examples include the following:

- **Planning and system design.** Identifying information and sources that best address a surveillance goal; identifying who will access information, by what methods and under what conditions; and improving analysis or action by improving the surveillance system interaction with other information systems.
- **Data collection.** Identifying potential bias associated with different collection methods (e.g., telephone use or cultural attitudes toward technology); identifying appropriate use of structured data compared with free text, most useful vocabulary, and data standards; and recommending technologies (e.g., global positioning systems (GPS) and radio-frequency identification (RFID)) to support easier, faster, and higher-quality data entry in the field.
- **Data management and collation.** Identifying ways to share data across different computing/technology platforms; linking new data

with data from legacy systems; and identifying and remedying data-quality problems while ensuring data privacy and security.

- **Analysis.** Identifying appropriate statistical and visualization applications; generating algorithms to alert users to aberrations in health events; and leveraging high-performance computational resources for large data sets or complex analyses.
- **Interpretation.** Determining the usefulness of comparing information from one surveillance program with other data sets (related by time, place, person, or condition) for new perspectives and combining data of other sources and quality to provide a context for interpretation.
- **Dissemination.** Recommending appropriate displays of information for users and the best methods to reach the intended audience; facilitating information finding, and identifying benefits for data providers.
- **Application to public-health programs.** Assessing the utility of having surveillance data directly flows into information systems that support public-health interventions and information elements or standards that facilitate this linkage of surveillance to action and improving access to and use of information produced by a surveillance system for workers in the field and healthcare providers.

The evolving field of surveillance informatics presents both challenges and opportunities. The challenges include finding efficient and effective ways of combining multiple sources of complex data and information into meaningful and actionable knowledge (e.g., for situational awareness). As these challenges are met, opportunities will arise for faster, better, and lower cost surveillance and interpretation of health events and trends. The domain of public-health informatics designs and evaluates methods appropriate for this complex environment.

Vision

High-value data, information, and knowledge are exchanged in a secure and timely manner for use in public-health surveillance tools that are powerful and sophisticated but user-friendly to accomplish the work of surveillance and response.

Challenges

Realizing this vision for 21st-century public-health surveillance requires attention to technology and process and to the specific needs (i.e., requirements) of the public-health community. The technology challenges for public-health surveillance are daunting. Public-health surveillance systems manage data that are high volume, heterogeneous, and distributed widely. In addition, data-quality concerns also might exist, occurring in both new and older legacy systems. Data from many information systems might not be shared easily or exchanged, as that might not have been a requirement of the system at the time of its development. Changing these systems in an environment of limited funding and time presents barriers that are at least as substantial as those for technologic and scientific concerns. Impediments include laws and regulations that preserve different data collection and sharing rules, privacy and security concerns, and academic and economic disincentives to sharing and collaboration.

Technology

Technology that seems the most innovative often relies on adopting and leveraging technology standards. Systems must have the ability not only to talk and listen but also to understand each other. Unfortunately, adopting only certain standards is insufficient. Both semantic (vocabulary) and syntactic (sentence structure) standards must be implemented and tested to ensure a system's validity. Certain types of errors are associated with data manipulation. Even highly structured data-collection techniques do not completely eliminate data errors. For example, providing data elements that can be selected from a drop-down list cannot prevent the entry of a male who is documented as receiving a Papanicolaou test. However, structured data collection techniques can simplify minimizing or identifying many such data-quality problems.

The standardization process that facilitates computer-readable forms of data, by its very nature, risks losing the richness of information found within unstructured documents (i.e., clinicians' notes or field observations). Accessing and integrating both structured and unstructured data is a major focus in health informatics. As public-health surveillance systems collect more and more structured data directly from clinical information systems, this capacity for structured and unstructured data access is increasingly important.

Economic pressures on healthcare and public health are diminishing the practicality of conducting active surveillance techniques (e.g., using detailed patient interviews, manual chart reviews, or manual data entry). In addition, the need for speed in the face of rapid global pandemics and bioterrorism makes the often incomplete ascertainment from passive reporting processes a substantial challenge. The application of informatics science can help ensure that 21st century systems are as valid as current methods while providing improved efficiency.

Transitioning Systems

The process of change is difficult, and transforming information systems and workflows is no exception. Initial investments of time, human resources, and capital are difficult to assemble. Transitioning to interconnected (i.e., interoperable) public-health surveillance information systems from multiple, stand-alone siloed systems involves unique challenges. For example, setting up automated data-collection streams from electronic health record (EHR) data sources is different from manual data abstraction from healthcare records. Concerns related to data quality, data standardization, process automation, workflow design, and system validation all need to be addressed. The need to use new and legacy systems in parallel for a period must be considered and planned for, including the challenging process of transitioning users off legacy systems. Challenges and resistance to change must be balanced by clearly defined desirable goals and objectives associated with the new surveillance system and informed by strong, systematic informatics analyses.

Leadership and Workforce

Because 21st-century surveillance crosses the lines of complex social and political systems, it can no longer rely solely on creative innovation among field personnel but requires senior leaders who can see the opportunities and have the resources to address the challenges. Optimistic and strong leadership for public-health informatics is critical to augment public-health surveillance sufficiently in the 21st century. Public-health leaders have the responsibility of examining their workforce and making conscious decisions to augment it with public-health informatics expertise. Leadership also requires the ability to assemble the appropriate set of stakeholders when addressing 21st-century public-health surveillance challenges. New challenges will, for example, require input and guidance from legal and privacy subject-matter specialists. Leadership is needed to devote adequate funding to implement short-term improvements and long-term visions of informatics-augmented public-health surveillance. The leadership challenge is complex considering the need to integrate siloed systems, which are often governed and funded independently (i.e., human immunodeficiency virus (HIV), tuberculosis (TB), lead poisoning). All members of the team, from senior management to the end-user, need to be invested in creating the most usable, goal-oriented system possible, identifying the ways electronic information can be managed and used for the maximum benefit.

Opportunities

Numerous opportunities are available to facilitate public-health informatics' impact on public-health surveillance. An important opportunity is the increasing adoption of EHRs and health information exchange (HIE) systems. The demonstration of meaningful use of EHRs, as articulated in the Centers for Medicare & Medicaid Services (CMS) final rule includes three public-health requirements: electronic submission to public-health agencies of immunization registry data, reportable lab results data, and syndromic surveillance data.

Electronic Health Records

The EHR and HIE systems collate information about individual patients from different information systems (e.g., registration, clinical record, laboratory, and imaging) and through information exchange or aggregation from across different provider entities. The adoption of the systems is being incentivized and facilitated by the Health Information Technology for Economic and Clinical Health (HITECH) Act in the United States.

Enacted as part of the American Recovery and Reinvestment Act (ARRA) of 2009 (4), the HITECH act authorized Medicaid and Medicare financial incentives for providers to adopt and use EHRs and authorized funding for the Office of the National Coordinator for Health Information Technology (ONC) to encourage health IT adoption, aid in standard-setting, build workforce, and support state- and regional-level development of HIE.

Opportunities are available to facilitate public-health informatics' impact on public-health surveillance. For example, hospitals now have an economic incentive to electronically transmit reportable laboratory results to public-health agencies (electronic-laboratory reporting). This can improve the speed and ascertainment completeness of reporting and also can affect the surveillance workflow and workload. As the semantics and the syntax of such electronic reports become more widely adopted (a process also accelerated by the HITECH Act), such information can flow more easily between computer applications and systems (i.e., interoperability). This interoperability creates the potential to eliminate data-reentry into case management applications, which can improve efficiency while reducing resource requirements and data-entry errors. As clinicians and public-health workers increasingly work in electronic environments using the same types of interoperable data, the opportunity for bidirectional communication around cases or clusters of conditions also can increase.

Technological Advancement

Electronic real-time data regarding the environment (e.g., water-quality data from supervisory control and data acquisition systems (DAQ)) and remote sensing systems (RSS) (continuous and/or automated collection and transmission) combined with the global positioning system and geographic information system revolutions also facilitate the overlay of environmental and person-centric information by time and place. As public participation in submitting information into the world wide web (WWW) increases (often labeled Web 2.0 and accelerated by the widespread adoption of smartphones and other wireless devices), the possibility exists to tap into information directly supplied by large numbers of persons (crowdsourcing) or derived from near-real-time information-seeking behaviors. Several of these types of data have been used to derive signals of important health trends faster and more broadly than more traditional case reporting systems (e.g., outbreak detection or monitoring by syndromic surveillance systems).

Public-Health Informaticians

One of the most valuable resources to be tapped is the diverse population of public-health professionals (formally trained or not) who have already made informatics a priority in their work. These include staff at the CDC and other federal agencies; state and local health departments, members of the Public Health Data Standards Consortium (PHDSC) and informatics leaders in several public-health associations, workers from all walks of public-health life who attend Public Health Information Network (PHIN) meetings, university scholars of public-health informatics, and staffs of nonprofit organizations, such as the Public Health Informatics Institute (PHII). Representatives of these groups come together to harmonize an ongoing agenda for public-health informatics at the Joint Public Health Informatics Taskforce (JPHIT), a coordinating body of several associations. By educating leaders and peers, testing innovations, and disseminating lessons learned, these persons and agencies are improving public-health surveillance (and ultimately health outcomes) by reducing costs, bridging silos, and improving access to timely, quality information.

Summing Up

These opportunities also represent a crisis: the move from manual reporting from traditional data sources to automated data collection from novel data sources has suddenly begun in earnest, and public-health agencies will need to keep pace or risk gradually losing old systems of health event ascertainment and failing to achieve the benefits of new electronic reporting. Several steps can help public-health agencies. The ONC-specified standards to accept surveillance information from healthcare providers should be adopted but will require changes to established surveillance and other information management systems. Public-health agencies with limited informatics support might find it valuable to work with academic centers or other agencies to facilitate their transition to the use of more standardized electronic data. Using this form of data should, in time, enable them to reduce labor while increasing the sophistication of their analyses in both surveillance systems and response systems. Active collaboration on new information systems and data collection initiatives can reap substantial benefits.

To achieve the vision, certain key points must be addressed. Stand-alone systems should be considered only when no other options are available. Existing systems (including commercial off-the-shelf solutions) should be used or modified wherever possible and existing data streams should be leveraged for multiple purposes. In the search for change, the Pareto principle is instructive—that there exists a 20 percent change that has the ability to solve 80 percent of the problem. Rather than delaying work by striving to develop an ideal system, small, incremental steps should be considered rather than immediate wholesale changes. Although time-consuming, planning for evaluations of surveillance systems can affect both time and resource savings. Combining disparate sources and forms of information can provide a richer picture of disease burden than individual data streams. Whenever possible, support staff should be enabled to sharpen their skills in the fundamentals of public-health informatics using local resources, online training, or national conferences. Even with the best planning, problems will occur; detecting them as early as possible and addressing them immediately is essential. Active participation in EHR/HIE initiatives will help ensure that public health is represented in planning as the overall healthcare system continues to change and evolve.

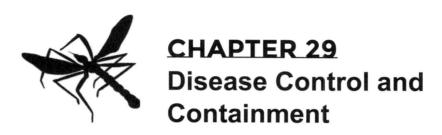

CHAPTER 29
Disease Control and Containment

Chapter Contents

Section 29.1

Standard Precautions for All Patient Care

This section includes text excerpted from "Standard Precautions," Centers for Disease Control and Prevention (CDC), June 18, 2018.

Standard precautions are the minimum infection prevention practices that apply to all patient care, regardless of suspected or confirmed infection status of the patient, in any setting where healthcare is delivered. These practices are designed to protect the dynamic host configuration protocol (DHCP) and prevent DHCP from spreading infections among patients. Standard Precautions include:

- Hand hygiene
- Use of personal protective equipment (e.g., gloves, masks, eyewear)
- Respiratory hygiene/cough etiquette
- Sharps safety (engineering and work practice controls)
- Safe injection practices (i.e., an aseptic technique for parenteral medications)
- Sterile instruments and devices
- Clean and disinfect environmental surfaces

Education and training are critical elements of standard precautions because they help DHCP make appropriate decisions and comply with recommended practices.

When standard precautions alone cannot prevent transmission, they are supplemented with transmission-based precautions. This second tier of infection prevention is used when patients have diseases that can spread through contact, droplet or airborne routes (e.g., skin contact, sneezing, coughing) and are always used in addition to standard precautions. Dental settings are not typically designed to carry out all of the transmission-based

Figure 29.1. Five Steps to Wash Your Hands the Right Way
*(Source: "Stop Germs! Wash Your Hands," Centers for Disease
Control and Prevention (CDC))*

precautions (e.g., airborne precautions for patients with suspected tuberculosis (TB), measles, or chickenpox) that are recommended for hospital and other ambulatory care settings. Patients, however, do not usually seek routine dental outpatient care when acutely ill with diseases requiring transmission-based precautions. Nonetheless, DHCP should develop and carry out systems for early detection and management of potentially infectious patients at initial points of entry to the dental setting. To the extent possible, this includes rescheduling nonurgent dental care until the patient is no longer infectious or referral to a dental setting with appropriate infection prevention precautions when urgent dental treatment is needed.

Hand Hygiene

Hand hygiene is the most important measure to prevent the spread of infections among patients and DHCP. Education and training programs should thoroughly address indications and techniques for hand hygiene practices before performing routine and oral surgical procedures.

For routine dental examinations and nonsurgical procedures, use water and plain soap (handwashing) or antimicrobial soap (hand antisepsis) specific for healthcare settings or use an alcohol-based hand rub. Although alcohol-based hand rubs are effective for hand hygiene in healthcare settings, soap and water should be used when hands are visibly soiled (e.g., dirt, blood, body fluids). For surgical procedures, perform a surgical hand scrub before putting on sterile surgeon's gloves. For all types of hand hygiene products, follow the product manufacturer's label for instructions.

Personal Protective Equipment

Personal protective equipment (PPE) refers to wearable equipment that is designed to protect DHCP from exposure to or contact with infectious agents. PPE that is appropriate for various types of patient interactions and effectively covers personal clothing and skin likely to be soiled with blood, saliva, or other potentially infectious materials (OPIM) should be available. These include gloves, face masks, protective eyewear, face shields, and protective clothing (e.g., reusable or disposable gown, jacket, laboratory coat). Examples of the appropriate use of PPE for adherence to standard precautions include:

- Use of gloves in situations involving possible contact with blood or body fluids, mucous membranes, nonintact skin (e.g., exposed skin that is chapped, abraded, or with dermatitis) or OPIM
- Use of protective clothing to protect skin and clothing during procedures or activities where contact with blood or body fluids is anticipated
- Use of mouth, nose, and eye protection during procedures that are likely to generate splashes or sprays of blood or other body fluids

The DHCP should be trained to select and put on appropriate PPE and remove PPE so that the chance for skin or clothing contamination is reduced. Hand hygiene is always the final step after removing and disposing of PPE. Training should also stress preventing further spread of contamination while wearing PPE by:

- Keeping hands away from the face
- Limiting surfaces touched
- Removing PPE when leaving work areas
- Performing hand hygiene

Respiratory Hygiene and Cough Etiquette

Respiratory hygiene and cough etiquette infection-prevention measures are designed to limit the transmission of respiratory pathogens spread by droplet or airborne routes. The strategies target primarily patients and individuals accompanying patients to the dental setting who might have undiagnosed transmissible respiratory infections, but also apply to anyone (including DHCP) with signs of illness including cough, congestion, runny nose, or increased production of respiratory secretions.

The DHCP should be educated on preventing the spread of respiratory pathogens when in contact with symptomatic persons. Respiratory hygiene/cough etiquette measures were added to standard precautions in 2007.

Sharps Safety

Most percutaneous injuries (e.g., needlestick, cut with a sharp object) among DHCP involve burs, needles, and other sharp instruments. Implementation of the Occupational Safety and Health Administration (OSHA) blood-borne pathogens standard has helped to protect DHCP from blood exposure and sharps injuries. However, sharps injuries continue to occur and pose the risk of blood-borne pathogen transmission to DHCP and patients. Most exposures in dentistry are preventable; therefore, each dental practice should have policies and procedures available addressing sharps safety. DHCP should be aware of the risk of injury whenever sharps are exposed. When using or working around sharp devices, DHCP should take precautions while using sharps, during the cleanup, and during disposal.

Engineering and work practice controls are the primary methods to reduce exposures to blood and OPIM from sharp instruments and needles. Whenever possible, engineering controls should be used as the primary method to reduce exposures to blood-borne pathogens. Engineering controls remove or isolate a hazard in the workplace and are frequently technology-based (e.g., self-sheathing anesthetic needles, safety scalpels, and needleless intravenous (IV) ports). Employers should involve those DHCP who are directly responsible for patient care (e.g., dentists, hygienists, dental assistants) in identifying, evaluating and selecting devices with engineered safety features at least annually and as they become available. Other examples of engineering controls include sharps containers and needle recapping devices.

When engineering controls are not available or appropriate, work-practice controls should be used. Work-practice controls are behavior-based and are intended to reduce the risk of blood exposure by changing the way

DHCP performs tasks, such as using a one-handed scoop technique for recapping needles between uses and before disposal. Other work-practice controls include not bending or breaking needles before disposal, not passing a syringe with an unsheathed needle by hand, removing burs before disassembling the handpiece from the dental unit, and using instruments in place of fingers for tissue retraction or palpation during suturing and administration of anesthesia.

All used disposable syringes and needles, scalpel blades, and other sharp items should be placed in appropriate puncture-resistant containers located close to the area where they are used. Sharps containers should be disposed of according to state and local regulated medical waste rules.

Safe Injection Practices

Safe injection practices are intended to prevent transmission of infectious diseases between one patient and another, or between a patient and DHCP during preparation and administration of parenteral (e.g., IV or intramuscular injection) medications. Safe injection practices are a set of measures DHCP should follow to perform injections in the safest possible manner for the protection of patients. DHCP most frequently handles parenteral medications when administering local anesthesia, during which needles and cartridges containing local anesthetics are used for one patient only and the dental cartridge syringe is cleaned and heat sterilized between patients. Other safe practices described here primarily apply to the use of parenteral medications combined with fluid infusion systems, such as for patients undergoing conscious sedation.

Unsafe practices that have led to patient harm include:

- Use of a single syringe—with or without the same needle—to administer medication to multiple patients
- Reinsertion of a used syringe—with or without the same needle—into a medication vial or solution container (e.g., saline bag) to obtain additional medication for a single patient and then using that vial or solution container for subsequent patients
- Preparation of medications in close proximity to contaminated supplies or equipment

Because of reports of transmission of infectious diseases by inappropriate handling of injectable medications, the Centers for Disease Control and Prevention (CDC) now considers safe injection practices to be a formal element of standard precautions.

Sterilization and Disinfection of Patient-Care Items and Devices

Instrument processing requires multiple steps using specialized equipment. Each dental practice should have policies and procedures in place for containing, transporting, and handling instruments and equipment that may be contaminated with blood or body fluids. Manufacturer's instructions for reprocessing reusable dental instruments and equipment should be readily available—ideally in or near the reprocessing area. Most single-use devices are labeled by the manufacturer for only a single-use and do not have reprocessing instructions. Use single-use devices for one patient only and dispose of appropriately.

Cleaning, disinfection, and sterilization of dental equipment should be assigned to DHCP with training in the required reprocessing steps to ensure reprocessing results in a device that can be safely used for patient care. Training should also include the appropriate use of PPE necessary for the safe handling of contaminated equipment.

Patient-care items (e.g., dental instruments, devices, and equipment) are categorized as critical, semicritical, or noncritical, depending on the potential risk for infection associated with their intended use.

- **Critical items,** such as surgical instruments and periodontal scalers, are those used to penetrate soft tissue or bone. They have the greatest risk of transmitting infection and should always be sterilized using heat.
- **Semicritical items** (e.g., mouth mirrors, amalgam condensers, reusable dental impression trays) are those that come in contact with mucous membranes or nonintact skin (e.g., exposed skin that is chapped, abraded, or has dermatitis). These items have a lower risk of transmission. Because the majority of semicritical items in dentistry are heat-tolerant, they should also be sterilized using heat.

If a semicritical item is heat-sensitive, DHCP should replace it with a heat-tolerant or disposable alternative. If none are available, it should, at a minimum, be processed using high-level disinfection.

Note: Dental handpieces and associated attachments, including low-speed motors and reusable prophylaxis angles, should always be heat sterilized between patients and not high-level or surface disinfected. Although these devices are considered semicritical, studies have shown that their internal surfaces can become contaminated with patient materials during use. If these devices are not properly cleaned and heat sterilized, the next patient may be exposed to potentially infectious materials.

Digital radiography sensors are also considered semi-critical and should be protected with a U.S. Food and Drug Administration (FDA)-cleared barrier to reduce contamination during use, followed by cleaning and heat-sterilization or high-level disinfection between patients. If the item cannot tolerate these procedures then, at a minimum, protect with an FDA-cleared barrier. In addition, clean and disinfect with a U.S. Environmental Protection Agency (EPA)-registered hospital disinfectant with intermediate-level (i.e., tuberculocidal claim) activity between patients. Because these items vary by manufacturer and their ability to be sterilized or high-level disinfected also vary, refer to manufacturer instructions for reprocessing.

Noncritical patient-care items (e.g., radiograph head/cone, blood pressure cuff, facebow) are those that only contact intact skin. These items pose the least risk of transmission of infection. In the majority of cases, cleaning, or if visibly soiled, cleaning followed by disinfection with an EPA-registered hospital disinfectant is adequate. Protecting these surfaces with disposable barriers might be a preferred alternative.

Cleaning to remove debris and organic contamination from instruments should always occur before disinfection or sterilization. If blood, saliva, and other contamination are not removed, these materials can shield microorganisms and potentially compromise the disinfection or sterilization process. Automated cleaning equipment (e.g., ultrasonic cleaner, washer-disinfector) should be used to remove debris to improve cleaning effectiveness and decrease worker exposure to blood. After cleaning, dried instruments should be inspected, wrapped, packaged, or placed into container systems before heat sterilization. Packages should be labeled to show the sterilizer used, the cycle or load number, the date of sterilization, and, if applicable, the expiration date. This information can help in retrieving processed items in the event of an instrument processing/sterilization failure.

The ability of a sterilizer to reach conditions necessary to achieve sterilization should be monitored using a combination of biological, mechanical, and chemical indicators. Biological indicators, or spore tests, are the most accepted method for monitoring the sterilization process because they assess the sterilization process directly by killing known highly resistant microorganisms (e.g., Geobacillus or Bacillus species). A spore test should be used at least weekly to monitor sterilizers. However, because spore tests are only performed periodically (e.g., once a week, once a day) and the results are usually not obtained immediately, mechanical and chemical monitoring should also be performed.

Mechanical and chemical indicators do not guarantee sterilization; however, they help detect procedural errors and equipment malfunctions. Mechanical monitoring involves checking the sterilizer gauges, computer displays, or printouts; and documenting the sterilization pressure, temperature, and exposure time in your sterilization records. Since these parameters can be observed during the sterilization cycle, this might be the first indication of a problem.

Chemical monitoring uses sensitive chemicals that change color when exposed to high temperatures or combinations of time and temperature. Examples include chemical indicator tapes, strips or tabs, and special markings on packaging materials. Chemical monitoring results are obtained immediately following the sterilization cycle, and therefore, can provide more timely information about the sterilization cycle than a spore test. A chemical indicator should be used inside every package to verify that the sterilizing agent (e.g., steam) has penetrated the package and reached the instruments inside. If the internal chemical indicator is not visible from the outside of the package, an external indicator should also be used. External indicators can be inspected immediately when removing packages from the sterilizer. If the appropriate color change did not occur, do not use the instruments. Chemical indicators also help to differentiate between processed and unprocessed items, eliminating the possibility of using instruments that have not been sterilized.

Note: A single-parameter internal chemical indicator provides information regarding only one sterilization parameter (e.g., time or temperature). Multiparameter internal chemical indicators are designed to react to ≥ 2 parameters (e.g., time and temperature; or time, temperature, and the presence of steam) and can provide a more reliable indication that sterilization conditions have been met.

Sterilization monitoring (e.g., biological, mechanical, chemical monitoring) and equipment maintenance records are an important component of a dental infection prevention program. Maintaining accurate records ensures cycle parameters have been met and establishes accountability. In addition, if there is a problem with a sterilizer (e.g., unchanged chemical indicator, positive spore test), documentation helps to determine if an instrument recall is necessary.

Ideally, sterile instruments and supplies should be stored in covered or closed cabinets. Wrapped packages of sterilized instruments should be inspected before opening and use to ensure the packaging material has not been compromised (e.g., wet, torn, punctured) during storage. The contents of any compromised packs should be reprocessed (i.e., cleaned, packaged, and heat-sterilized again) before use on a patient.

Environmental Infection Prevention and Control

Policies and procedures for routine cleaning and disinfection of environmental surfaces should be included as part of the infection prevention plan. Cleaning removes large numbers of microorganisms from surfaces and should always precede disinfection. Disinfection is generally a less-lethal process of microbial inactivation (compared with sterilization) that eliminates virtually all recognized pathogenic microorganisms but not necessarily all microbial forms (e.g., bacterial spores).

The emphasis for cleaning and disinfection should be placed on surfaces that are most likely to become contaminated with pathogens, including clinical contact surfaces (e.g., frequently touched surfaces, such as light handles, bracket trays, switches on dental units, computer equipment) in the patient-care area. When these surfaces are touched, microorganisms can be transferred to other surfaces, instruments or to the nose, mouth, or eyes of DHCP or patients. Although hand hygiene is the key to minimizing the spread of microorganisms, clinical contact surfaces should be barrier protected or cleaned and disinfected between patients. EPA-registered hospital disinfectants or detergents/disinfectants with label claims for use in healthcare settings should be used for disinfection. Disinfectant products should not be used as cleaners unless the label indicates the product is suitable for such use. DHCP should follow manufacturer recommendations for use of products selected for cleaning and disinfection (e.g., amount, dilution, contact time, safe use, and disposal). Facility policies and procedures should also address prompt and appropriate cleaning and decontamination of spills of blood or other potentially infectious materials. Housekeeping surfaces, (e.g., floors, walls, sinks) carry less risk of disease transmission than clinical contact surfaces and can be cleaned with soap and water or cleaned and disinfected if visibly contaminated with blood.

Section 29.2

Transmission-Based Precautions

This section includes text excerpted from
"Transmission-Based Precautions," Centers for
Disease Control and Prevention (CDC), January 7,
2016. Reviewed January 2020.

Transmission-based precautions are the second tier of basic infection control and are to be used in addition to Standard Precautions for patients who may be infected or colonized with certain infectious agents for which additional precautions are needed to prevent infection transmission.

Contact Precautions

Contact precautions should be used for patients with known or suspected infections that represent an increased risk for contact transmission.

- **Ensure appropriate patient placement** in a single patient space or room if available in acute care hospitals. In long-term and other residential settings, make room placement decisions balancing risks to other patients. In ambulatory settings, place patients requiring contact precautions in an exam room or cubicle as soon as possible.
- **Use personal protective equipment (PPE) appropriately,** including gloves and gowns. Wear a gown and gloves for all interactions that may involve contact with the patient or the patient's environment. Donning PPE upon room entry and properly discarding before exiting the patient room is done to contain pathogens.
- **Limit transport and movement of patients** outside of the room to medically-necessary purposes. When transport or movement is necessary, cover or contain the infected or colonized areas of the patient's body. Remove and dispose of contaminated PPE and perform hand hygiene prior to transporting patients on contact precautions. Do not clean PPE to handle the patient at the transport location.
- **Use disposable or dedicated patient-care equipment** (e.g., blood pressure cuffs). If common use of equipment for multiple patients is unavoidable, clean and disinfect such equipment before use on another patient.
- **Prioritize cleaning and disinfection of the rooms** of patients on contact precautions ensuring rooms are frequently cleaned and disinfected (e.g., at least daily or prior to use by another patient if outpatient setting) focusing on frequently-touched surfaces and equipment in the immediate vicinity of the patient.

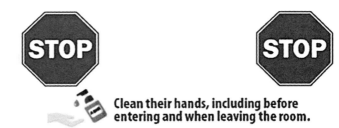

Clean their hands, including before
entering and when leaving the room.

PROVIDERS AND STAFF MUST ALSO:

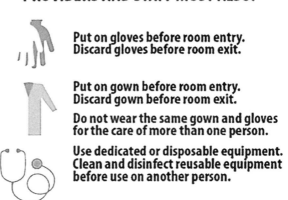

Put on gloves before room entry.
Discard gloves before room exit.

Put on gown before room entry.
Discard gown before room exit.

Do not wear the same gown and gloves
for the care of more than one person.

Use dedicated or disposable equipment.
Clean and disinfect reusable equipment
before use on another person.

Figure 29.2. Contact Precautions That Everyone
Should Follow

Droplet Precautions

Use droplet precautions for patients known or suspected to be infected
with pathogens transmitted by respiratory droplets that are generated by a
patient who is coughing, sneezing, or talking.

- **Source control:** put a mask on the patient.
- **Ensure appropriate patient placement in a single room if possible.**
  In acute care hospitals, if single rooms are not available, utilize the
  recommendations for alternative patient placement considerations in
  the Guideline for Isolation Precautions. In long-term care and other
  residential settings, make decisions regarding patient placement on a
  case-by-case basis considering infection risks to other patients in the
  room and available alternatives. In ambulatory settings, place patients
  who require droplet precautions in an exam room or cubicle as soon

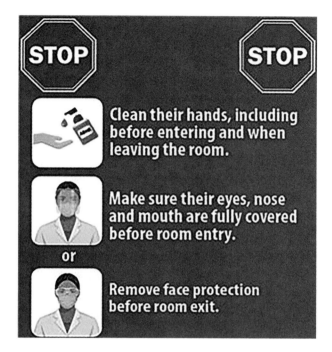

Figure 29.3. Droplet Precautions That Everyone
Should Follow

as possible and instruct patients to follow respiratory hygiene/cough
etiquette recommendations.

- **Use personal protective equipment (PPE) appropriately.** Don
mask upon entry into the patient room or patient space.
- **Limit transport and movement of patients** outside of the room to
medically-necessary purposes. If transport or movement outside of
the room is necessary, instruct the patient to wear a mask and follow
respiratory hygiene/cough etiquette.

Air-Borne Precautions

Use Air-borne precautions for patients known or suspected to be infected
with pathogens transmitted by the airborne route (e.g., tuberculosis,
measles, chickenpox, disseminated herpes zoster).

- **Source control:** put a mask on the patient.

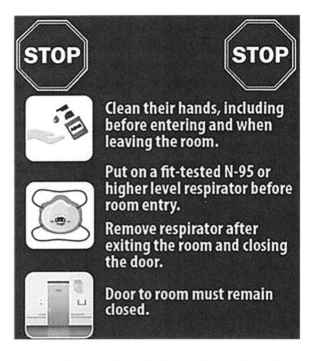

Figure 29.4. Air-Borne Precautions That
Everyone Should Follow

- **Ensure appropriate patient placement in an air-borne infection isolation room (AIIR)** constructed according to the *Guideline for Isolation Precautions*. In settings where Airborne Precautions cannot be implemented due to limited engineering resources, masking the patient and placing the patient in a private room with the door closed will reduce the likelihood of air-borne transmission until the patient is either transferred to a facility with an AIIR or returned home.
- **Restrict susceptible healthcare personnel from entering the room** of patients known or suspected to have measles, chickenpox, disseminated zoster, or smallpox if other immune healthcare personnel are available.
- **Use personal protective equipment (PPE)** appropriately, including a fit-tested NIOSH-approved N95 or higher level respirator for healthcare personnel.

- **Limit transport and movement of patients** outside of the room to medically-necessary purposes. If transport or movement outside an AIIR is necessary, instruct patients to wear a surgical mask, if possible, and observe respiratory hygiene/cough etiquette. Healthcare personnel transporting patients who are on air-borne precautions do not need to wear a mask or respirator during transport if the patient is wearing a mask and infectious skin lesions are covered.
- **Immunize susceptible persons as soon as possible following unprotected contact** with vaccine-preventable infections (e.g., measles, varicella or smallpox).

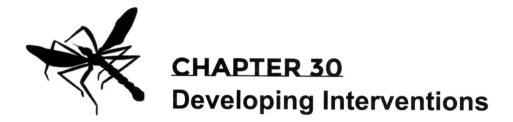

CHAPTER 30
Developing Interventions

Guiding Principles for Interventions

Public-health officials who have the responsibility and legal authority for making decisions about interventions should consider certain key principles: selecting the appropriate intervention, facilitating the implementation of the intervention, and assessing the effectiveness of the intervention.

During Epidemiologic-Field Investigations of Acute Public-Health Problems

- As soon as an acute public-health problem is detected, public-health responsibility and societal expectations exist to intervene as soon as possible to minimize preventable morbidity and mortality.
- Public-health interventions should be scientifically driven on the basis of established facts and data, current investigation findings, and knowledge from previous investigations and studies. Although salient sociopolitical forces (e.g., public fear or political outcry) might create pressures for rapid public-health interventions, the interventions must be based on evidence. However, adopting certain intervention components might be necessary to make them more acceptable and responsive to the needs of

This chapter includes text excerpted from "Developing Interventions," Centers for Disease Control and Prevention (CDC), December 13, 2018.

the affected community, potentially affected persons, elected officials, and the media.

- For any given problem, the type(s) and the number of interventions to be implemented will vary, depending on the nature of the acute problem, including its cause, mode of spread, and other factors.
- The type(s) and the number of interventions used might evolve as a function of incremental gains in information developed during the investigation.
- Most public-health interventions demand—and even might be potentiated by—open, two-way communication between involved government agencies and the public.

Determinants for Employing Interventions

Field epidemiologists must consider multiple crucial determinants during the course of making a decision about whether a scientifically rational basis exists for employing an intervention and when selecting one or more specific interventions optimally matched to the public-health problem. These determinants, which might be both interrelated and not mutually exclusive, encompass a constellation of factors (e.g., specific knowledge of causative etiologic agent(s) and of reservoirs or mode(s) of acquisition or spread) and recognition of other causal determinants as reflected, in part, by assessing the investigation's ability to address the causation criteria. This chapter examines three highly interrelated key determinants: severity of the problem, levels of certainty about key epidemiologic factors, and causation criteria. Additionally, it considers the sociopolitical context and its possible role in determining interventions.

The Severity of the Problem

The severity of a specific problem is a principal determinant of the urgency and course of a field investigation and of any early intervention. The greater the severity, the sooner a public-health intervention is expected. The primary determinants of severity are the consequences of the event and the probability of the event occurring. Consequences to consider include the most common symptoms and syndrome caused, duration of illness, complications including hospitalization and case-fatality rates, need for treatment, and economic impact. The consequences, even more than the probability, tend to drive the perception of the importance of intervening.

One example is botulism, which is a low-probability but high-consequence event. Virtually all the U.S. cases trigger extensive epidemiologic investigations because identifying the food or beverage source can prevent additional intoxications, and identifying exposed or ill persons enables the administration of life-saving antitoxin. Similarly, clusters of a healthcare-associated infection—especially among postsurgical or immunocompromised patients—are often investigated because of the potential for serious complications and greatly prolonged hospitalization, the possibility of iatrogenic illness as an avoidable medical event, and the immediate need to resolve questions about the safety of continuing to admit patients to the hospital

Levels of Certainty about Agents, Sources, and Modes of Spread

In addition to severity, a spectrum of other factors influences the aggressiveness, extent, and scientific rigor of an epidemiologic field investigation. In the prototypic investigation, control measures are formulated only after other steps have been implemented. In practice, however, control measures might be appropriate or warranted at any step in the sequence. For most outbreaks of acute disease, the scope of an investigation is dictated by the levels of certainty about:

- The etiology of the problem (e.g., the specific pathogen or toxic agent)
- The source or mode of spread (e.g., waterborne, airborne, or vectorborne)
- When the problem is identified initially, the levels of certainty about the etiology, source, and mode of spread can range from known to unknown.

These basic dichotomies are illustrated in Figure 30.1 by four examples that represent the extremes. In certain situations, control measures follow policy or practice guidelines; in others, interventions are appropriate only

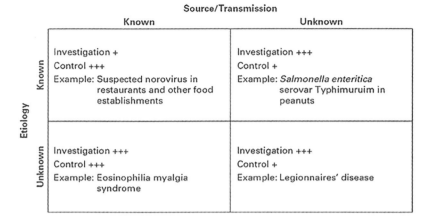

Figure 30.1. Basic Dichotomies

Relative emphasis of investigative and control efforts (intervention options) in disease outbreaks as influenced by levels of certainty about etiology and source or mode of transmission. Investigation means the extent of the investigation; control means the basis for rapid implementation of control or intervention measures at the time the problem is initially identified. Plus signs indicate the level of response indicated, ranging from + (low) to +++ (high).

after exhaustive epidemiologic investigation. Preliminary control measures often can start on the basis of limited initial information and then be modified as investigations proceed.

For example, a suspected norovirus outbreak associated with a restaurant or food preparation establishment might warrant a spectrum of interventions, including:

- Promptly excluding food service employees symptomatic with vomiting or diarrhea
- Temporarily closing the restaurant
- Replacing all food items
- Sanitizing all surfaces and equipment
- Monitoring food-handling practices until more specific information are available from the epidemiologic investigation
- Educating food handlers about norovirus containment
- Providing training and education about health codes for restaurant owners

In such an instance, the response will be based on knowledge of possible continuing sources of norovirus or some other enteric pathogen, exposure in a restaurant, and removal of those sources. Although this sort of prompt and appropriate response addresses the possibility of continued transmission on the basis of known agent-specific facts and experience, epidemiologists sometimes need to extend the investigation, depending on the circumstances and needs (e.g., when a trace-back is indicated to identify a continuing primary source for a restaurant-associated outbreak, such as shellfish or lettuce that was contaminated before being harvested)

More commonly, a degree of uncertainty exists about the etiology or sources and the mode of spread. For most gastrointestinal outbreaks, selecting control measures depends on knowing whether transmission has resulted from the person-to-person, foodborne, or waterborne spread and, if either of the two latter modes, on identifying the source. For example, an outbreak of *Salmonella enterica* serovar Typhimurium across multiple states during 2008 required extensive multipronged epidemiologic field investigations and analytic (case-control) studies before peanut butter and peanut butter—containing products were identified as the transmission vehicles. The converse situation—involving a presumed source but unknown etiology—is illustrated by the nationwide outbreak of eosinophilia-myalgia syndrome (EMS) in the United States in 1989. During that outbreak, L-tryptophan, a nonprescription dietary supplement, initially was implicated as the source of the exposure, and contaminants in specific brands were eventually implicated through laboratory analysis. In the interim, epidemiologists issued recommendations preventing further exposures and cases. Finally, as illustrated by the Legionnaires' disease outbreak in 1976, an extensive field investigation can fail to identify the cause, the source, and mode of spread in time to control the acute problem but still can enable advances in knowledge that ultimately lead to preventive measures.

Causation and the Field Investigation

In his seminal article, The *Environment and Disease: Association or Causation?* on criteria for assessing causal associations in epidemiology, British epidemiologist and statistician Austin Bradford Hill concluded with a call for basing action on weighing the strength of the epidemiologic evidence against the severity of the consequences of delaying action and of taking premature action. These same concerns commonly confront epidemiologists during field investigations. The criteria specified by Hill—temporality, the strength of association, biological gradient, consistency, plausibility, coherence, experiment, and analogy—provide a useful framework for assessing the strength of epidemiologic evidence developed during a field investigation. Assessing causality at each step in an investigation is important not only for assessing the strength of evidence developed up to that point but also in helping to identify what evidence is missing or requires further attention and for planning additional approaches (e.g., data gathering and analysis) essential for supporting decisions regarding interventions.

Such criteria as strength of association, dose-response, and temporality can increase confidence in initiating actions. Moreover, at any step in the investigation, evidence that satisfies a specific criterion might be unavailable. Nonetheless, field investigators should try to collect data for examining causality by using as many criteria as is feasible. Although a single criterion might not be convincing in a given context or fully accepted on the basis of the interpreter's viewpoint, a combination of well-assessed criteria pointing to a common exposure can strengthen confidence and facilitate support for directed interventions.

Epidemiology—in particular, field epidemiology—is a relatively young scientific discipline in the medical world, acquiring academic, and then public, acceptance only gradually over the past five to six decades. Among certain sectors—for example, the legal profession, private enterprise, and even regulatory agencies—acceptance of epidemiologic conclusions have been slower, in part because of the nature of causation in epidemiology: epidemiologic evidence establishes associations, not hard, irrefutable proof. Meanwhile, epidemiologic evidence often is the first basis for implicating a causative agent or mode of spread before the results of more in-depth and lengthier scientific investigations become available to support decision-making about interventions. Moreover, and lamentably, epidemiologic evidence that compels epidemiologists to take prompt action might not readily convince others whose cooperation is necessary for initiating action. For example, years elapsed after field studies had clearly implicated antecedent aspirin use as a risk factor for Reye syndrome (RS) before industry and the U.S. Food and Drug Administration (FDA) accepted the association and issued warnings to that effect. The story of toxic shock syndrome further illustrates the reluctance of some to accept epidemiologic evidence in the face of an acute public health problem on the scale of a nationwide epidemic. These examples underscore the practical challenges in balancing the need to assess causality through the process of scientific inquiry with the potentially conflicting need to intervene quickly to protect the public's health.

During an outbreak, multiple groups of persons might be exposed, affected, or involved in some respects. Because of differences in knowledge, beliefs, and perceived impact of the outbreak, each group might draw different conclusions about causality from the same information. For example, in a suspected restaurant-associated foodborne illness outbreak, restaurant patrons, the public, owners and management, media, attorneys, and public health officials are each likely to have a different threshold for judging the degree of association between eating food from the restaurant and illness. In this situation, the public health field epidemiologist's concerns might focus especially on the criteria of strength of association and dose-response effect between exposure to a certain food item and illness, whereas a restaurant patron's primary concern is simply plausibility. In contrast, attorneys— who either are representing plaintiff-patrons who putatively acquired their illnesses as a result of restaurant exposure or are defending a restaurant epidemiologically associated with a foodborne illness epidemic—will approach such a problem by using a legal framework for causation, which varies from epidemiologic causation. In civil cases, the plaintiff's attorney, in particular, must meet a preponderance-of-evidence standard of proof, which means that the factfinder (i.e., the judge or jury) must believe that the plaintiff's version of events is more probable than not for the plaintiff to prevail; this standard also has been analogized to a probability of 0.51 or greater

Sociopolitical Context

Field investigations often occur in the public limelight, whether intentionally or not. When a problem is perceived as severe (e.g., a death has occurred) and possibly ongoing, the public might demand information and action. In addition, when interest is intense among politicians, including executive branch leaders (e.g., governors and mayors), such leaders might wish to be visible and demonstrate their interest in protecting the public. For example, a school child's death from meningitis might lead to political pressure to close the school. A hospital patient's death from Legionnaires' disease might lead to political pressure to consider closing the hospital.

As part of the deliberation about when and how to intervene, effective and continuous communication with all concerned entities is essential. These entities need to be aware of the possibilities, the ongoing risks (if any), and how best to address them given the level of information available. An essential component of any intervention is effective communication with political leaders and the public. Such communication will assist in enabling the use of scientific factors as the determinants for selecting the intervention(s) to protect the public against disease and should help minimize the potential for unnecessary, costly, and misleading interventions. Nonetheless, the evidence-based perspective might not be the only one eventually considered in the choice of interventions. During the 2014 to 2015 Ebola virus disease (EVD) epidemic in parts of West Africa, many U.S. jurisdictions, often for political reasons, implemented strict quarantine and health monitoring for persons who had traveled to an affected country, despite these persons having no history of exposure to anyone with Ebola virus infection.

Intervention Options

Interventions for preventing and controlling public-health problems — including infectious disease outbreaks and noninfectious diseases, injuries, and disabilities — can be approached through different classification schemes. Examples of these approaches include:

- Interventions targeting specific aspects of the relation between the host, environment, and disease-or injury-causing agent
- Primary, secondary, and tertiary prevention options
- Haddon's injury prevention model, which keys on intervention strategies at the prevent, event, and postevent phases

In addition to the specific nature of the etiologic agent, decision-makers might need to consider other factors, including:

- The agent's reservoir or source
- The mode of spread or transmission
- Host-related risk factors
- Environmental and other mediating factors
- A priori evidence of the effectiveness of the intervention
- Operational and logistical feasibility
- Legal authority necessary to support implementing the measure

In this chapter, the model used to systematically identify and characterize the spectrum of intervention options for outbreaks and other acute health threats focus on two basic biological and environmental dimensions:

- Interventions that can be directed at the source(s) of most infectious and other disease-causing agents
- Interventions that can be directed at persons susceptible to such agents

The first category—interventions directed at the source—includes measures that would eliminate the disease-causing agent's presence as a risk factor for susceptible populations (e.g., seizing and destroying contaminated foods or temporarily barring an infected person from preparing or serving food). Both categories encompass some of the same options and thus are not completely mutually exclusive. For example, during the 2016 to 2017 Zika virus infection outbreak, men returning from travel to epidemic areas were advised to use condoms when having sex with susceptible pregnant or potentially pregnant women, as well as for pregnant or potentially pregnant susceptible women to use condoms with any male partner who might have been exposed to the virus to decrease the women's risk for exposure.

During the EVD epidemic in 2014 to 2015, public-health officials in the United States used a combination of intervention measures directed at persons in whom EVD was diagnosed (isolation), at their close contacts (active monitoring, quarantine, or restrictions on travel), at those providing healthcare to them (training in the correct use of special protective gear and active monitoring), and at those arriving from selected countries (screening or active monitoring).

Selection from measures listed below and other alternatives might be considered at any stage of a field investigation. During the early stages, interventions based on established guidelines for disease control can be applied. For example, as indicated earlier in this chapter, excluding symptomatic employees and removing all possible existing sources of an enteric pathogen, such as norovirus from a food preparation facility can be done regardless of the actual source of the outbreak. If at a subsequent point, the nature of the risk for infection is more sharply defined, then additional, tailored corrective measures can be directed at the source and/or mode of spread.

Selected Public Health Intervention Options for Outbreaks and Other Acute Health Threats

These interventions are grouped according to those that can be directed at the source(s) of most infectious and other disease-causing agents and those that can be directed at persons susceptible to such agents.

Interventions directed at the source:

- Treat infected or affected persons and animals.
- Isolate infected persons, including cohorts, if needed.
- Use barrier methods (e.g., face masks, condoms).
- Monitor exposed persons for signs of illness.
- Quarantine contaminated sites or sources.
- Implement cordon sanitaire, close public places, and prevent gatherings to freeze or limit movement and minimize the likelihood of mixing groups by exposure or infection status.
- Use contact tracing, partner notification, and treatment.
- Seize or destroy contaminated food, property, animals, or other sources.
- Clean and disinfect contaminated surfaces and other environmental repositories.
- Modify the affected environment through vector control.
- Modify the affected environment by restricting or controlling dangerous drugs or contaminants.

- Modify behavior to reduce risks to self or others.
- Deter through civil suits or criminal prosecution.

Interventions directed at susceptible persons or animals:
- Administer postexposure prophylaxis.
- Immunize or vaccinate in advance.
- Exclude unvaccinated persons from cohorts of vaccinated persons.
- Use barrier methods (e.g., face masks, condoms).
- Implement cordon sanitaire, close public places, and prevent gatherings to freeze or limit movement and minimize the likelihood of mixing groups by exposure or infection status.
- Modify behavior to reduce risks to self or others.
- Use shelter-in-place (i.e., reverse quarantine).
- Issue press releases, health alerts, and other information about risk reduction.

Challenges and Evolving Approaches in Interventions

Although this chapter has explored a science-based foundation for identifying, selecting, and implementing public-health interventions, field investigators also must contend with a spectrum of new and evolving concerns that challenge decision-making about interventions. This chapter briefly addresses three such concerns.

The dilemma public-health officials face in selecting and implementing interventions when science-based information might be limited regarding their appropriateness or effectiveness. For certain infectious diseases and other public-health problems, recent efforts to plan for selecting and using different interventions have encountered controversy or other challenges because of limitations in the availability of science-based information about their benefits versus their societal costs. For example, during deliberations about what measures might be most effective for responding to an influenza A (H5N1) pandemic, many persons have questioned whether sufficient science-based evidence exists to support the widespread use of some relatively draconian social distancing measures.

The paramount importance of increasing an affected community's understanding of the nature of the public health problem and the rationale for the recommended intervention(s). An influential trend in selecting and implementing interventions is the increasing role of community involvement. For example, for the past several decades, public health agencies have had to innovatively modify their responses to such problems as outbreaks of multidrug-resistant tuberculosis, clusters of cases of human immunodeficiency virus (HIV) infection, resurgent and antibiotic-resistant sexually transmitted diseases (STDs), and meningococcal disease among men who have sex with men. For some public-health problems, traditional methods for investigation and contact evaluation have been supplanted by newer social network approaches—interventions that require increased involvement of community representatives. In such settings, community support is essential for the success of the investigation and longer-term prevention and control measures; conversely, failure to obtain community trust and support can disable or constrain the impact of an investigation. This can be especially true when problems disproportionately affect groups who are marginalized and who otherwise might be initially reluctant to work with public health officials. The need for obtaining community trust also implicates the important role of health and risk communications, as well as the importance of explaining to the community both the rationale for and potential limitations of an intervention (e.g., why the intervention might not work or be 100% effective). Community representatives can also help disseminate information to persons most at risk through blogs, social media, mobile phone applications, or other nontraditional communication channels. The increasing role of community involvement in and support for public-health interventions applies not only to infectious diseases but also to preventing and controlling environmental hazards, including substance abuse, injuries, and other noninfectious disease problems.

The sometimes complex nature of making a decision about when to terminate an acute intervention or how to institutionalize or to sustain it for a longer period. This final challenge encompasses the need to assess the effectiveness of each intervention and make decisions about whether and when to terminate or sustain it. At the earliest possible moment, data being generated by the epidemiologic investigation should be used to assess the effectiveness of each intervention. Such information also guides decision-making regarding modification or termination of already implemented interventions and the selection and the use of additional or new measures. A decision to leave an intervention in place long term or permanently might be made in situations where the public-health risk cannot be eliminated and remains an ongoing threat (e.g., ban on use of lead-based paint or sustaining a recommendation to vaccinate men who have sex with men against meningococcal disease after an outbreak is over because of sustained higher risk.

Summing Up

Epidemiologic field investigations are usually initiated in response to epidemics or the occurrence of other acute diseases, injury, or environmental-health problems. Under such circumstances, the primary objective of the field investigation is to use the scientific principles of epidemiology to determine a rational and appropriate response for ending or controlling the problem. Key factors that influence decisions about the timing and choice of public-health interventions include a carefully crafted balance among:

- The severity of the problem
- The levels of scientific certainty of the findings
- The extent to which causal criteria have been established
- The intervention's operational and logistical feasibility
- The public and political perceptions of what is the best course of action
- Legal considerations

This chapter has examined essential factors epidemiologists and other public-health officials must consider when making decisions about selecting and implementing public-health interventions during epidemiologic-field investigations. Taking these factors into account, the following actions should be reconsidered at each progressive stage of the field investigation:

- Define the scope of the public health problem with available information by assessing:
  - The severity of the illness, injury, or environmental hazard
  - The nature of the suspected etiologic agent

- The number of possible susceptible persons and the extent of their exposure
- Possible reasons for the outbreak
- Determine whether possible reasons for the outbreak might be ongoing, and, for all potentially ongoing reasons and exposures for which intervention(s) might be offered, consider what empiric interventions can be used to reduce or eliminate any ongoing risk for exposure or illness.
- For each potential intervention, consider the costs and benefits of implementing the intervention at that stage of the investigation in the absence of additional information.
- Implement all reasonable empiric interventions.
- Communicate the rationale for implementing or not implementing interventions at any point to persons within the community who have been exposed or affected, as well as others who might need to know.
- Continuously assess the effectiveness of and modify the interventions as new investigation information becomes available.

Adherence to these and other steps during epidemiologic-field investigations can be integral to helping attain and optimize a scientifically rational basis for selecting and implementing public-health interventions for controlling or terminating a problem.

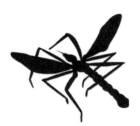

CHAPTER 31
Pharmacological Interventions: Medical Countermeasures

Medical countermeasures, or MCMs, are the U.S. Food and Drug Administration (FDA)-regulated products (biologics, drugs, devices) that may be used in the event of a potential public-health emergency stemming from a terrorist attack with a biological, chemical, or radiological/nuclear material, or a naturally occurring emerging disease.

The MCMs can be used to diagnose, prevent, protect from, or treat conditions associated with chemical, biological, radiological, or nuclear (CBRN) threats, or emerging infectious diseases.

The MCMs can include:

- **Biologic products,** such as vaccines, blood products, and antibodies
- **Drugs,** such as antimicrobial or antiviral drugs
- **Devices,** including diagnostic tests to identify threat agents, and personal-protective equipment (PPE), such as gloves, respirators (face masks), and ventilators

How Medical Countermeasures Are Accessed and Used in Emergencies

Depending on the emergency and public-health need, during a public-health emergency, MCMs may be provided by the Strategic National

This chapter includes text excerpted from "What Are Medical Countermeasures?" U.S. Food and Drug Administration (FDA), December 19, 2018.

Stockpile (SNS), which is overseen by the Assistant Secretary for Preparedness and Response (ASPR), or through state and local stockpiles or other pharmaceutical caches. MCMs are usually dispensed or administered by healthcare workers and public-health responders under official federal, state, and/or local emergency-response plans.

In some cases, at the time of a public-health emergency, MCMs may be approved by the FDA and will be used in approved ways during a response. Some MCMs may not be approved yet, or they may be approved but not for the indication under consideration during the emergency.

Because of its role in regulating medical products, and the nature of some of these products, the FDA may need to use special authorities to allow the use of such MCMs in impacted populations during or in anticipation of emergencies. Mechanisms the FDA can use to allow the emergency use of MCMs include the emergency use authorization (EUA) authority and several authorities related to the emergency use of approved MCMs.

The Animal Rule

Before a medical product can be approved by the FDA, the sponsor must demonstrate efficacy—that the product works. In some cases, such as developing MCMs for potential bioterror threats, human challenge studies (exposing people to the threat agent) would not be ethical or feasible. In these cases, the FDA may grant approval based on well-controlled animal studies when the results of those studies establish that the drug or biological product is reasonably likely to produce clinical benefit in humans. The product sponsor must still demonstrate the product's safety in humans.

The FDA's Role in Supporting the Development of Medical Countermeasures

Through the Medical Countermeasures Initiative (MCMi), the FDA works with partners at all levels of government—local, state, national and international—to support MCM-related public-health preparedness and response efforts. The FDA coordinates MCM-related efforts across HHS and the U.S. Government (USG) interagency partners. It also works with nongovernment organizations, universities and research centers, and industry to further the development of MCMs for public-health emergency preparedness.

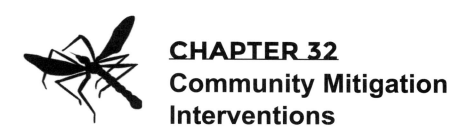

CHAPTER 32
Community Mitigation Interventions

Chapter Contents

Quarantine, Isolation, and Social Distancing

This section contains text excerpted from the following sources: Text in this section begins with excerpts from "Quarantine and Isolation," Centers for Disease Control and Prevention (CDC), September 29, 2017; Text under the heading "Social Distancing" is excerpted from "Social Distancing," Centers for Disease Control and Prevention (CDC), March 7, 2017.

Isolation and quarantine help protect the public by preventing exposure to people who have or may have a contagious disease.

- **Isolation** separates sick people with a contagious disease from people who are not sick.
- **Quarantine** separates and restricts the movement of people who were exposed to a contagious disease to see if they become sick.

The U.S. Quarantine Stations, located at ports of entry and land-border crossings, use these public-health practices as part of a comprehensive quarantine system that serves to limit the introduction of infectious diseases into the United States and to prevent their spread.

History of Quarantine
The Middle Ages

The practice of quarantine began during the 14th century in an effort to protect coastal cities from plague epidemics. Ships arriving in Venice from infected ports were required to sit at anchor for 40 days before landing. This practice, called "quarantine," was derived from the Italian word "quaranta giorni" which means 40 days.

Early American Quarantine

When the United States was first established, little was done to prevent the importation of infectious diseases. Protection against imported diseases fell under local and state jurisdiction. Individual municipalities enacted a variety of quarantine regulations for arriving vessels.

State and local governments made sporadic attempts to impose quarantine requirements. Continued outbreaks of yellow fever finally prompted Congress to pass federal quarantine legislation in 1878. This legislation, while not conflicting with states' rights, paved the way for federal involvement in quarantine activities.

Late Nineteenth Century

Outbreaks of cholera from passenger ships arriving from Europe prompted a reinterpretation of the law in 1892 to provide the federal government more authority in imposing quarantine requirements. The following year, Congress passed legislation that further clarified the federal role in quarantine activities. As local authorities came to realize the benefits of federal involvement, local quarantine stations were gradually turned over to the U.S. government. Additional federal facilities were built and the number of staff was increased to provide better coverage. The quarantine system was fully nationalized by 1921 when the administration of the last quarantine station was transferred to the United States government.

Public-Health Service Act

The Public Health Service Act of 1944 clearly established the federal government's quarantine authority for the first time. The act gave the U.S. Public Health Service (PHS) responsibility for preventing the introduction, transmission, and spread of communicable diseases from foreign countries into the United States.

Reorganization and Expansion

This PHS cutter ship was used to transport quarantine inspectors to ships flying the yellow quarantine flag. The flag was flown until quarantine and customs personnel inspected and cleared the ship to dock at the port.

Originally part of the Treasury Department, Quarantine and PHS, its parent organization, became part of the Federal Security Agency (FSA) in 1939. In 1953, PHS and Quarantine joined the Department of Health, Education, and Welfare (HEW). Quarantine was then transferred to the agency now known as the "Centers for Disease Control and Prevention (CDC)" in 1967. The CDC remained part of HEW until 1980 when the department was reorganized into the U.S. Department of Health and Human Services (HHS).

When the CDC assumed responsibility for Quarantine, it was a large organization with 55 quarantine stations and more than 500 staff members. Quarantine stations were located at every port, international airport, and major border crossing.

From Inspection to Intervention

After evaluating the quarantine program and its role in preventing disease transmission, the CDC trimmed the program in the 1970s and changed its focus from routine inspection to program management and intervention. The new focus included an enhanced surveillance system to monitor the onset of epidemics abroad and a modernized inspection process to meet the changing needs of international traffic.

By 1995, all U.S. ports of entry were covered by only seven quarantine stations. A station was added in 1996 in Atlanta, Georgia, just before the city hosted the 1996 Summer Olympic Games. Following the severe acute respiratory syndrome (SARS) epidemic of 2003, the CDC reorganized the quarantine station system, expanding to 18 stations with more than 90 field employees.

Quarantine Now

The Division of Global Migration and Quarantine (DGMQ) is part of the CDC's National Center for Emerging and Zoonotic Infectious Diseases (NCEZID) and is headquartered in Atlanta. Quarantine stations are located in Anchorage, Atlanta, Boston, Chicago, Dallas, Detroit, El Paso, Honolulu, Houston, Los Angeles, Miami, Minneapolis, New York, Newark, Philadelphia, San Diego, San Francisco, San Juan, Seattle, and Washington, D.C.

Under its delegated authority, the DGMQ is empowered to detain, medically examine, or conditionally release individuals and wildlife suspected of carrying a communicable disease.

The list of quarantinable diseases is contained in an executive order of the President and includes cholera, diphtheria, infectious tuberculosis, plague, smallpox, yellow fever, viral hemorrhagic fevers (such as Marburg, Ebola, and Congo-Crimean), and SARS.

Many other illnesses of public-health significance, such as measles, mumps, rubella, and chickenpox, are not contained in the list of quarantinable illnesses but continue to pose a health risk to the public. Quarantine Station personnel respond to reports of ill travelers aboard airplanes, ships, and land-border crossings to make an assessment of the public-health risk and initiate an appropriate response.

Social Distancing

Social distancing is a measure to increase the physical space between people and reduce the frequency of contact. It includes canceling events, such as large gatherings, and closing/restricting access to buildings, and applies to groups, not just individuals. Discourage visits to medical departments and hospital emergency departments by the "worried well" and by those with symptoms of uncomplicated flu, as such visits encourage the spread of pandemic flu virus. However, those having signs of severe disease and those in high-risk groups, per the CDC guidance, should seek prompt medical attention. Healthcare facilities could also restrict or limit visitors in their facilities during an outbreak

Social distancing is a measure to increase the physical space between people and reduce the frequency of contact. It includes canceling events, such as large gatherings, and closing/restricting access to buildings, and applies to groups, not just individuals.

Discourage visits to medical departments and hospital emergency departments by the "worried well" and by those with symptoms of uncomplicated flu, as such visits encourage the spread of pandemic flu virus. However, those having signs of severe disease and those in high-risk groups, per the CDC guidance, should seek prompt medical attention.

Healthcare facilities could also restrict or limit visitors to their facilities during an outbreak.

Exclude/segregate persons with influenza-like illness (ILI):

- Urge employees with ILI to stay home; promptly exclude from work people with ILI; separate sick employees while on-site (designate rooms to do so).

Employees should be familiar with the training and education addressing these social distancing policies and measures. For pandemics with severe disease, the aim is to reduce the frequency and types of face-to-face contact between employees, customers, and patients. Measures might include canceling nonessential meetings, avoiding hand-shaking, closing venues, such as child-care centers and cafeterias, and changes in office layout, use of shared equipment and seating during meetings. Plan for the use of remote communication (e.g., telephone/web-based meetings and business functions) and needed IT infrastructure and give priority to personnel at high medical risk for influenza complications (i.e., those with chronic medical conditions or who are pregnant). Observe travel restrictions and advice to travelers from public-health authorities.

Section 32.2

Movement Restrictions and Travel Notice

This section contains text excerpted from the following sources: Text under the heading "Travel Epidemiology" is excerpted from "Travel Epidemiology," Centers for Disease Control and Prevention (CDC), June 21, 2019; Text under the heading "Travel Health Notices" is excerpted from "Travel Health Notices," Centers for Disease Control and Prevention (CDC), December 23, 2019.

Travel Epidemiology

Travelers are epidemiologically important population because of their mobility, their potential for exposure to diseases outside their home country, and the possibility that they may serve as a conduit for disease from one country to another. In the past 10 years, for example, travelers have faced newly emerging threats, including Ebola, chikungunya, and Zika. Evolving epidemiology of the disease, the increasing prevalence of antimicrobial drug resistance, and the development of new vaccines and prophylactic treatments have each contributed to creating the ongoing need for surveillance of international travelers.

The risk of travel-related illnesses varies depending on destination and traveler characteristics. Existing information regarding the actual risk for travelers (often expressed as a number of events per 100,000 travelers) is limited for several reasons. It is difficult to obtain an accurate numerator (number of cases of disease among travelers) and denominator (number of travelers overall or travelers to a specific destination who are susceptible to infection). To calculate a true risk for a traveler, scientific studies would have to document the number of travelers susceptible to that disease or condition and the number of those affected during a specific period of time. If the illness is mild, the traveler may never seek healthcare, or clinicians might not perform diagnostic tests to identify the cause accurately. Furthermore, because travelers often visit multiple destinations, it could be difficult to determine the location where the exposure occurred and attribute risk to that location.

Frequently quoted studies on the incidence of infection in travelers use a variety of methodologic designs, each with its own strengths and weaknesses, making findings difficult to compare or combine. These studies have examined, for the most part, only a few key diseases or conditions, combining all travelers regardless of destination. Many have been single-clinic or single-destination studies that lead to conclusions that are not generalizable to groups of travelers with different local, national, or cultural backgrounds.

Healthcare providers must understand the epidemiologic features of the traveling population to guide pretravel recommendations and posttravel evaluations. The characteristics of travel-related diseases must be considered, including mode of transmission, incubation period, signs and symptoms, duration of illness, and diagnostic testing. The presence, frequency, seasonality, and geographic distribution of the disease need to be assessed; these might change over time because of outbreaks, emergence or reemergence in new areas or populations, successful public-health interventions, or other factors.

Data on disease incidence in local populations could identify the most important diseases to monitor within a country, but the relevance of such data to travelers—who have different risk behaviors, eating habits, accommodations, knowledge of preventive measures, and activities—is usually limited. Surveillance data that focus on travelers or on illnesses that affect travelers, are, therefore, more useful in describing travel-related disease patterns and risks.

Two existing networks provide data on the demographics of the U.S. international travelers and the acquisition of travel-related illness. Global TravEpiNet (GTEN) is a consortium of health clinics across the United States that provide pretravel-health consultations; data from GTEN provide a snapshot of the types of travelers seeking pretravel healthcare and their travel practices, as well as longitudinal cohort data on risk and acquisition of travel-associated conditions. The GeoSentinel Global Surveillance Network, a worldwide data collection and communication network composed of the International Society of Travel Medicine (ISTM) travel and tropical medicine clinics, collects posttravel-illness surveillance data. GeoSentinel analyzes this data to describe the relationships between travel and travel-related illness in specific subpopulations of travelers.

Familiarity with the epidemiology and prevalence of travel-related infections, coupled with demographic information on travelers and their particular travel details, can help clinicians provide optimal health-related information and advice. Clinical networks and surveillance systems provide epidemiologic data on new and prevalent global-infectious disease threats. Improved collaboration between travel-health providers and the travel-health clinical networks is needed to further expand and develop the evidence base in this field; this will allow for better-informed preparation before travel and enhanced clinical awareness of travel epidemiology for clinicians seeing patients before and after travel.

Travel-Health Notices

Travel-health notices inform travelers and clinicians about current health issues that impact travelers' health, such as disease outbreaks, special events or gatherings, and natural disasters, in specific international destinations.

Warning level 3. Avoid all nonessential travel to this destination. The outbreak is of high risk to travelers and no precautions are available to protect against the identified increased risk.

Alert level 2. Practice enhanced precautions for this destination. The travel-health notice describes additional precautions added or defines a specific at-risk population.

Watch level 1. Practice usual precautions for this destination, as described in the travel-health notice and/or on the destination page (wwwnc.cdc.gov/travel/destinations/list). This includes being up-to-date on all recommended vaccines and practicing appropriate mosquito avoidance.

Section 32.3
Guidelines for Air Travel Restrictions

This section includes text excerpted from "Travel
Restrictions to Prevent the Spread of Disease,"
Centers for Disease Control and Prevention (CDC),
May 21, 2019.

A disease is just a flight away. To protect America's health, the Centers for Disease Control and Prevention (CDC) partners with the Department of Homeland Security (DHS) to prevent the spread of serious contagious diseases during travel. The CDC uses a Do Not Board list to prevent travelers from boarding commercial airplanes if they are known or suspected to have a contagious disease that poses a threat to the public's health. Sick travelers are also placed on a Lookout list so they will be detected if they attempt to enter the United States by land or sea. These tools can be used for anyone who poses a threat to the public's health.

Local and state public-health officials can request the CDC's assistance if a person who poses a public-health threat intends to travel. The CDC helps ensure these people do not travel while contagious.

Placing People on the Lists
The criteria for adding people to the Do Not Board and Lookout lists are:
- Known or believed to be infectious with, or at risk for, a serious contagious disease that poses a public-health threat to others during travel; and any of the following three:
  - Not aware of diagnosis or not following public-health recommendations
  - Likely to travel on a commercial flight involving the United States or travel internationally by any means
  - Need to issue travel restriction to respond to a public-health outbreak or to help enforce a public-health order

Criteria number one plus one of the three subsets must be met for a person to be placed on the Do Not Board and Lookout lists.

Once a person is placed on these lists, airlines will not issue a boarding pass to the person for any commercial flight within, arriving to, or departing from the United States.

To date, the Do Not Board and Lookout lists have been used for people with suspected or confirmed infectious tuberculosis (TB), including multidrug-resistant tuberculosis (MDR-TB) and measles. However, travel restrictions can also be used for other suspected or confirmed contagious diseases that could pose a public-health threat during travel, including viral hemorrhagic fevers such as Ebola.

Preventing people with contagious diseases from traveling also helps to make sure they get or continue medical treatment, such as for infectious TB.

Taking People off the Lists

Once public-health authorities confirm a person is no longer contagious, the person is removed from the lists (typically within 24 hours). Also, the CDC reviews the records of all persons on the lists every two weeks to determine whether they are eligible for removal.

FAQs for Public Health Do Not Board and Lookout Lists

What Is the Do Not Board List?

The CDC established the Do Not Board list in June 2007, in collaboration with the DHS, to prevent commercial air travel by people who are contagious with certain diseases of public-health concern, such as infectious TB and measles. Travelers on the Do Not Board list (a public-health list) are not part of the No-Fly list, which is used for law enforcement purposes.

How Does the Do Not Board List Work?

A person on the do not board list is prevented from obtaining a boarding pass for any flight into, out of, or within the United States. The Transportation Security Administration (TSA) enforces this list for commercial-air travel.

What Is a Public-Health Lookout List?

The public-health Lookout prompts a public-health review of a person's infectious disease status before they are admitted into the United States. Customs and Border Protection (CBP) enforces this tool to put the person in contact with public-health authorities to ensure appropriate isolation, if indicated, and other public-health management. Having a public-health Lookout attached to a person's name does not prevent travel or necessarily deny entry into the United States. A public-health Lookout is issued to complement the Do Not Board, alerting the DHS when a person who has been placed on this list tries to enter the United States at any port of entry (seaport, airport, land border).

Why Are Both Tools Needed?

The public health Do Not Board and Lookout lists are two different but complementary tools for controlling travel. TSA administers the Do Not Board, which prevents infected persons from flying. The public-health Lookout list is managed by Customs and Border Protection (CBP) and prevents people from crossing the U.S. border. Since its inception in 2007, both lists have been primarily used for TB cases.

What Authority Does the United States Government Have to Put People on the Do Not Board List?

Under the Aviation and Transportation Security Act (ATSA) (49 U.S.C. 114), TSA may take actions necessary to mitigate threats to aviation and transportation security, including denying boarding to travelers the CDC identifies as likely posing a public-health threat to passengers or crew.

What Diseases Do These Restrictions Cover?

Most public health Do Not Board and Lookout cases have been for infectious TB, with a very small number for measles. However, these border-health tools can be used for any communicable diseases that pose a serious public-health threat.

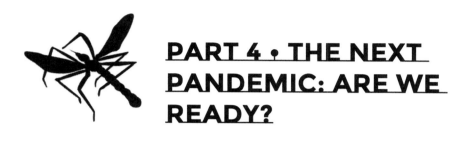

PART 4 • THE NEXT PANDEMIC: ARE WE READY?

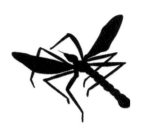

CHAPTER 33
Getting Ahead of the Next Pandemic

When a deadly mystery illness was detected in Liberia in April 2017, first responders were on the ground within 24 hours. Through the Ministry of Health's quick action and collaboration with global partners, the cause of the outbreak was identified as meningococcal disease and contained with only 31 cases and 13 deaths. In stark contrast, when Ebola struck Liberia just 3 years ago, it took the country months to mount an effective response and thousands of lives were lost as responders raced to control the growing epidemic.

The difference between these two outbreaks is just one example of the progress made since 2014 to advance the Global Health Security Agenda's (GHSA) goal to strengthen countries' response capacities. GHSA is a global effort to save lives and reduce the impact of disease threats—whether naturally occurring or manmade—by stopping them at their source.

An article released in the Centers for Disease Control and Prevention (CDC) *Emerging Infectious Diseases* (EID) journal details early results of the CDC's global health security work through collaboration with 17 partner countries. *Implementing the GHSA in 17 Countries: Contributions by the Centers for Disease Control and Prevention* shows how the CDC is accelerating progress toward a world more prepared for public-health threats. Part of EID's new

This chapter includes text excerpted from "Getting Ahead of the Next Pandemic: Is the World Ready?" Centers for Disease Control and Prevention (CDC), October 26, 2017.

Global Health Security Supplement, the article outlines the CDC-supported progress during the first two years of GHSA implementation.

With supplemental funding from the U.S. government of $582 million over 5 years (FY 2015 to 2019), the CDC is supporting Liberia and 16 other GHSA countries in strengthening core public-health systems to rapidly detect, respond, and prevent the spread of disease and limit the impact of outbreaks on families, communities, and whole economies. These efforts include strengthening:

- **Surveillance** systems to rapidly detect and report cases
- **Laboratory networks t**o accurately identify the cause of illness
- **A workforce of disease detectives and rapid responders** to identify, track, and contain outbreaks
- **Emergency operations systems** to coordinate an effective response

"These core areas are a platform for a functioning public-health system in any country and are critical for effective disease detection and response," said Rebecca Bunnell, Ph.D., deputy director for science, policy, and communication in the CDC's Division of Global Health Protection (DGHP) and senior author of the article. "From meningococcal disease in Liberia to yellow fever in Uganda, outbreaks can be contained and pandemics prevented when countries have these core capabilities in place."

A Timely Look at Progress toward Global-Health Security Agenda Milestones

The GHSA partner countries, including the United States, meet in Kampala, Uganda, for the fourth High-Level GHSA Ministerial Meeting to discuss sustaining and extending these critical efforts.

"In a world more interconnected than ever—where emerging diseases continually threaten people's health and drug resistance continues to grow—ensuring the safety and security of all people requires strong, diverse partnerships and a global commitment to GHSA beyond 2018," said Rebecca Martin, Ph.D., director of the CDC's Center for Global Health (CGH).

The CDC report describes progress to meet GHSA milestones and concludes that, overall, GHSA partner countries (Phase I) were successful in expanding their capacity for combating public-health threats. The analysis found more than 675 advancements across the 17 countries as a result of the CDC's GHSA work, including these:

- **Disease surveillance.** Thirteen countries (76%) expanded surveillance systems for three or more syndromes (for example, severe acute respiratory syndrome (SARS), acute flaccid paralysis (AFP), acute hemorrhagic fever (AHF), and acute watery diarrhea with dehydration) that signal possible public-health emergencies.
- **Laboratory systems.** Sixteen countries (94%) acquired new diagnostic equipment and capabilities (such as specimen test kits) to detect priority pathogens, such as influenza, polio, human immunodeficiency viruses (HIV), tuberculosis (TB), typhoid fever, and cholera.
- **Workforce development.** All 17 countries participated in three-month Frontline Field Epidemiology Training Programs (FETP) designed to put disease detectives on the ground who know how to identify, track, and contain outbreaks. These included new Frontline programs in 14 countries.
- **Emergency management and response.** All 14 countries trained emergency operations center staff in basic public-health emergency management, giving them the necessary skills to coordinate an efficient and effective response.

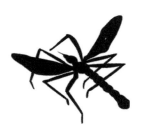

CHAPTER 34
The 1918 Flu Pandemic: Why It Matters 100 Years Later

One hundred years ago, an influenza (flu) pandemic swept the globe, infecting an estimated one-third of the world's population and killing at least 50 million people.

The pandemic's death toll was greater than the total number of military and civilian deaths from World War I, which was happening simultaneously. The 1918 pandemic was caused by an influenza A (H1N1) virus. The pandemic is commonly believed to have occurred in three waves. The unusual flu-like activity was first identified in the U.S. military personnel during the spring of 1918. Flu spread rapidly in military barracks where men shared close quarters. The second wave occurred during the fall of 1918 and was the most severe. The third wave of illness occurred during the winter and spring of 1919.

Here are the 5 things you should know about the 1918 pandemic and why it matters 100 years later.

The 1918 Flu Virus Spread Quickly

Five hundred million people were estimated to have been infected by the 1918 H1N1 flu virus. At least 50 million people were killed around the world, including an estimated 675,000 Americans. In fact, the 1918

This chapter includes text excerpted from "The 1918 Flu Pandemic: Why It Matters 100 Years Later," Centers for Disease Control and Prevention (CDC), May 14, 2018.

pandemic actually caused the average life expectancy in the United States to drop by about 12 years for both men and women.

In 1918, many people got very sick, very quickly. In March of that year, outbreaks of flu-like illnesses were first detected in the United States. More than 100 soldiers at Camp Funston in Fort Riley, Kansas, became ill with the flu. Within a week, the number of flu cases quintupled. There were reports of some people dying within 24 hours or less. 1918 flu illness often progressed to organ failure and pneumonia, with pneumonia the cause of death for most of those who died. Young adults were hit hard. The average age of those who died during the pandemic was 28 years old.

No Prevention and No Treatment for the 1918 Pandemic Virus

In 1918, as scientists had not yet discovered flu viruses, there were no laboratory tests to detect or characterize these viruses. There were no vaccines to help prevent flu infection, no antiviral drugs to treat flu illness, and no antibiotics to treat secondary bacterial infections that can be associated with flu infections. Available tools to control the spread of flu were largely limited to nonpharmaceutical interventions (NPIs), such as isolation, quarantine, good personal hygiene, use of disinfectants, and limits on public gatherings, which were used in many cities. The science behind these was very young and applied inconsistently. City residents were advised to avoid crowds and instructed to pay particular attention to personal hygiene. In some cities, dance halls were closed. Some streetcar conductors were ordered to keep the windows of their cars open in all but rainy weather. Some municipalities moved court cases outside. Many physicians and nurses were instructed to wear gauze masks when with flu patients.

Illness Overburdened the Healthcare System

An estimated 195,000 Americans died during October alone. In the fall of 1918, the United States experienced a severe shortage of professional nurses during the flu pandemic because large numbers of them were deployed to military camps in the United States and abroad. This shortage was made worse by the failure to use trained African American nurses. The Chicago chapter of the American Red Cross (ARC) issued an urgent call for volunteers to help nurse the ill. Philadelphia was hit hard by the pandemic with more than 500 corpses awaiting burial, some for more than a week. Many parts of the United States had been drained of physicians and nurses due to calls for military service, so there was a shortage of medical personnel to meet the civilian demand for healthcare during the 1918 flu pandemic. In Massachusetts, for example, Governor McCall asked every able-bodied person across the state with medical training to offer their aid in fighting the outbreak.

As the numbers of sick rose, the Red Cross put out desperate calls for trained nurses as well as untrained volunteers to help at emergency centers. In October of 1918, Congress approved a $1 million budget for the United States Public Health Service (USPHS) to recruit 1,000 medical doctors and more than 700 registered nurses.

At one point in Chicago, physicians were reporting a staggering number of new cases, reaching as high as 1,200 people each day. This, in turn, intensified the shortage of doctors and nurses. Additionally, hospitals in some areas were so overloaded with flu patients that schools, private homes, and other buildings had to be converted into makeshift hospitals, some of which were staffed by medical students.

Major Advancements in Flu Prevention and Treatment since 1918

The science of influenza has come a long way in 100 years! Developments since the 1918 pandemic include vaccines to help prevent the flu, antiviral drugs to treat flu illness, antibiotics to treat secondary bacterial infections, such as pneumonia, and a global influenza surveillance system with 114 World Health Organization (WHO) member states that constantly monitors flu activity. There also is a much better understanding of nonpharmaceutical interventions—such as social distancing, respiratory and cough etiquette and hand hygiene—and how these measures help slow the spread of flu.

There is still much work to do to improve the United States and global readiness for the next flu pandemic. More effective vaccines and antiviral drugs are needed in addition to better surveillance of influenza viruses in birds and pigs. The CDC also is working to minimize the impact of future flu pandemics by supporting research that can enhance the use of community mitigation measures (i.e., temporarily closing schools, modifying, postponing, or canceling large public events, and creating physical distance between people in settings where they commonly come in contact with one another). These nonpharmaceutical interventions continue to be an integral component of efforts to control the spread of flu, and in the absence of flu vaccine, would be the first line of defense in a pandemic.

Risk of a Flu Pandemic Is Ever-Present, but the CDC Is on the Frontlines Preparing to Protect Americans

Four pandemics have occurred in the past century: 1918, 1957, 1968, and 2009. The 1918 pandemic was the worst of them. But the threat of a future flu pandemic remains. A pandemic flu virus could emerge anywhere and spread globally.

The CDC works tirelessly to protect Americans and the global community from the threat of a future flu pandemic. The CDC works with domestic and global public health and animal health partners to monitor human and animal influenza viruses. This helps the CDC know what viruses are spreading, where they are spreading, and what kind of illnesses they are causing. The CDC also develops and distributes tests and materials to support influenza testing at state, local, territorial, and international laboratories so they can detect and characterize influenza viruses. In addition, the CDC assists global and domestic experts in selecting candidate viruses to include in each year's seasonal flu vaccine and guides prioritization of pandemic vaccine development. The CDC routinely develops vaccine viruses used by manufacturers to make flu vaccines. The

CDC also supports state and local governments in preparing for the next flu pandemic, including planning and leading pandemic exercises across all levels of government. An effective response will diminish the potential for a repeat of the widespread devastation of the 1918 pandemic.

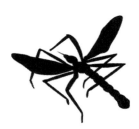

CHAPTER 35
Viruses of Special Concern

A novel influenza A virus is one that has caused a human infection but is different from current seasonal human influenza A viruses that circulate among people. Novel influenza A viruses are usually influenza A viruses that circulate among animals. Some novel influenza A viruses are believed to pose a greater pandemic threat than others and are more concerning to public-health officials because they have caused serious human illness and death and also have been able to spread in a limited manner from person-to-person. Novel influenza A viruses are of extra concern because of the potential impact they could have on public health if they gain the ability to spread easily from person-to-person, which might cause the next influenza pandemic. Human infection with a novel influenza A virus is a nationally notifiable condition reportable to the Centers for Disease Control and Prevention (CDC).

Avian Influenza A Viruses

Avian influenza A viruses do not normally infect humans, however, sporadic human infections have occurred. Illness in humans caused by avian influenza A virus infections have ranged from mild to severe (e.g., pneumonia).

This chapter includes text excerpted from "Viruses of Special Concern," Centers for Disease Control and Prevention (CDC), April 29, 2018.

Several subtypes of avian influenza A viruses are known to have infected people (H5, H6, H7, H9, H10 viruses). Highly pathogenic Asian avian influenza A(H5N1) and low pathogenic Asian A(H7N9) viruses account for the majority of human infections with avian influenza A viruses.

Human infections with avian influenza A viruses have most often occurred after exposure to infected poultry or their secretions or excretions, such as through direct or close contact, including visiting a live poultry market.

Avian Influenza A H5 Viruses

Among H5 avian influenza A viruses, Asian highly pathogenic avian influenza (HPAI) A (H5N1) viruses have caused the most human infections. Asian H5N1 viruses are circulating among poultry in Asia and the Middle East and human infections with these viruses have been reported in 17 countries since 2003. Human infections are often associated with severe pneumonia and mortality greater than 50 percent. Probable, limited, nonsustained human-to-human spread of Asian H5N1 viruses has been reported in several countries. (HPAI H5 viruses detected in birds and poultry in the United States are different and have not caused human infections.)

The World Health Organization (WHO) tracks the number of reported, confirmed human infections with HPAI H5N1 viruses.

On January 8, 2014, the first case of human infection with the Asian HPAI H5N1 virus in the Americas was reported in Canada in a traveler returning from China. (No human infections with Asian H5N1 virus have been reported in the United States.)

Sporadic human infections with HPAI H5N6 viruses also have been reported in China, resulting in severe illness and high mortality.

Avian Influenza A H7 Viruses

Among H7 viruses, low pathogenic Asian lineage avian influenza A H7N9 viruses have caused the most reported human infections; with most of them occurring in China. The first human infections with H7N9 viruses were reported by WHO on April 1, 2013, and sporadic human infections continue to be reported in China. In late 2016, some low pathogenicity Asian H7N9 viruses developed mutations that made them highly pathogenic in poultry. These HPAI H7N9 Asian viruses continue to be associated with human infections in China. Many Asian H7N9 virus-infected patients have had a severe respiratory illness. During the past five annual epidemics of Asian H7N9 virus infections in people, the mortality rate in hospitalized patients has averaged about 40 percent. Probable, limited, nonsustained human-to-human spread of Asian H7N9 viruses also has been reported in China. Since the implementation of a large-scale H5-H7 poultry vaccination program in September 2017, few human infections with Asian H7N9 viruses have been reported.

In January 2015, the Government of Canada and the Ministry of Health in British Columbia reported the first two cases of human infection in North America with the Asian H7N9 virus in a husband and wife who had traveled to China. Cases of Asian H7N9 virus infection associated with travel to China also have been reported in Hong Kong, Taiwan, and Malaysia.

Avian Influenza A H9 Viruses

Sporadic human infections with some low pathogenicity H9N2 viruses also have been reported in China, Hong Kong, Bangladesh, and Egypt. Most H9N2 virus infections in people have occurred in children after poultry exposures. H9N2 virus infection of humans generally causes mild upper respiratory tract illness.

Swine Influenza and Variant Influenza A Viruses

Sporadic human infections with swine influenza A viruses circulating among pigs can occur. When this happens, these viruses are called "variant viruses." They also can be denoted by adding the letter "v" to the end of the influenza A virus subtype designation.

Illness associated with variant virus infection has been mostly mild with symptoms similar to those of seasonal flu. Like seasonal influenza, however, serious illness, resulting in hospitalization and death, is possible. In general, variant viruses have been associated with less severe illness and much lower mortality than human infection with avian influenza A viruses. Most commonly, human infections with variant viruses occur in people with exposure to infected pigs (e.g., children who have direct or close contact with pigs at a fair or workers in the swine industry), but limited, nonsustained spread from person to person of some variant viruses has been detected.

Human infections with H1N1v, H3N2v, and H1N2v viruses have been detected in the United States.

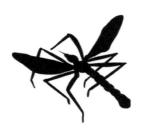

CHAPTER 36
Getting Your Household Ready for Pandemic Flu

Chapter Contents

Section 36.1

Keep Yourself and Members of Your Household Healthy by Planning for Pandemic Flu

This section includes text excerpted from "Get Your Household Ready for Pandemic Flu," Centers for Disease Control and Prevention (CDC), April 2017.

Influenza can spread quickly from sick people to others who are nearby at home, school, work, and public events. Seasonal influenza, also known as the "flu," is a contagious respiratory illness caused by flu viruses that infect the nose, throat, and lungs. Flu mostly spreads by droplets containing flu viruses traveling through the air (up to six feet) when a sick person coughs or sneezes. Less often, people also might get the flu by touching surfaces or objects with flu viruses on them and then touching their eyes, nose, or mouth.

The best way to prevent the flu is by getting a flu vaccine. The Centers for Disease Control and Prevention (CDC) recommends a yearly flu vaccine for everyone six months and older. Vaccination can reduce flu illnesses, doctors' visits, and missed work and school due to flu illness, as well as prevent flu-related hospitalizations. The CDC also recommends that people practice everyday preventive actions (or personal National Provider Identifiers (NPIs)) at all times to protect themselves and their loved ones from the flu and other respiratory infections.

Millions of people in the United States get sick with the flu each year, and thousands of people are hospitalized; these numbers may increase during a flu pandemic. Flu pandemics are much less common but can occur at any time. Do not let your household be caught by surprise! Just as you prepare for seasonal flu, you should prepare for pandemic flu. Create an emergency plan to prepare your household for a flu pandemic. Taking action now can help protect you and the health of those you care about.

Pandemic Flu Is Not Seasonal Flu

A flu pandemic occurs when a new flu virus that is different from seasonal flu viruses emerges and spreads quickly between people, causing illness worldwide. Most people will lack immunity to the pandemic flu virus. Pandemic flu can be more severe, causing more deaths than seasonal flu. Because it is a new virus, a vaccine may not be available right away. A pandemic could, therefore, overwhelm normal operations in schools, workplaces, and other community settings.

National Provider Identifiers Can Help Slow the Spread of Flu

When a new flu virus emerges, it can take up to six months before a pandemic flu vaccine is widely available. When a vaccine is not available, NPIs are the best way to help slow the spread of flu. They include personal, community, and environmental actions. These actions are most effective when used together.

You play a key role in flu readiness. Safeguard your health and the health of your household members by making a pandemic flu plan now.

Personal National Provider Identifiers

Personal NPIs are everyday preventive actions that can help keep people from getting and spreading the flu. These actions include staying home when you are sick, covering your coughs and sneezes with a tissue, and washing your hands often with soap and water.

Community National Provider Identifiers

Community NPIs are strategies organizations and community leaders can use to help limit face-to-face contact. These strategies may include making sick-leave policies more flexible in workplace settings, temporarily dismissing schools, avoiding close contact with others, and canceling large public events.

Environmental National Provider Identifiers

Environmental NPIs are surface cleaning measures that remove germs from frequently touched surfaces and objects.

Section 36.2

Take Action to Help Slow the Spread of Flu and Illness

This section includes text excerpted from "Get Your Household Ready for Pandemic Flu," Centers for Disease Control and Prevention (CDC), April 2017.

The Centers for Disease Control and Prevention (CDC) has developed recommended actions for preventing the spread of flu in household settings. Practice everyday preventive actions at all times. Plan for additional community National Provider Identifiers (NPI) actions that may be recommended by public-health officials, if a flu pandemic occurs.

Everyday Preventive Actions

Everyone should always practice good personal-health habits to help prevent the flu.

- **Stay home when you are sick.** Stay home for at least 24 hours after you no longer have a fever or signs of a fever without the use of fever-reducing medicines.
- **Cover your coughs and sneezes with a tissue.**
- **Wash your hands often with soap and water for at least 20 seconds.** Use at least a 60 percent alcohol-based hand sanitizer if soap and water are not available.
- **Clean frequently touched surfaces and objects.**

National Provider Identifiers Reserved for a Flu Pandemic

Everyone should be prepared to take these additional actions if recommended by public-health officials.*

- For everyone: Avoid close contact with others. Keep a distance of at least three feet.

- Stay home if someone in your house is sick.
- For sick persons: Create a separate room for sick household members.
- Use a facemask, at home or out in public.
- Avoid sharing personal items.
- Postpone or cancel your attendance at large events.

These additional actions might be recommended for severe, very severe, or extreme flu pandemics.

What Are the Symptoms of Flu?

- Fever*
- Cough
- Sore throat
- Runny or stuffy nose
- Body aches
- Headache
- Chills
- Fatigue
- Sometimes vomiting and diarrhea

Signs of fever include chills, feeling very warm, flushed appearance, or sweating.

When Should You Seek Emergency Care?

Emergency Symptoms for Children*

- Fast breathing or trouble breathing
- Bluish skin color
- Not drinking enough fluids
- Not waking up or not interacting
- Being so irritable that the child does not want to be held
- Flu-like symptoms that improve but then return with a fever and a worse cough
- Fever with a rash

Additional emergency signs for infants include being unable to eat, no tears when crying, and significantly fewer wet diapers than normal.

Emergency Symptoms for Adults

- Difficulty breathing or shortness of breath
- Pain or pressure in the chest or abdomen
- Sudden dizziness
- Confusion
- Severe or persistent vomiting
- Flu-like symptoms that improve but then return with a fever and a worse cough

Good Health Habits Start at Home

Teach children to correctly practice good personal-health habits at all times. Young children may need your help doing this! Tell them about the importance of not sharing personal items, such as water bottles, lip gloss, or food.

Section 36.3

Before a Flu Pandemic Occurs: Plan

This section includes text excerpted from "Get Your Household Ready for Pandemic Flu," Centers for Disease Control and Prevention (CDC), April 2017.

Did You Know That School Dismissals May Happen If a Flu Pandemic Occurs?

A flu pandemic can last for several months. Public-health officials may recommend community actions based on the severity of the pandemic that limits exposure, such as temporarily dismissing schools early in a pandemic. Dismissing schools can help slow the spread of disease before pandemic flu becomes widespread in the community. School authorities also may decide to dismiss schools if too many students or staff are absent. School dismissals and other National Provider Identifiers (NPI) recommendations may be challenging to plan for and implement in your household. However, you may be asked to follow such recommendations for the safety and well-being of your household members.

Developing a household plan for pandemic flu will help ensure flu readiness. The details of your plan should be based on the needs and daily routine of your household, including alternative arrangements for the child, elder, and pet care.

Create an Emergency Plan of Action for Pandemic Flu

Talk with the People Who Need to Be Included in Your Plan

Meet with household members, other relatives, and friends to discuss what should be done if a flu pandemic occurs and what the needs of each person will be.

Plan Ways to Care for Those at Greater Risk for Serious Complications

Certain people are at greater risk for serious complications if they get the flu, including during a flu pandemic. Flu can worsen their health conditions, and the services they rely on may not be available. The Centers for Disease Control and Prevention (CDC) will recommend actions to help keep people who are at high risk for flu complications healthy if a pandemic occurs.

Get to Know Your Neighbors

Talk with them about pandemic flu and emergency planning. If your neighborhood has a website or social media page, consider joining it to stay connected to neighbors, information, and resources.

Identify Organizations in Your Community That Can Offer Assistance

Create a list of community and faith-based organizations that you and your household can contact in the event you lack access to information, healthcare services, support, and resources. Consider including organizations that provide mental health or counseling services, food, and other supplies.

Create an Emergency Contact List

Ensure that your household has a current list of emergency contacts for family, friends, neighbors, carpool drivers, healthcare providers, teachers, employers, the local public-health department, and other community resources.

Practice Good Personal-Health Habits and Plan for Home-Based Actions to Prevent Spreading Flu

Practice and Teach Everyday Preventive Actions Now

Get yourself and your household members in the routine of practicing everyday preventive actions to prevent the spread of respiratory illnesses, such as flu. Avoid close contact with people who are sick. Practicing other good health habits, such as getting plenty of rest, exercising, drinking plenty of fluids, eating healthy foods, and managing stress can also help stop the spread of germs and prevent the flu.

Plan to Have Extra Supplies of Important Items on Hand

Do plan to have extra supplies of important items on hand. For example, keep on hand extra supplies, such as soap, hand sanitizer with at least 60 percent alcohol, tissues, and disposable facemasks. If you or your household members have a chronic condition and regularly take prescription drugs, talk to your healthcare provider, pharmacist, and insurance provider about keeping an emergency supply of medications at home. These supplies can always be used for a different emergency and then restocked.

Note: Keep hand sanitizer out of the reach of small children. Consumption of alcohol-based hand sanitizers can lead to alcohol poisoning. Small children should only use alcohol-based hand sanitizer under adult supervision.

Have a Separate Room for Sick Household Members

Choose a room in your home that can be used to separate sick household members from those who are healthy. If possible, also choose a bathroom for the sick person to use. Plan to clean these rooms daily.

Be Prepared for Your Child's School or Child Care Facility to Be Temporarily Dismissed

Learn about the Emergency Operations Plan at Your Child's School or Child Care Facility

During a flu pandemic, local public-health officials may recommend schools be dismissed temporarily to help slow the spread of flu. School authorities also may decide to dismiss school if too many students or staff are absent. Understand the local School Board's plan for continuing education and social services during school dismissals, such as student meal programs. If your child attends a college or university, encourage your child to learn about the school's plan for pandemic flu.

Plan Alternative Child Care Arrangements

Determine how your children will be cared for should schools be dismissed during a flu pandemic.

Plan for Changes at Your Workplace

Learn about your employer's emergency operations plan. Discuss sick-leave policies and telework options for sick workers or those needing to stay home to care for a sick household member. Join the emergency planning team at your workplace (if possible).

Section 36.4

During a Flu Pandemic: Take Action

This section includes text excerpted from "Get Your
Household Ready for Pandemic Flu," Centers for
Disease Control and Prevention (CDC), April 2017.

Did You Know That People May Be Able to Spread the Flu to Others before Knowing They Are Sick as Well as While They Are Sick?

Knowing when someone is sick with the flu is not always easy. Adults may be able to spread the flu to other people beginning one day before symptoms occur and up to five to seven days after becoming sick. Children can spread the flu for longer than seven days. Flu symptoms start one to four days after the virus enters the body. That means you may be able to pass on the flu to someone else before you know you are sick, as well as while you are sick. Some people can be infected with the flu virus, but have no symptoms at all. During this time, they may still spread the virus to others. During a pandemic, you can take action to protect yourself and others by:

- Staying home when you are sick with flu symptoms
- Keeping away from others who are sick
- Limiting face-to-face contact with others (as much as possible)

If you or your household members are at high risk for flu complications, please consult with your healthcare provider for more information. Early action to stop the spread of flu will help keep you and your household members healthy.

Put Your Emergency Plan into Action
Stay Informed about the Local Flu Situation

Get up-to-date information about local flu activity from public-health officials. An early sign that you may need to take steps to protect your family is increased flu-related absenteeism at your child's school. Be aware of temporary school dismissals in your area, as this may affect your family's daily routine.

Avoid Close Contact with Others

Flu viruses can travel through the air up to six feet. During a pandemic, public-health officials may recommend that people keep a distance of at least three feet to help slow the spread of flu. Avoid close contact with people who are sick.

Stay Home If You Become Sick

Even if you do not have a fever, stay home if you have flu symptoms. If you have a fever, stay home for at least 24 hours after your fever is gone without the use of fever-reducing medicines, such as acetaminophen. When seeking medical care or other necessities, wear a facemask and keep your distance from others as much as possible. Seek emergency care if flu symptoms become severe. Public-health officials also may recommend that you stay home for at least 3 days, if a member of your household is sick, to avoid spreading the flu to others.

Continue Practicing Everyday Preventive Actions

Cover your coughs and sneezes with a tissue, and wash your hands often with soap and water for at least 20 seconds. If soap and water are not available, use a 60 percent alcohol-based hand sanitizer. Avoid sharing personal items, such as food, drinks, or lip gloss. Clean frequently touched surfaces and objects with regular soap and water or U.S. Environmental Protection Agency (EPA)-approved products. Always follow product labels when using disinfectants.

Use the Separate Room and Bathroom You Prepared for Sick Household Members

Provide sick household members with clean disposable facemasks to wear at home. Clean the sick room and bathroom daily. Use soap and water, bleach and water solution, or EPA-approved household products.

Stay in Touch with Others by Phone or E-Mail

If you live alone and become sick during a flu pandemic, you may need to ask for help. If you have a chronic disease condition and live alone, ask your friends, family, and healthcare providers to check on you during a pandemic.

Inform Your Workplace about Changes in Your Schedule

Notify your workplace as soon as possible if your schedule changes. Ask to work from home or take leave if you or someone in your household gets sick with flu symptoms, or if your child's school is temporarily dismissed.

Manage Your Children's Activities during a Pandemic

Notify your children's child care facility or school if they are sick with the flu. Talk with their teachers about classroom assignments and activities they can do from home.

Keep track of school dismissals in your community. Read or watch media sources that report school dismissals. Stay in close contact with children who are at a college or university, and be aware of what steps their schools are taking to protect students. If schools are temporarily dismissed, use alternative child care arrangements.

Keep routines at home as normal as possible. If schools are dismissed, try to keep children busy with activities and exercises at home. Keep educational materials, such as books and videos, on hand. Ensure that children keep up with school work. Watch your children's health closely. If your children are in the care of someone else, urge caregivers to watch for flu-like symptoms.

Discourage children and teens from gathering in other public places while school is dismissed. If they must be in groups for childcare or other reasons, keep them in small groups of six or fewer. Make sure groups consist of the same children each day. If children show flu-like symptoms, separate them from others immediately.

Make Smart Decisions about Attending Large Events

Decide Whether to Attend Large Events

Public-health officials may recommend postponing or canceling large events, such as sporting events, conferences, worship services, and other community events. Stay up-to-date about event cancellations before you leave home. Find out if there are other ways to enjoy the event without leaving home, such as watching it on TV or online.

Know Your Risk for Getting and Spreading the Flu at the Event

Stay home if you do not feel well or are more likely to get very sick with the flu. The number of people that will be attending, their ages, and where the event will be located can affect your risk of getting sick.

If You Decide to Attend a Public Event, Practice Good Health Habits

Try to keep at least 3 feet of distance between you and others at the event. Avoid close contact, such as shaking hands, hugging, and kissing, with other people. Wash hands often, or use at least a 60 percent alcohol-based hand sanitizer when soap and water are not available. Avoid surfaces that are touched often, such as doorknobs and handrails.

Stay Connected on Social Media

Many public-health departments will use social media, such as Facebook and Twitter, to communicate timely and accurate pandemic flu information to the public.

Section 36.5

After a Flu Pandemic Has Ended: Follow Up

This section includes text excerpted from "Get Your Household Ready for Pandemic Flu," Centers for Disease Control and Prevention (CDC), April 2017.

Did You Know That Most People Have Never Heard of Pandemic Flu or National Provider Identifiers?

Remember, a flu pandemic can last for several months. The impact on individuals, households, and communities can be great. When public-health officials determine the pandemic has ended in your community, take time to improve your household's emergency plan. As public-health officials continue to plan for pandemic flu, you and your household also have a responsibility. Your ongoing commitment to pandemic flu planning will be the key to successfully preventing the spread of flu during a pandemic.

Evaluate the Effectiveness of Your Emergency Plan of Action

Discuss and note the lessons learned. Were your flu-prevention actions effective at home, school, work, and public gatherings? Talk about problems found in your plan and effective solutions. Identify additional resources for you and your household. Review your plan each year before school begins and replenish the necessary supplies.

Start community discussions about emergency planning. Be creative and tell your story on social media, blogs, discussion boards, and community meetings. Let others know about the flu-readiness actions that worked for you and your household. Promote the importance of practicing good personal-health habits.

Continue to practice everyday preventive actions.

Congratulations on Planning for a Flu Pandemic

A flu pandemic can occur at any time, and having a plan in place is very important. Your emergency plan will help you and members of your household respond more quickly and effectively when an actual emergency occurs.

Be Ready for Any Type of Emergency

Your preparedness efforts should not end with the flu. Review and update your plan to include action steps you and your household can take during other emergencies and natural disasters, such as earthquakes, hurricanes, and tornados.

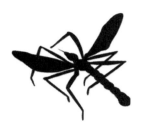

CHAPTER 37
The National Pandemic Strategy

Chapter Contents

About National Pandemic Strategy

This section includes text excerpted from "National Pandemic Strategy," Centers for Disease Control and Prevention (CDC), June 15, 2017.

In 1997, avian influenza A(H5N1) viruses first spread from poultry directly to infect humans in Hong Kong, resulting in the deaths of 6 of 18 infected persons. Concerned about the possibility that this A(H5N1) virus could easily infect humans and eventually spread from person-to-person, the World Health Organization (WHO) and the United States government increased pandemic preparedness planning. Since 2000, the world has experienced a pandemic and there have been other instances of novel influenza A viruses infecting people, including avian and swine influenza A viruses. An influenza pandemic could place extraordinary demands on public health and healthcare systems as well as on essential community services. Preparing for such a threat is an important priority.

In 2005, officials at the U.S. Department of Health and Human Services (HHS) developed a Pandemic Influenza Plan to coordinate and improve efforts to prevent, control, and respond to A(H5N1) viruses as well as other novel influenza A viruses of animal (e.g., from birds or pigs) with pandemic potential. Although it is impossible to predict when the next pandemic will occur, the U.S. government has developed three tools to guide national, state and local planning and response.

Section 37.2
Pandemic Intervals Framework

This section includes text excerpted from "Pandemic Intervals Framework (PIF)," Centers for Disease Control and Prevention (CDC), November 3, 2016. Reviewed January 2020.

The Pandemic Intervals Framework (PIF) describes the progression of an influenza pandemic using six intervals. This framework is used to guide influenza pandemic planning and provides recommendations for risk assessment, decision-making, and action in the United States. These intervals provide a common method to describe a pandemic activity that can inform public-health actions. The duration of each pandemic interval might vary depending on the characteristics of the virus and the public health response.

In addition to describing the progression of a pandemic, certain indicators and assessments are used to define when one interval moves into another. The Centers for Disease Control and Prevention (CDC) uses two tools; the Influenza Risk Assessment Tool (IRAT) and the Pandemic

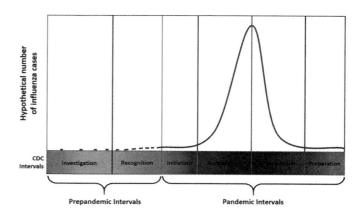

Figure 37.1. Preparedness and Response Framework for Novel Influenza A Virus Pandemics: CDC Intervals

Table 37.1. Description of the Six Pandemic Intervals

Interval	Description
1. Investigation of cases of novel influenza A virus infection in humans	When novel influenza A viruses are identified in people, public-health actions focus on targeted monitoring and investigation. This can trigger a risk assessment of that virus with the Influenza Risk Assessment Tool (IRAT), which is used to evaluate if the virus has the potential to cause a pandemic.
2. Recognition of the increased potential for ongoing transmission of a novel influenza A virus	When increasing numbers of human cases of novel influenza A illness are identified and the virus has the potential to spread from person-to-person, public-health actions focus on control of the outbreak, including treatment of sick persons.
3. Initiation of a pandemic wave	A pandemic occurs when people are easily infected with a novel influenza A virus that has the ability to spread in a sustained manner from person-to-person.
4. Acceleration of a pandemic wave	The acceleration (or "speeding up") is the upward epidemiological curve as the new virus infects susceptible people. Public-health actions at this time may focus on the use of appropriate nonpharmaceutical interventions in the community (e.g., school and child-care facility closures, social distancing), as well the use of medications (e.g., antivirals) and vaccines, if available. These actions combined can reduce the spread of the disease, and prevent illness or death.
5. Deceleration of a pandemic wave	The deceleration (or "slowing down") happens when pandemic influenza cases consistently decrease in the United States. Public-health actions include continued vaccination, monitoring of pandemic influenza A virus circulation and illness, and reducing the use of nonpharmaceutical interventions in the community (e.g., school closures).
6. Preparation for future pandemic waves	When pandemic influenza has subsided, public-health actions include continued monitoring of pandemic influenza A virus activity and preparing for potential additional waves of infection. It is possible that a second pandemic wave could have a higher severity than the initial wave. An influenza pandemic is declared ended when enough data shows that the influenza virus, worldwide, is similar to a seasonal influenza virus in how it spreads and the severity of the illness it can cause.

Severity Assessment Framework (PSAF,) to evaluate the pandemic risk that a new influenza A virus can pose. The results from both of these assessments are used to guide federal, state, and local public-health decisions.

Section 37.3

Influenza Risk Assessment Tool

This section includes text excerpted from "Influenza Risk Assessment Tool (IRAT)," Centers for Disease Control and Prevention (CDC), October 9, 2019.

What Is the Influenza Risk Assessment Tool?

The Influenza Risk Assessment Tool (IRAT) is an evaluation tool developed by the Centers for Disease Control and Prevention (CDC) and external influenza experts that assesses the potential pandemic risk posed by influenza A viruses that circulate in animals but not in humans. The IRAT assesses potential pandemic risk based on two different scenarios: "emergence" and "public-health impact."

"Emergence" refers to the risk of a novel (i.e., new in humans) influenza virus acquiring the ability to spread easily and efficiently in people. "Public-health impact" refers to the potential severity of human disease caused by the virus (e.g., deaths and hospitalizations) as well as the burden on society (e.g., missed workdays, strain on hospital capacity and resources, and interruption of basic public services) if a novel influenza virus were to begin spreading efficiently and sustainably among people.

The IRAT uses 10 scientific criteria to measure the potential pandemic risk associated with each of these scenarios. These 10 criteria can be grouped into three overarching categories: "properties of the virus," "attributes of the population," and "ecology and epidemiology of the virus." Influenza subject matter experts evaluate novel influenza viruses based on each of these 10 criteria. Each of the 10 criteria is then weighted statistically based on its significance to each of the two scenarios. A composite score for each virus is then calculated based on the given scenario. These composite scores provide a means to rank and compare influenza viruses to each other in terms of their potential pandemic risk for each of the two scenarios.

The IRAT is an evaluative tool, not a predictive tool. Flu is unpredictable, as are future pandemics.

What Is the Purpose of the Influenza Risk Assessment Tool?

The IRAT is intended to do the following:

- Prioritize and maximize investments in pandemic preparedness by helping to determine which novel (new) influenza viruses to develop vaccines against and capitalizing on surveillance efforts and in-country capacity building activities.
- Identify key gaps in information and knowledge which can be the basis to prompt additional studies. For example, if the information is not available for one of the 10 criteria used by the IRAT additional studies could be done or resources allocated to provide the needed information.
- Document in a transparent manner the data and scientific process used to inform management decisions associated with pandemic preparedness.
- Provide a flexible means to easily and regularly update the risk assessment of novel influenza viruses as new information becomes available.
- Be an effective communications tool for policymakers and the influenza community.
- Provide a means to weigh the 10 evaluation criteria differently depending on whether the intent of the risk assessment is to measure the ability of an influenza virus to "emerge" as a pandemic capable virus (i.e., become capable of efficient human-to-human spread) or "impact" the human population if it did emerge.

What Are the Evaluation Criteria Used by the Influenza Risk Assessment Tool?

The IRAT consists of 10 evaluation criteria grouped within 3 overarching categories. These categories and criteria are described as follows:

- The "properties of the virus" category contain 4 of the 10 evaluation criteria, including:
  - **Genomic analysis** is a measure of the extent of genetic diversity or the presence of known molecular signatures important for human infections and disease.
  - **"Receptor binding"** refers to the host preference (e.g., animal or human) of an influenza virus as well as the types of tissues and cells the virus is best suited to infecting (e.g., nose tissue and cells versus deep lung tissue and cells). Some influenza viruses are better adapted to infecting humans as opposed to animals.
  - **Transmission in lab animals** is a measure of the ability of an influenza virus to transmit efficiently in animals in laboratory studies. Some influenza viruses can transmit through the air via small infectious droplets expelled through coughs or sneezes, whereas other influenza viruses may only spread through direct contact with an infected host.
  - **"Antiviral treatment options"** refer to the predicted effectiveness of influenza antiviral medications, such as oseltamivir, zanamivir, and M2 blockers.
- The "attributes of the population" category contain three of the 10 evaluation criteria, including:
  - **"Existing population immunity"** refers to whether the human population has any existing immune protection against the novel influenza virus being evaluated. Susceptibility to infection and severity of illness associated with specific influenza viruses may depend on age, geographic area, or genetic factors.
  - **Disease severity** and **pathogenesis** measures the severity of illness caused by a particular influenza virus in people and/or animals.
  - **Antigenic relatedness** is a measure of how similar an influenza virus not circulating in humans is to seasonal influenza vaccines,

prepandemic candidate vaccine viruses, and stockpiled prepandemic vaccines.
- The "ecology and epidemiology" category contains the final three evaluation criteria, including:
  - **Global distribution (animals)** measures how widespread an influenza virus is in animals, the rate of spread over time, and any management factors that may affect the distributions.
  - **"Infection in animal species"** refers to what kinds of animals are impacted by the influenza virus and the likelihood of human contact with these animals. For example, are influenza infections occurring in wild birds or domestic birds?
  - **"Human infections"** refers to evidence and frequency of human infections with an influenza virus not currently capable of sustained human-to-human transmission. If evidence exists, under what circumstances are human infections occurring? For example, how frequently and easily does transmission occur after direct and prolonged contact between humans and infected animals?

How Are the Influenza Risk Assessment Tools 10 Evaluation Criteria Ranked and Weighted?

Each of the 10 evaluation criteria provided in the IRAT tool is used by influenza experts to generate point scores estimating the potential pandemic risk associated with that criterion. The point scores fall into 3 general classifications of risk: low risk, moderate risk, and high risk.
- **"Low risk"** is associated with a point score between 1 and 3
- **"Moderate risk"** is associated with a point score between 4 to 7
- **"High risk"** is associated with a point score between 8 to 10

Each of the 10 evaluation criteria also is weighted according to importance to each of the 2 scenarios: emergence and public-health impact.

Potential Emergence Risk

The first scenario is: "What is the risk that a novel virus has the potential for sustained human-to-human transmission?" The evaluation criteria may be ranked and weighted as follows (with the first criterion receiving the highest rank and weight score, and the last criterion receiving the lowest rank and weight score).

- Human infections
- Transmission in lab animals
- Receptor binding
- Existing population immunity
- Infection in animal species
- Genomic analysis
- Antigenic relatedness
- Global distribution (animals)
- Disease severity and pathogenesis
- Antiviral treatment options

Potential Impact Risk

The second scenario is: "If the virus were to achieve sustained human-to-human transmission, what is the risk that a novel virus has the potential for significant impact on public health?" The same evaluation criteria could be ranked and weighted as follows (with the first criterion receiving the highest rank and weight score, and the last criterion receiving the lowest rank and weight score).

- Disease severity and pathogenesis
- Existing population immunity
- Human Infections
- Antiviral treatment options
- Antigenic relatedness
- Receptor binding
- Genomic analysis
- Transmission in lab animals
- Global distribution (animals)
- Infection in animal species

Does the Influenza Risk Assessment Tools Get Updated?

In 2018, the CDC Influenza Division coordinated a review of the IRAT with the objectives of identifying any need for updating or replacing evaluation criteria and further refining their definitions for clarity. The review resulted in a confirmation of all 10 evaluation criteria and a refinement of the technical definitions of each criterion. A scored virus was re-evaluated with the updated IRAT as a validation approach. The conclusion of the validation exercise was that the revised IRAT achieved scores similar to the original version, provided risk element definitions of greater clarity, and, therefore, is suitable for future evaluations.

What Influenza Viruses Have Been Assessed Using the Influenza Risk Assessment Tool?

The IRAT is an evaluation tool conceived by the CDC and further developed with assistance from global animal and human health influenza experts. The IRAT is used to assess the potential pandemic risk posed by influenza A viruses that are not currently circulating in people. Input is provided by the U.S. government animal and human health influenza experts.

Does the Influenza Risk Assessment Tool Have Any Limitations?

Yes. The IRAT cannot predict the next pandemic and is not intended to do so. Furthermore, the IRAT is not intended to eliminate the need for subject matter expertise. In fact, subject matter experts are needed to carefully analyze the 10 criteria of the IRAT to make determinations of pandemic risk and to rank the importance of the criteria according to the specific risk question or situation. Lastly, the IRAT is not intended to make exact risk estimates. For example, many risk assessments generate a quantitative measure that describes the likelihood of exposure or disease risk. The IRAT focuses on the perceived pandemic potential of novel influenza viruses as estimated by subject matter experts using the IRAT evaluation criteria and available data.

Section 37.4

Pandemic Severity Assessment Framework

This section includes text excerpted from "Pandemic Severity Assessment Framework (PSAF)," Centers for Disease Control and Prevention (CDC), November 3, 2016. Reviewed January 2020.

Once a novel influenza A virus is identified and is spreading from person-to-person in a sustained manner, public-health officials use the Pandemic Severity Assessment Framework (PSAF) to determine the impact of the pandemic, or how "bad" the pandemic will be. There are two main factors that can be used to determine the impact of a pandemic. The first is clinical severity, or how serious is the illness associated with infection. The second factor is transmissibility, or how easily the pandemic virus spreads from person-to-person. These two factors combined are used to guide decisions about which actions the Centers for Disease Control and Prevention (CDC) recommends at a given time during the pandemic.

The framework is divided into two parts. The first part is the initial assessment, which happens early during a pandemic. At this time, activity may be detected in pockets or certain communities across the country so information and understanding about the pandemic virus will be limited. By studying the information that is available, the CDC can produce a preliminary assessment of the potential impact of the pandemic (e.g., low to moderate transmissibility and moderate to high clinical severity). However, that assessment may change as the pandemic evolves and more information is known.

The results of these assessments can be compared to past pandemics (or even seasonal influenza epidemics), creating a quick comparative snapshot of the potential impact of the pandemic. For example, using the PSAF, the 1918 pandemic can be characterized as one with very high transmissibility and very high clinical severity whereas the 2009 H1N1 pandemic can be characterized as one with moderate transmissibility and clinical severity for the overall population. The results help public-health officials and healthcare professionals make timely and informed decisions, and to take appropriate actions.

The PSAF is one of two assessment tools developed by the CDC to guide and coordinate actions among federal, state, local, and tribal entities involved in pandemic response.

Section 37.5

Allocating and Targeting Pandemic Influenza Vaccine during an Influenza Pandemic

This section includes text excerpted from "Interim Updated Planning Guidance on Allocating and Targeting Pandemic Influenza Vaccine during an Influenza Pandemic," Centers for Disease Control and Prevention (CDC), October 24, 2018.

Effective allocation and administration of the pandemic influenza vaccine will play a critical role in preventing influenza and reducing its effects on health and society during a future pandemic. Although the timing and severity of a future pandemic and characteristics of the next pandemic influenza virus strain are not known, it is important to plan and prepare. The overarching aim of the national pandemic influenza vaccination program is to vaccinate all persons in the United States who choose to be vaccinated, prior to the peak of disease. The U.S. government's goal is to have a sufficient pandemic influenza vaccine available for an effective domestic response within four months of a pandemic declaration. Additionally, plans are to have first doses available within 12 weeks of the President or the Secretary of Health and Human Services declaring a pandemic. To meet these timelines, the U.S. government is investing significant resources to create and evaluate new vaccine development approaches and production technologies. Prepandemic influenza vaccine stockpiles of the bulk vaccine against viruses with pandemic potential are also being established and maintained.

Despite these investments, there are other issues to consider. Stockpiled pandemic vaccine availability will depend on the degree to which they match the circulating pandemic strain and other properties, and manufacturing capacity. In a pandemic, a novel virus has not circulated in humans, and it is assumed that the majority of the population may not have immunity to the virus, causing more people to become ill. Rates of severe illness, complications, and death may be much higher than seasonal flu and more widely distributed. The greater frequency and severity of the disease will increase the burden on the healthcare system, the risk of ongoing transmission in the community, and may increase rates of absenteeism and disruptions in the availability of critical products and services in healthcare and other sectors. Similarly, homeland and national security and critical infrastructure (e.g., transportation and power supply) could be threatened if illness among critical personnel reduces their capabilities.

Given that the influenza vaccine supply will increase incrementally as the vaccine is produced during a pandemic, targeting decisions may have to be made. Such decisions should be based on vaccine supply, pandemic severity and impact, the potential for disruption of community critical infrastructure, operational considerations, and publicly articulated pandemic vaccination program objectives and principles. The overarching objectives guiding vaccine allocation and use during a pandemic are to reduce the impact of the pandemic on health and minimize disruption to society and the economy. Specifically, the targeting strategy aims to protect those who will: maintain homeland and national security, are essential to the pandemic response and provide care for persons who are ill, maintain essential community services, be at greater risk of infection due to their job and those who are most medically vulnerable to severe illness such as young children and pregnant women.

Recognizing that demand may exceed supply at the onset of a pandemic, federal, state, tribal, and local governments, communities, and the private sector have asked for updated planning guidance on who should receive vaccination early in a pandemic.

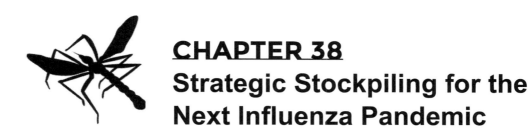

CHAPTER 38
Strategic Stockpiling for the Next Influenza Pandemic

Historical Context

Preparations for the next influenza pandemic have captured a remarkable amount of attention, effort, and fiscal funding since 2004 when the scientific and public-health communities became increasingly concerned about the emergence of a novel influenza virus (H5N1) infecting humans in Eurasia. Many feared the occurrence of an outbreak on the scale of the 1918 to 1919 pandemic, during which one-third of the world's population became infected and as many as 100 million people died.

Numerous guidance documents call for stockpiling certain supplies that might be needed to care for influenza patients during a pandemic. Just-in-time supply chains and standard operating procedures may be insufficient to meet demand as the number of cases increase. Healthcare systems have been challenged to determine the medical supplies that should be procured. Despite the publication of numerous pandemic planning recommendations, little or no guidance has been available about this topic.

In December 2005, the U.S. Department of Veterans Affairs (VA), which has governance over the largest integrated healthcare system in the United States, directed its medical centers to make detailed pandemic

This chapter includes text excerpted from "Stockpiling Supplies for the Next Influenza Pandemic," Centers for Disease Control and Prevention (CDC), July 19, 2010. Reviewed January 2020.

influenza preparations. This directive was ushered in by a guidance document that broadly defined the goals and expectations of individual VA medical centers and provided a framework for planning and preparedness. Steps taken by medical centers, including decisions about stockpiling items, were determined by leaders at the local level.

To help the healthcare system prepare for a pandemic, a multidisciplinary group of experts drawn from the VA system was empaneled to help bridge the gap between policy and procedure. Among the most challenging tasks was the development of a prioritized list detailing supplies and the essential quantities that should be stockpiled. This chapter aims to provide a detailed example of a healthcare system's approach to building a cache of supplies for the next influenza pandemic and to help identify critical gaps in knowledge that must be addressed for adequate preparedness.

Steps toward Preparedness

The 1,400 medical facilities in the national VA healthcare system are decentralized into 23 Veterans Integrated Service Networks (VISNs), each representing a specific region of the nation. The concepts described in this chapter are based on actions taken by staff in VISN 8, which includes southern Georgia, most of Florida, and all of Puerto Rico, and provides healthcare for around 500,000 veterans. Regional network offices help integrate the activities of the medical facilities included in each VISN. Local medical center leaders are primarily responsible for the activities at each hospital and its affiliated outpatient clinics.

Committee Formation

The VISN 8 leadership appointed a multidisciplinary team to a pandemic influenza planning committee (PIPC) that was tasked to ensure a coordinated and consistent planning and response effort across the VISN.

During a pandemic, the first priority would be to provide the best possible care to patients while maximizing healthcare worker safety. Essential and relatively affordable patient care supplies and medications meant for basic life support (e.g., intravenous fluids, oxygen, and antimicrobial drugs) would be purchased first, and more expensive, technologically advanced life support (e.g., mechanical ventilation) equipment would be purchased when additional funds become available. Vaccines and antiviral drugs would not be relied upon as primary means of intervention because their availability and effectiveness during a pandemic remain uncertain. Although plans to acquire, store, distribute, and administer these countermeasures supplies would be made when possible and necessary, these plans would not be relied upon as primary countermeasures in most pandemic scenarios.

Agreeing on Assumptions to Key Questions

The PIPC members recognized that the uncertainty surrounding a pandemic would require a series of assumptions and that any assumption would include some guesswork. To minimize errors, available historical data and guidance from governmental institutions were used to estimate the effect on our healthcare system.

How Many Persons Should We Expect Would Seek Healthcare at Our Facilities?

Most tools estimate the effect on healthcare facilities based on population size, but the research team was dealing with a subpopulation of veterans that may seek care at the VA facilities or at any other community resource. In addition, VA facilities may open their doors to nonveterans during a pandemic. The team decided, arbitrarily, to define their universe of patients as the number of individually enrolled persons who sought care at VA facilities during the previous fiscal year. This figure enabled them to calculate system and facility needs in a standardized fashion.

Once the number of patients was established, they used the U.S. Department of Health and Human Services (HHS) 1918-scale pandemic model and FluSurge version 2.0 software to estimate the number of persons who would be expected to seek care, be hospitalized, admitted to an intensive care unit (ICU), or be treated with mechanical ventilation. The only modification to the DHHS model was in the proportion of the population likely to contract influenza. The model calls for 40 percent disease incidence for children, 20 percent for healthy adults, and a somewhat higher incidence for elderly persons. Therefore, 25 percent seemed a reasonable number for the VA, an institution that does not provide healthcare to children. Calculations were based on the population likely to request care, not on the physical or personnel capacity of the facilities. It was their assertion that physical capacity would be increased and standards of healthcare would be lowered, as necessary, during a pandemic to permit serving as many people as possible. The team did acknowledge that alternate sites of care might become available during a pandemic. However, they viewed this possibility as too unpredictable to include in their assumption model.

What Length of Hospital Stay Would Be Required by the Patients?

Length-of-stay figures were needed to calculate supply needs because resource use is more accurately calculated by patient-days of care instead of a number of admissions. The team used some of the assumptions made by FluSurge version 2.0 as follows: average length of stay (not in ICU) of 5 days per patient, an additional 10 days for those requiring an ICU stay, and an average time receiving mechanical ventilation of 10 days.

What Personal Protective Equipment Would Be Needed to Care for Patients with Pandemic Influenza?

Among the gaps in knowledge regarding pandemic influenza is the mechanism of human-to-human transmission of influenza. The Institute of Medicine's (IOM) recommendation to consider all transmission routes probable and consequential was accepted. Precautions against standard, contact, droplet, and airborne transmission were incorporated into the plan. The team assumed that the sole use of disposable N95 respirators would be prohibitively expensive or otherwise not possible because of global shortages. Instead, they decided that staff with prolonged periods of exposure (e.g., physicians, nurses, respiratory technicians, selected housekeepers) would be issued and that just-in-time fit testing, a reusable elastomeric half-face mask with 3 sets of filters, would be used. They estimated that they would need around 1,000 of these masks and reusable goggles for every 50,000 patients served (on the basis of the size and catchment population of one of their medium-size facilities). Disposable masks would be limited to the beginning of the pandemic and to personnel with infrequent exposure. Using these principles, they calculated the workload, supplies, and medication required to care for typical influenza patients. Accordingly, estimates were produced for the average needs of influenza patients requiring >1 types of services, including outpatient, inpatient medical ward, or ICU settings with or without mechanical ventilation.

Calculating Supply and Medication Needs

The team estimated the per patient encounter needs by staff category and the number of healthcare worker contacts per patient, per day, for each type of healthcare setting. In a similar fashion, supply needs were estimated per patient encounter (for outpatients) or per patient-day of care (for inpatients). The ascertained supply and medication needs were combined in a spreadsheet to estimate the needs of each facility and for their network. Spreadsheet formulas enabled the needs of each facility or healthcare system to be easily modified by using the number of individually enrolled patients.

Prioritizing Supply Needs

Because limited financial resources were available, the PIPC was asked to establish a prioritization scheme. Although every item on the list was considered important, each was subcategorized into purchase priority A, B, and C; A was the most important. To arrive at the category level, the following scheme was used. Category A was personal protective equipment, basic life-support items (intravenous fluids, oxygen), and first-line antimicrobial drugs. Category B was second-line antimicrobial drugs, ventilator supplies, sedatives, nebulizers and β-agonists, home care packs, and morgue packs. Category C was disposable ventilators, proton pump inhibitors, and vasopressors. Antiviral medications and vaccines were not included in this list because it was expected that the VA would acquire and maintain a centralized cache of oseltamivir, and vaccine availability and effectiveness were unknown.

Compromising

The calculated cost of purchasing all essential items for a population of 500,000 amounted to approximately $11 million. Despite efforts to prioritize the items into 3 categories, the calculated cost of category A items far exceeded the funds available. The PIPC debated the best approach and recommended that the available funds be used to purchase a percentage of category A items and that future funds would be used to purchase additional category A items and decreasing percentages of category B and category C items. For example, the funds available at that time were sufficient to purchase 12.5 percent of category A items. Upon the availability of future funding, perhaps an additional 7.5 percent of category A items would be purchased along with 5 percent of category B items and 2.5 percent of category C items.

Ordering Items

Purchasing items in large quantities through a prenegotiated agreement enabled a discount off retail prices. However, despite this contract, back-order delays occurred (and would be expected to occur during a pandemic) for several key items. One supplier of personal protective equipment indicated that shipment would be delayed by six to nine months, affirming predictions of shortages of personal protective equipment. This experience underscored making purchases well in advance of the date when the items were expected to be used for patient care.

Storing Items

Storage of supplies proved to be among the most resource-intensive components of cache-building. Although initial wishes were to store a cache on the campus of each medical center, the space necessary was too large for most VA institutions to accommodate. After extensive discussion and careful analysis of options, a decision was made to store pandemic supplies in a 10,000-square-foot, temperature-controlled, leased warehouse. Quoted costs for space ranged from $10 to $14 per square foot per year ($100,000 to $140,000 per year for 10,000 square feet). The recommended location was near an airport to ensure efficient transport of supplies either by a tractor-trailer or by air cargo. A back-up emergency generator was included to maintain air-conditioning in the event of a power failure.

Many items purchased for the cache had expiration dates. Although most items had multiple-year shelf lives, some shelf lives were as short as one year. The variability of manufacturer-ascribed expiration dates and other reasons for supply rotation led to the recognition that the cache would become a dynamic component of medical system supplies. Items would need to be inspected regularly and rotated through the storage facility on a regular basis. To meet this need, a human resource commitment of one full-time employee equivalent would be necessary for logistics management of the inventory. Duties of this person would include inspecting the inventory, assisting with incoming and outgoing deliveries, rotating items into the routinely used supplies of the medical system to ensure use before expiration, and prodding physical security for the inventory. This person would also be charged with developing and maintaining a plan for transportation and deployment of the inventory in the event of a pandemic. In addition, each medical facility would also be required to provide an employee to help manage the inventory and who would report to the cache in the event of a pandemic.

Summing Up

Despite the numerous uncertainties posed by pandemic influenza, the types and quantities of essential items that should be stockpiled can be estimated by using a reasoned approach. What is offered in this chapter is a method to calculate the components of a stockpile by using assumptions that are drawn from previous pandemics. This method enables the modification of figures, making them scalable and adaptable to any size population. By following the logic of the proposed calculations, it should be possible to modify the assumptions and other figures as needed for almost any community or healthcare system.

CHAPTER 39

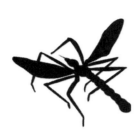

Global Health Security: Prevent, Detect, and Respond to Global Health Threats

Chapter Contents

About Global Health Security

This section includes text excerpted from "About Global
Health Security," Centers for Disease Control and
Prevention (CDC), August 19, 2019.

More than 70 percent of the world remains underprepared to prevent,
detect, and respond to a public-health emergency. Through the Global
Health Security Agenda (GHSA), the Centers for Disease Control
and Prevention (CDC) works with countries to strengthen public-
health systems and contain outbreaks at the source, before they spread
into regional epidemics or global pandemics. Public-health threats,
health emergencies, and infectious diseases do not recognize or respect
boundaries. Effective and functional public-health systems in all countries
reduce the risk and opportunity for health threats to affect the United
States.

What Global Health Security Does

In the fight against infectious diseases, no nation can stand alone. When
it takes less than 36 hours for an outbreak to spread from a remote village
to any major city in the world, protecting everyone's health and national
security means making sure other countries have the knowledge and
resources to stop threats before they can spread beyond their borders.
Together, everyone must build these first lines of defense to better prevent,
detect, and respond to disease.

Protecting Americans' health includes strengthening global health
security. The Division of Global Health Protection (DGHP) leads the
Centers for Disease Control and Prevention (CDC) global health security
efforts, working with the partner countries to help build the core public-
health capacities that are needed to identify and contain outbreaks before
they become epidemics that could affect everyone.

Why Global Health Security Is Important

From avian flu to Zika, to drug-resistant bacteria, the world faces a host of dangerous pathogens and potential epidemics. New diseases, such as the middle-east respiratory syndrome-coronavirus (MERS-CoV) and influenza H7N9, can emerge without warning and quickly spread. In this globally connected world, their effects have unprecedented reach.

A changing world means the risk is greater than ever. The ease of global travel means there are more opportunities for disease to spread; the increasing urbanization of the world means that there is more potential for diseases to emerge and strike in densely populated areas, and the disturbing but real threat of disease used as an instrument of terror requires the nation to have faster, more thorough, and more adaptive capabilities.

Outbreaks can be stopped effectively and lives can be saved, even when the disease is fast-moving and deadly. Investments in core areas of public health have already made a difference in stopping deadly outbreaks, such as Ebola in Nigeria, polio in Mali, yellow fever in Angola, and avian flu in Cameroon. However, across the globe, dangerous gaps in public-health systems still exist. About 70 percent of the world's countries report that they are not fully prepared for an outbreak.

Outbreaks can start anywhere and spread across the globe almost overnight, with devastating results. In 2003, an outbreak of severe acute respiratory syndrome (SARS) infected approximately 8,100 people, killed more than 700, and reached more than two dozen countries, heightening the world's awareness that we must all work together to stop diseases from spreading.

The 2014 to 2016 Ebola epidemic in West Africa is the most recent—and tragic—example of the urgent need for all countries to strengthen their public-health systems. This epidemic was the first time Ebola spread into urban areas, and it reached 10 countries and killed more than 11,000 people before its end, disrupting global travel and trade and costing the world billions. It is estimated that the next global pandemic could cost the world upwards of $60 billion.

How Global Health Security Does It

The Global Health Security Agenda (GHSA) aims to close gaps in preparedness and accelerate progress toward a world safe and secure from infectious disease threats. This work is critical to protecting health in the United States and around the world and is focused on:

- **Disease surveillance and outbreak response,** including establishing routine surveillance for priority diseases and developing information technology tools and systems
- **Emergency management,** ensuring countries have the knowledge and resources they need, including emergency operations centers that can mount a fast, coordinated response when outbreaks happen
- **Safe laboratory systems and diagnostics,** building the capacity to identify disease threats close to the source and inform decision-making
- **Developing the workforce,** training frontline responders, laboratorians, disease detectives, emergency managers, and other health professionals who are responsible for taking the lead when crisis strikes

Building global health security cannot be accomplished alone. Key CDC programs; other U.S. government agencies; ministries of health; and international organizations, all of them are involved to accomplish global health security goals. World-class experts from across the CDC are sent into the field, where they share knowledge and gain on-the-ground experience that better prepares us to handle health threats at home in the United States. They build on the work already being done in countries to be as efficient and effective as possible.

Section 39.2

Why Global Health Security Matters

This section includes text excerpted from "Why Global Health Security Matters," Centers for Disease Control and Prevention (CDC), February 13, 2014. Reviewed January 2020.

Disease Threats Can Spread Faster and More Unpredictably than Ever Before

People are traveling more. Food and medical product supply chains stretch across the globe. Biological threats (such as Middle-East respiratory syndrome coronavirus, or MERS-CoV) and drug-resistant illnesses pose a growing danger to people everywhere, whether diseases are naturally occurring, intentionally produced, or the result of a laboratory accident. Nowadays in this interconnected world, poorly treated cases of tuberculosis (TB) or pneumonia in Asia and Africa have shown up in U.S. hospitals within days.

Emerging global disease threats have created the opportunity to forge new global solutions such as the International Health Regulations (IHR), signed by all 194 member states of the World Health Organization (WHO). Substantial investments have been made to combat infectious disease threats. There is a greater global health security capacity than ever before.

Global Health Security Provides Protection from Infectious Disease Threats

A disease threat anywhere can mean a threat everywhere. It is defined by:

- The emergence and spread of new microbes
- Globalization of travel and trade
- Rise of drug resistance
- The potential use of laboratories to make and release—intentionally or not—dangerous microbes

As dangerous new threats are emerging, familiar microbes (such as TB) are becoming resistant to drugs that once kept them at bay. There are strains of organisms spreading that are resistant to most available antibiotics. Nowadays, in communities across the United States, someone in a nursing home or a hospital is fighting an infection that doctors have limited or no tools to treat. The Global Health Security (GHS) initiative will lead to earlier detection and more effective control of these resistant germs before they spread to the United States.

Global Health Security Is Economically Smart

Countries better insulated from disease threats mean safer environments for Americans to travel to and do business. Healthier countries are more stable and prosperous—they are more viable trading partners.

Pandemic disease threats and ineffective responses can have a devastating impact on public health and the global economy.

- Severe acute respiratory syndrome (SARS) cost $30 billion in only 4 months. GHS means safer nations, more stable economies, and fewer failed states.
- Acquired immunodeficiency syndrome (AIDS) has imposed an economic burden worldwide and has taken an especially heavy toll in low-income countries. A sizeable portion of that cost is a result of AIDS spreading silently for decades before detection and response.
- Pandemic influenza can cause rapid and widespread death and disruption, stressing commerce and national economies.

Global Health Security Strengthens Public-Health Systems

The Centers for Disease Control and Prevention (CDC) strengthens other global health programs—such as maternal and child health, flu prevention, and immunization—through the cross-cutting global health security activities around the world. These activities include helping build better lab systems; create faster and more accurate data sharing; establish and improve emergency operations centers that can respond more quickly to all public-health crises, and support nationwide surveillance systems that enable real-time disease tracking and reporting.

Section 39.3

The Global Health Security Agenda

This section includes text excerpted from "The Global Health Security Agenda," Centers for Disease Control and Prevention (CDC), January 27, 2016. Reviewed January 2020.

In partnership with the U.S. government sister agencies, other nations, international organizations, and public and private stakeholders, the Centers for Disease Control and Prevention (CDC) seeks to accelerate progress toward a world safe and secure from infectious disease threats and to promote global health security as an international security priority, to:

- Prevent and reduce the likelihood of outbreaks—natural, accidental, or intentional
- Detect threats early to save lives
- Respond rapidly and effectively using multi-sectoral, international coordination and communication

The United States will work with partner countries on nine specific objectives to prevent, detect, and effectively respond to infectious disease threats.

Prevent

- Prevent the emergence and spread of antimicrobial drug-resistant organisms and emerging zoonotic diseases, and strengthen international regulatory frameworks governing food safety.

- Promote national biosafety and biosecurity systems.
- Reduce the number and magnitude of infectious disease outbreaks.

This is achieved through the following objectives:
- Preventing the emergence and spread of drug-resistant microbes and emerging zoonotic diseases and strengthening international regulatory frameworks governing food safety:
  - Act to reduce the individual and institutional factors that enable antimicrobial resistance and the emergence of disease threats that move from animals to humans. These are known as "zoonotic diseases."
  - Increase surveillance and early detection of drug-resistant microorganisms and novel zoonotic diseases
  - Strengthen supply chains
  - Promote safe practices in livestock production and the marketing of animals
  - Promote the appropriate and responsible use of antibiotics in all settings, including developing strategies to improve food safety
- Promoting national biosafety and biosecurity systems
  - Promote the development of ways for countries to manage biological materials needed for diagnosis, research, and biosurveillance. This effort involves identifying, securing, safety monitoring, and storing dangerous microbes in a minimal number of facilities. It is also necessary to advance safe and responsible conduct for handling microbes.
- Reducing the number and magnitude of infectious disease outbreaks
  - Establish effective programs for vaccination against epidemic-prone diseases and infection control in hospitals.

Detect
- Launch, strengthen and link global networks for real-time biosurveillance.
- Strengthen the global norm of rapid, transparent reporting and sample sharing.

- Develop and deploy novel diagnostics and strengthen laboratory systems.
- Train and deploy an effective biosurveillance workforce.

Respond

- Develop an interconnected global network of Emergency Operations Centers (EOC) and multisectoral response to biological incidents.
- Improve global access to medical and nonmedical countermeasures during health emergencies.

This is achieved through the following objectives:
- Developing an interconnected global network of Emergency Operations Centers and multisectoral response to biological incidents:
  - Promote the establishment of emergency operations centers
  - Create/strengthen trained, functioning, multi-sectoral rapid response teams with access to a real-time information system and capacity to attribute the source of an outbreak
- Improving global access to medical and nonmedical countermeasures during health emergencies:
  - Strengthen capacity to produce or procure personal protective equipment, medications, vaccines, and technical expertise
  - Enhance capacity to plan for and deploy nonmedical countermeasures
  - Strengthen policies and operational frameworks to share public and animal health and medical personnel and countermeasures with partners

Section 39.4

International Health Regulations: Enhancing Global Health Capacity

This section includes text excerpted from "International Health Regulations (IHR)," Centers for Disease Control and Prevention (CDC), August 19, 2019.

With the signing of the revised International Health Regulations (IHR) in 2005, the international community agreed to improve the detection and reporting of potential public-health emergencies worldwide. IHR (2005) better addresses global health security concerns and is a critical part of protecting global health. The regulations require that all countries have the ability to detect, assess, report and respond to public-health events.

The Centers for Disease Control and Prevention (CDC) is working with countries around the globe to help meet IHR (2005) goals. The CDC's global programs address over 400 diseases, health threats, and conditions that are major causes of death, disease, and disability. These global programs are run by world leaders in epidemiology, surveillance, informatics, laboratory systems, and other essential disciplines. Through partnerships with other countries' ministries of health, the CDC is improving the quantity and quality of critical public-health services.

About International Health Regulations
International Health Regulations Basics

With trade and travel expanding on a global level, the opportunity for greater disease transmission also increases. The public health and economic impact due to infectious diseases can cause great harm to humans and severely damage a country's resources. IHR (2005) is coordinated by the World Health Organization (WHO) and aims to keep the world informed about public-health risks and events. As an international treaty, the IHR (2005) is legally binding; all countries must report events of international public-health importance. Countries reference IHR (2005) to determine how to prevent and control global health threats while keeping international travel and trade as open as possible.

International Health Regulations (2005) requires that all countries have the ability to do the following:

- **Detect:** Make sure surveillance systems and laboratories can detect potential threats
- **Assess:** Work together with other countries to make decisions in public-health emergencies
- **Report:** Report specific diseases, plus any potential international public health emergencies, through participation in a network of National Focal Points (NFP)
- **Respond:** Respond to public-health events

The IHR (2005) also includes specific measures countries can take at ports, airports and ground crossings to limit the spread of health risks to neighboring countries, and to prevent unwarranted travel and trade restrictions.

International Health Regulations: Made for Today's Health Threats

In an interconnected society, it is more important than ever to make sure all countries are able to respond to and contain public-health threats.

In 2003, severe acute respiratory syndrome (SARS) threatened global health, showing us how easily an outbreak can spread. Recently, the Ebola epidemic in West Africa and outbreaks of Middle East respiratory syndrome-coronavirus (MERS-CoV) have shown that people are only as safe as the most fragile state. All countries have a responsibility to one another to build healthcare systems that are strong and that work to identify and contain public-health events before they spread.

While previous regulations required countries to report incidents of cholera, plague, and yellow fever, IHR (2005) is more flexible and future-oriented, requiring countries to consider the possible impact of all hazards, whether they occur naturally, accidentally, or intentionally. In spite of broader global agreement to the importance of IHR (2005), only about 1/3 of the countries in the world currently have the ability to assess, detect, and respond to public-health emergencies. These gaps in global preparedness leave Americans and the rest of the world vulnerable.

And global health security is not just a health issue; a crisis such as SARS or Ebola can devastate economies and keep countries from developing. The World Bank Group estimates that Guinea, Liberia, and Sierra Leone together would have lost at least $1.6 billion in foregone economic growth in 2015 as a result of the Ebola epidemic. The impact of this kind of economic devastation reaches farther and wider than ever.

Protecting People

One of the most important aspects of IHR (2005) is the requirement that countries detect and report events that may constitute a potential public-health emergency of international concern (PHEIC).

Under IHR (2005), a PHEIC is declared by the WHO if the situation meets two of four criteria:

- Is the public-health impact of the event serious?
- Is the event unusual or unexpected?
- Is there a significant risk of international spread?
- Is there a significant risk of international travel or trade restrictions?

Once a WHO member country identifies an event of concern, the country must assess the public-health risks of the event within 48 hours. If the event is determined to be notifiable under the IHR, the country must report the information to WHO within 24 hours.

Some diseases always require reporting under the IHR, no matter when or where they occur, while others become notifiable when they represent an unusual risk or situation.

Always notifiable:

- Smallpox
- Poliomyelitis due to wild-type poliovirus
- Human influenza caused by a new subtype
- SARS

Other potentially notifiable events:
- May include cholera, pneumonic plague, yellow fever, viral hemorrhagic fever, and West Nile fever, as well as any others that meet the criteria laid out by the IHR
- Other biological, radiological, or chemical events that meet IHR criteria

Since IHR (2005) was put into place, four PHEICs have been declared by WHO:
- H1N1 influenza (2009)
- Polio (2014)
- Ebola (2014)
- Zika virus (2016)

When a PHEIC is declared, the WHO helps coordinate an immediate response with the affected country and with other countries around the world.

Global International Health Regulations Participation

The IHR represents an agreement between 196 countries, including all WHO the Member States, to work together for global health security.

In the United States, the CDC works with state and local reporting and response networks to receive information at the federal level and then respond to events of concern at the local and federal levels. The U.S Department of Health and Human Services (HHS) has assumed the lead role in carrying out the reporting requirements for IHR (2005). The Health and Human Services' Secretary's Operations Center (SOC) is the National Focal Point (NFP) responsible for reporting events to WHO. The CDC works with other federal agencies to support IHR (2005) implementation.

Monitoring and Evaluation Framework
How to Assess Health Security Capacity

Being adequately prepared to manage these infectious disease outbreaks is a challenge for many countries. The IHR (2005) Monitoring and Evaluation

Framework (MEF) provides a roadmap for assessing a country's health security capacity, enabling them to identify areas for improvement.

The IHR MEF is composed of four processes:

- States Parties Self-Assessment Annual Reporting (SPAR)
- Joint External Evaluations (JEE)
- After Action Reviews (AAR)
- Simulation Exercises (SimEx)

The SPAR is a mandatory process under IHR (2005); the JEE, AAR, and SimEx are voluntary. Together, these provide a comprehensive approach to assessing a country's health security capacity and developing recommendations for how to address associated gaps.

Additionally, results of the JEE and other country-based assessments can be used to guide the development of National Action Plans for Health Security (NAPHS). The NAPHS aims to address gaps in a country's health security capacity through a system that aligns with the JEE's recommendations.

When used together, these processes can help governments improve their preparedness against infectious disease threats, gain domestic support for health security work, and direct partners to the areas where more support is needed. To support IHR MEF activities within countries, the CDC serves as a major contributor to global public-health efforts to prevent, detect, and respond to public-health risks.

Joint External Evaluation

The joint external evaluation (JEE) is a voluntary and comprehensive process to evaluate country capacity across 19 technical areas, to address infectious disease risks through a coordinated response.

The JEE process brings together experts from around the world to help a country assess its strengths and weaknesses and identify recommendations to improve its health security capacity. Multisectoral collaboration, through processes, such as the JEE, is key to strengthening health systems—this means engaging not just health partners, but other government sectors, such as environmental, agricultural, defense, and finance.

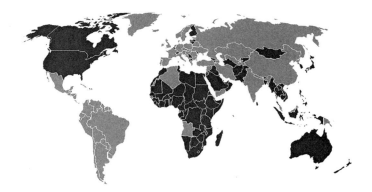

Figure 39.1. Joint External Evaluation Countries Map

Through the JEE, countries are able to:
• Identify the most critical gaps within their health systems
• Prioritize opportunities for enhanced preparedness and response
• Engage with current and prospective donors and partners to effectively target resources

The CDC has collaborated with WHO on developing and refining the JEE process and tools since its inception in 2016. As of July 2019, 100 JEEs have been completed, representing over half of the UN member states that committed to achieving the goals of the IHR 2005. The CDC has provided assistance in over 60 percent of the JEEs conducted throughout the world and helps countries who have completed this process translates JEE findings and recommendations into action.

Joint Assessments Map

After a JEE is completed, the external experts work with their country counterparts to produce a written report, which includes the scores and all-important priority actions. This section serves as a guide for the country on how to build health security capacity within each technical area. The associated priority actions can feed directly into a National Action Plan for Health Security (NAPHS) and other post-JEE planning processes. JEE

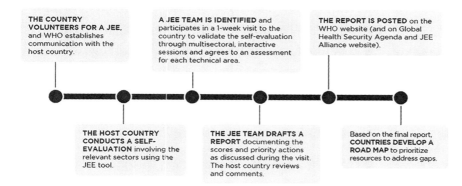

THE COUNTRY VOLUNTEERS FOR A JEE, and WHO establishes communication with the host country.

A JEE TEAM IS IDENTIFIED and participates in a 1-week visit to the country to validate the self-evaluation through multisectoral, interactive sessions and agrees to an assessment for each technical area.

THE REPORT IS POSTED on the WHO website (and on Global Health Security Agenda and JEE Alliance website).

THE HOST COUNTRY CONDUCTS A SELF-EVALUATION involving the relevant sectors using the JEE tool.

THE JEE TEAM DRAFTS A REPORT documenting the scores and priority actions as discussed during the visit. The host country reviews and comments.

Based on the final report, COUNTRIES DEVELOP A ROAD MAP to prioritize resources to address gaps.

Figure 39.2. Joint External Evaluation Process

results are also published online so that partners can work with countries in a more coordinated fashion to address health security gaps.

Section 39.5
Zoonotic Disease Programs for Enhancing Global Health Security

This section includes text excerpted from "Zoonotic Disease Programs for Enhancing Global Health Security," Centers for Disease Control and Prevention (CDC), November 20, 2017.

Zoonotic disease pathogens such as rabies virus have been causing outbreaks in humans for thousands of years. In fact, most infectious diseases in humans originate in animals, and the frequency of such transmissions has been increasing over time. Researchers have found that 75 percent of emerging infectious organisms pathogenic to humans are zoonotic in origin. The zoonotic diseases include globally devastating diseases such as Ebola virus disease (EVD), Middle-East respiratory syndrome (MERS), highly pathogenic avian influenza, severe acute respiratory syndrome (SARS), and bovine spongiform encephalopathy (BSE). These and other zoonotic diseases affect many countries, resulting in high morbidity and mortality rates in humans and animals, cause disruptions of regional and global trade, and strain national and global public-health resources. Newly emerging health threats are associated with substantial economic costs, including direct and indirect impacts on the healthcare system, costs associated with the actual response, and overall disruption of economic activity.

The World Bank estimated that six major zoonotic disease epidemics from 1997 to 2009 resulted in an economic loss of >$80 billion. Experiences from most recent outbreaks indicate that detecting and effectively responding to emerging epidemics requires a multisectoral approach. In 2010, recognizing the need for multidisciplinary collaboration to address health threats at the human-animal–ecosystem interface, the World Health Organization (WHO), Food and Agriculture Organization (FAO), and World Organisation for Animal Health (OIE) formalized their collaboration and identified three priority areas of work together, two of which are zoonotic diseases (rabies and zoonotic influenza). Endemic zoonotic diseases have the dual impact of causing illness and death in humans and animals as well as substantial economic loss in resource-poor societies where livestock farming is a major engine of economic growth at the household and national levels. Fortunately, proven control and prevention strategies exist for many zoonotic diseases that are most prevalent in affected communities (e.g., rabies, anthrax, brucellosis).

To better prevent, detect, and respond to global infectious disease threats, the U.S. government and other partners developed the Global Health Security Agenda (GHSA) with initial implementation in one country in Africa and Asia in 17 phases. GHSA is intended to make progress in the implementation of WHO International Health Regulations, the Office of Indian Education (OIE) Veterinary Services Pathway, and other similar frameworks for achieving an adequate level of preparedness to tackle emerging-health threats in animals and humans. To build the necessary infrastructure and human capital, the U.S. government and global partners allocated funds to advance GHSA across 11 action packages that included zoonotic diseases. This section describes specific steps to prevent, detect, and respond to endemic zoonotic diseases and how to leverage them to detect and effectively respond to emerging and re-emerging zoonotic health threats, and thereby enhance global health security. Some of the steps have been implemented in several GHSA phase 1 countries.

Approaches for One Health Zoonotic Disease Program Implementation

Mitigating the impact of endemic and emerging zoonotic diseases of public-health importance requires multisectoral collaboration and interdisciplinary partnerships. Collaborations across sectors relevant to zoonotic diseases, particularly among human and animal (domestic and wildlife) health disciplines, are essential for quantifying the burden of zoonotic diseases, detecting and responding to endemic and emerging zoonotic pathogens, prioritizing the diseases of greatest public-health concern, and effectively launching appropriate prevention, detection, and response strategies. Multisectoral approaches under a One Health umbrella are more expedient and effective and lead to efficient utilization of limited resources.

Prioritization of Zoonotic Diseases

Developing strategies to prevent, detect, and respond to zoonotic diseases is challenging in resource-poor settings where there are other competing public-health priorities. In addition, effective mitigation of their impact requires multi-sectoral collaborations and interdisciplinary partnerships that may take time to establish. Therefore, having all relevant sectors jointly identify zoonotic diseases of greatest concern is an essential first step for many countries. Multi-sectoral partnerships are easier to create if participants from multiple sectors, including humans, animals (domestic and wildlife), and environmental health develop a prioritized list of zoonotic diseases to work on together and commit to sharing public- and animal-health resources. Engagement of different sectors early in the process facilitates collaboration during program implementation and ensures program ownership. In addition, systems developed to address the prioritized diseases can be leveraged to tackle other zoonotic infections and emerging health threats.

To help identify high-priority zoonotic diseases for multi-sectoral engagement, the One Health office at the Centers for Disease Control and Prevention (CDC) developed the One Health Zoonotic Disease Prioritization tool, a semiquantitative tool for prioritization with equal input from represented sectors, irrespective of whether reliable surveillance data are available. The tool is designed to bring together a multidisciplinary team of professionals from the human, animal, and environmental-health agencies and other relevant sectors with a common goal of developing country-specific criteria for ranking zoonotic diseases of greatest national concern. The tool has been used to select zoonotic diseases for further programmatic activity in multiple countries in the implementation of the zoonotic disease action package of GHSA. Typically, the prioritization is performed by trained facilitators during a workshop with voting members from multiple ministries covering human, animal, and environmental health and from multinational organizations (e.g., FAO, WHO, OIE), academic institutions, and other partners working in the area of zoonotic diseases (e.g., the CDC, U.S. Agency for International Development (USAID)). The country's government ministries should select participants. In countries that have conducted prioritization workshops, the CDC provided training to in-country workshop facilitators to promote country ownership of the process. Minimizing the role of external facilitators helps to retain objectivity in the process and allow decision making by the host country representatives.

Assessing the Burden of Zoonotic Diseases

Accurately estimating the burden of zoonotic diseases is a critical step in both identifying public- and animal-health priorities and assessing the impact of prevention and control strategies, including potential economic effects on the food supply, such as with avian and swine influenza viruses. Metrics for human zoonotic disease burden may include numbers of cases of illness, hospitalizations, deaths, disability, or quality-adjusted life years, and economic impacts such as healthcare-associated costs and lost productivity.

Some of these metrics can also be used to assess animal health burden. In countries where zoonotic disease data may not be readily available, the burden of different zoonotic diseases could be better ascertained by conducting studies in selected regions. Such studies may focus on zoonotic diseases selected in the prioritization process or diseases that are deemed more prevalent on the basis of limited epidemiologic or clinical data. Estimation of disease burden should involve studies in humans and affected or implicated animal species. Conducting ecologic and wildlife studies may be necessary to define risk to humans from selected zoonotic pathogens in animal reservoirs or arthropod vectors. Investigators should consider using existing databases or laboratory specimens, such as banked sera collected as part of human immunodeficiency virus (HIV) indicator surveys, to quantify the potential risks to humans of some zoonotic diseases.

Zoonotic Disease Surveillance in Animals and Humans

Rapid and effective response to endemic and emerging zoonotic diseases relies heavily on timely and efficient surveillance and reporting system. Surveillance in animals and humans is critical for early identification and possible prediction of future outbreaks, allowing for preemptive action. Components of effective surveillance include establishing event-based and indicator-based surveillance, and adequate laboratory capacity in both public health and animal health laboratory systems. Training epidemiologists and the establishment of effective laboratory systems are critical for a successful zoonotic disease surveillance program.

An effective surveillance system may require the following: standard case definitions for priority zoonotic diseases under surveillance, based on existing guidance from global human and animal health organizations such as WHO, CDC, HIV, and FAO; evaluation of existing national surveillance systems to determine their timeliness, effectiveness, and usefulness; new or refined surveillance and reporting systems and linkages to share data between public-health and animal-health agencies and other relevant sectors; evaluation of potential electronic disease reporting mechanisms, including the use of smartphone technologies; establishment of surveillance data dissemination platforms (which may include regular reports and publications) to provide awareness and feedback to human and animal health agencies and other stakeholders; evaluation of available diagnostic tests and appropriate testing capabilities in central and regional public-health and animal-health laboratories; and establishment of a national emergency-management system, such as an Emergency Operations Center (EOC), to assist in coordinated-zoonotic disease surveillance, response to zoonotic disease outbreaks, and prevention and control efforts across relevant sectors.

Laboratory Systems

Timely, accurate, and reliable laboratory tests are critical for building outbreak response capacities, identify etiologies of disease, and to monitor endemic and emerging zoonotic diseases in humans, domestic and food animals, and wildlife. Well-functioning and separate national public health and animal health laboratory systems are essential to identify etiologic agents so that appropriate prevention, detection, and response strategies can be implemented. Laboratories should be an integral part of the public-health infrastructure with a system for rapid testing of prioritized samples and timely sharing of results. Successful and sustainable laboratory systems require strategic interagency planning across sectors and building on existing capacities in the country to standardize laboratory methods, prioritize laboratory resources, and develop information-sharing channels. A requirement for ensuring testing quality is the commitment from the top levels of management to provide the necessary resources to sustain the functional roles of the laboratory in an environment that supports quality and safety. The roles and responsibilities of all human and animal laboratory staff need to be defined, documented and communicated, and written policies and procedures should be available and understood. In addition, all laboratory staff should be trained on these policies and procedures to ensure they are executed in a consistent and reliable manner. Accurate and reliable test results depend on having a sample that has been collected, stored, and transported correctly; sample requirements vary by the disease and suspected pathogen. Laboratories should be designed to optimize workflow, support the quality of testing, and protect the safety of laboratory staff and the community. Regularly conducted proficiency testing helps to monitor the quality and performance of the laboratory.

Critical human and animal laboratory systems that countries need to establish or expand include central and regional laboratory capacity; specimen referral systems for rapid, safe, and reliable specimen transport; laboratory training programs that promote workforce development and retention; and affordable, flexible laboratory accreditation schemes to ensure lab quality. Opportunities for mentoring relationships with reference laboratories or private partnerships should be encouraged. Laboratories may assist in determining disease burden and characterization of human, animal, and ecologic drivers of disease spillover from animals to humans to optimize models for predicting disease emergence (e.g., risk mapping).

Outbreak Response Using One Health Approach

A successful zoonotic disease outbreak response requires:

- The ability to detect the outbreak using established surveillance systems including event-based reporting
- Adequate laboratory capability to confirm the outbreak etiology
- A workforce trained to respond and perform descriptive and analytical epidemiology for animal and human diseases
- The ability to implement appropriate control and prevention measures
- Outbreak and emergency-management system in place to coordinate multisectoral response activities at the national to subnational levels

The involvement of all relevant stakeholders is crucial, including those in human, animal, and environmental health sectors. Outbreak response activities are best supported by an overarching operations framework that clearly identifies the roles and responsibilities of key institutions and officials for all relevant sectors and provides direction for coordination of activities at the local and national levels. Countries should establish functional cross-sector coordination and communication pathways before an outbreak occurs. Multisectoral collaboration is easier during an emergency if agencies had already been collaborating in joint priority-setting and actively working together to address prioritized zoonotic diseases.

Early detection of an impending human outbreak may in some instances be achieved through the detection of an increase in disease in animal populations, such as livestock and wildlife populations. Detection of an outbreak or an increase in a case count of a zoonotic disease by the wildlife, livestock, or public-health agency should trigger enhanced surveillance by the other agencies. This detection can only occur if there is effective communication between the different sectors. Outbreak response protocols or national strategies should be developed for priority zoonotic diseases that specifically address coordination of activities, data sharing (including how to integrate animal, human, and environmental health information), trigger points or threshold for action, and roles and responsibilities of each stakeholder. Establishing joint training opportunities for animal and human-health workers will facilitate information sharing and enhance collaboration for effective prevention, detection, and response programs. When possible, joint simulation exercises can be conducted to demonstrate the proficiency of response and adequate interagency and multisectoral collaboration.

Prevention and Control of Zoonotic Diseases

The prevention and control strategies of zoonotic diseases will vary by disease and the availability of proven interventions. Some of the zoonotic diseases most prevalent in resource-limited areas are vaccine-preventable (e.g., rabies, brucellosis, anthrax). Therefore, the implementation of routine immunization programs may be needed for disease prevention. Depending on the disease, this may be primarily human vaccination or vaccination of livestock or other domestic animals. For some diseases, such as highly pathogenic avian influenza, prevention and control may involve large-scale culling and effective biosecurity programs. For diseases, such as anthrax and rabies, preemptive vaccination of animals will prevent outbreaks in the animal population while at the same time protecting humans. In others (e.g., Rift Valley fever (RVF)), disease outbreaks in animals may be the first signal to start the implementation of prevention programs such as ring vaccination of animals. Waiting until an outbreak is detected in humans can be costly to the lives of animals and humans and can strain limited public-health resources.

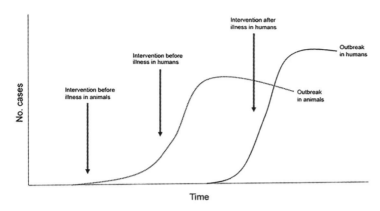

Figure 39.3. Opportunities for Intervention to Prevent and Control Endemic and Emerging Zoonotic Diseases

Effective human and animal disease surveillance systems are critical for early detection and response, for planning prevention and control programs, and to evaluate the effectiveness of control and prevention strategies. Timely and effective communication and collaboration between human- and animal-health agencies are essential to developing disease prevention and control strategies involving both human and animal populations. As part of an effective response, countries should consider developing and evaluating communication strategies to educate human and animal healthcare providers and the general population on zoonotic disease transmission and prevention. Community education programs may include safe farming and biosecurity measures, animal slaughtering practices, understanding animal contact, and exposure risks, and use of personal prevention measures to avoid or reduce exposure to vector-borne and other zoonotic diseases. Livestock and poultry are key sources of food and livelihood, and important economically for trade; prevention strategies that target zoonotic diseases associated with food animals must be compatible with the needs of the communities that are economically dependent on those animals.

Communicating effectively regarding prevention strategies will also enhance engagement in future outbreak control efforts because the communities will better understand the reasons behind any intervention.

Similarly, a well-informed population can serve as an early alert system, notifying appropriate authorities about possible cases of the disease in humans or animals. For zoonotic diseases with potential domestic and food animal reservoirs, important strategies in disease control can include animal vaccination, vector control, test and treat, or cull programs, and effective biosecurity measures. The development and implementation of cost-effectiveness and cost-benefit models to evaluate and refine disease prevention and control methods and programs will ensure effective use of resources; evaluations may include the negative effects culling has on societal well-being and livelihood of farmers.

Research Conclusion

Effective zoonotic disease prevention, detection, and response require close collaboration, including well-defined roles and responsibilities among the animal, human, and environmental health sectors. Such collaborations can help reduce illness and deaths in animals and humans and minimize their social and economic impact at the household and national levels. In most countries, animal health and human health decision-makers are located within different ministries. Establishing multisectoral One Health partnerships across agencies and with interdisciplinary personnel at the national, subnational, and local levels (including government departments responsible for health, agriculture, veterinary services, environment, and laboratories) can strengthen zoonotic disease detection and response activities. These structures must be in place before an outbreak, epidemic, or pandemic occurs to have an effective, coordinated public- and animal-health response. Countries that lack a well-functioning coordination mechanism could fail to rapidly detect and effectively respond to emerging health threats, which could spread to other countries and threaten global health security.

Countries should consider convening regular cross-sectoral meetings to build multi-sectoral and interdisciplinary relationships, encourage transparency, and combine efforts across agencies. Developing mutually agreed-upon standard operating procedures is essential. Identifying designated points of contact ensures improved coordination across sectors, allowing for a quicker collaborative response to zoonotic disease outbreaks. Additional benefits of establishing a formal, multisectoral coordination mechanism include identifying high-priority research areas and developing training opportunities for interdisciplinary outbreak response teams. Multisectoral collaborations should also be established at subnational levels. Identifying One Health focal points at the local, district, and regional levels are critical and the list of these designated contacts should be shared among sectors. These approaches will enhance cross-sectoral utilization of limited resources while leveraging each sector's capabilities for improved prevention, detection, and the response of zoonotic diseases.

In some countries, formal, national collaborative One Health coordinating mechanisms were established to facilitate multi-sectoral engagement. Examples include the Zoonotic Disease Unit in Kenya, the Zoonotic Disease Secretariat in Cameroon, and the Guidelines for Coordinated Prevention and Control of Zoonotic Diseases in Vietnam. The creation of such mechanisms with dedicated financial and human resources will facilitate outbreak detection and response, prevention and control of high-priority endemic zoonotic diseases, and early detection and response to emerging health threats. They also allow countries to develop shared visions to maximize impact and build in measurements for success and help design an overall plan for the sustainability of cross-sectoral collaborations.

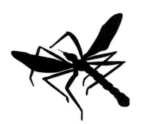

CHAPTER 40
A Look Back at Progress since the 2009 H1N1 Pandemic

In 2009, a novel H1N1 influenza (flu) virus emerged to cause the first flu pandemic in 40 years. The 2009 H1N1 pandemic was estimated to be associated with 151,700 to 575,400 deaths worldwide during the first year it circulated. This H1N1 virus has continued to circulate seasonally to this day. The Centers for Disease Control and Prevention (CDC) and its many partners have made great strides in the fields of influenza surveillance, prevention, and treatment since 2009, benefiting both the annual response to seasonal flu epidemics, as well as the global capacity to respond to the next pandemic.

Gene Sequencing Technology

During the pandemic, owing in part to the preparedness work done prior to 2009, the CDC and public-health laboratories were able to use molecular testing technology, "with its pinpoint accuracy and revolutionary speed" to detect cases, and monitor the spread of the virus and its characteristics, including watching for emerging drug resistance, for example. In the wake of the 2009 pandemic, numerous retrospective analyses deemed the use of this technology to be one of the response's key successes.

This chapter includes text excerpted from "Ten Years of Gains: A Look Back at Progress Since the 2009 H1N1 Pandemic," Centers for Disease Control and Prevention (CDC), July 31, 2019.

Since the pandemic, the CDC's ability to map the complete influenza virus genome has improved exponentially, thanks to considerable leaps forward in gene sequencing technology, sometimes referred to as Next Generation Sequencing or Advanced Molecular Detection (AMD) technology. Where previous technologies revealed the genes of the predominant influenza virus in a respiratory specimen, it is now possible to see the gene sequences of all of the influenza particles in a single specimen, thereby giving deeper insight into how influenza viruses may change, for example, by mutating inside a single patient to become resistant to antiviral drugs.

In 2012 the CDC's influenza laboratory transitioned from a characterization-first approach to a sequence-first approach so now all flu viruses undergo full sequencing as a first step when they arrive at the CDC. This change has reduced public-health response time to flu outbreaks and also served to greatly expand the global repositories of influenza gene sequence data. Meanwhile, ongoing technological improvements by device manufacturers and the CDC's innovative protocols have brought the gene sequencing cost per virus down from about $180.00 in 2012 to $25.00 per virus in 2019, with additional improvements in the works to bring the cost down even further.

In 2009, the CDC sequenced influenza virus genomes primarily for the identification of vaccine reference viruses. Now, the CDC performs "next-generation sequencing" on close to 7,000 influenza viruses annually, and has submitted more than 30,000 flu virus genomes to public databases.

Influenza Public-Health Laboratory Tests
Reverse Transcription-Polymerase Chain Reaction

Since 2009, the widespread adoption by public-health laboratories of the testing technique called "real-time Reverse transcription-polymerase Chain Reaction" (rRT-PCR) with the CDC's flu rRT-PCR test kits has directly enhanced the nation's pandemic preparedness in a number of ways. For one, the widespread use of both has led to the standardization of influenza testing across the nation's public health laboratories. Relative to the other diagnostic methods widely used by laboratories to reveal the type and subtype of flu virus in a sample, rRT-PCR produces more-reliable results and produces those results faster than most other laboratory techniques.

The CDC's primary rRT-PCR test for influenza viruses (called the "CDC Human Influenza Virus Real-Time RT-PCR Diagnostic Panel") is an internationally recognized reference method for the detection of influenza. This means the performance of other detection methods is often measured against the performance of the CDC's rRT-PCR flu test.

The adaptability of the rRT-PCR test allows laboratories to quickly adjust how specimens are processed in outbreak and pandemic situations to avoid backlogs and unnecessary use of resources. The CDC provides algorithms that help to ensure that as more specimens are tested, reagents are conserved, thereby maximizing their public-health benefit and further reducing the possibility of supply shortages.

Although laboratories have the option of using other rRT-PCR tests, the use of the CDC test in lieu of commercially manufactured rRT-PCR tests takes the pressure off individual laboratories of ensuring their tests are able to detect the newest emerging viruses.

The CDC uses gene sequence data to update its influenza diagnostic kits and reagents, which are used around the world by public-health laboratories as the gold-standard for detecting influenza, in large part because of the CDC's rapid response in updating the kits and reagents each time a novel virus emerges. For example, in 2012 the United States. experienced a rapid uptick in human infections with swine influenza viruses (called "variant virus infections") associated with exposure to infected pigs. The CDC quickly confirmed the CDC rRT-PCR test kit's ability to detect those swine viruses appearing in people, and then issued guidance to laboratories on how to interpret rRT-PCR test results when testing specimens from patients with known pig exposure. Since then, the CDC has monitored how the diagnostic kit has performed in detecting variant infections and has updated guidance and virus-specific assay materials (called "reagents") to make sure the tests are able to detect these viruses as they have evolved.

In April 2013, shortly after the first influenza A(H7N9) human infections in China were reported and within days of China the CDC sharing gene sequences of the H7N9 virus, U.S. CDC quickly modified and then quality-checked the CDC's existing H7 rRT-PCR test and drafted protocols and guidance for its use. On April 22, 2013, the U.S. Food and Drug Administration (FDA) issued an Emergency Use Authorization and the H7 rRT-PCR test with test components and the CDC guidance were made available to public-health laboratories so they would be able to test for H7N9 viruses too.

Advances in Tests Used in Clinical Settings

Compared to ten years ago, clinicians now have more tests available for the detection of influenza viruses in respiratory specimens, including a wider selection of highly accurate molecular assays (some rapid, some not), and improved rapid influenza antigen detection tests (RIDTs).

Rapid and accurate diagnosis of influenza virus infection facilitates timely patient management for seasonal influenza as well as pandemic influenza. Influenza testing has been used to inform decisions on the use of antiviral drugs for treatment, to avoid misuse of antibiotics for treatment, and to reduce the need for other diagnostic tests. Influenza testing can also be helpful in informing recommendations for sick people living with others who are at high risk of developing serious influenza complications.

The need for better rapid influenza tests and clear rapid test guidance for clinicians became apparent during the 2009 H1N1 pandemic when false-negative rapid antigen detection test results contributed to delays and missed opportunities in treating pandemic flu virus-infected patients with antiviral drugs; and delays in implementing infection control measures for such patients.

Shortly after the pandemic, the CDC and partners began working to address issues with rapid antigen detection tests available at the time, reaching an important milestone in 2017 when RIDTs were reclassified by the FDA and held to higher standards.

In June 2014, a new kind of rapid influenza test was approved by the FDA (the Alere (TM) I Influenza A&B test by Alere Scarborough, Inc D/B/A Binax, Inc, now owned by Abbott and called the "ID NOWTIM Influenza A&B") which detects flu A and B viruses by detecting the PB2 flu virus gene in respiratory specimens. This approval marked the beginning of a new category of tests, referred to as rapid influenza molecular assays.

Rapid influenza molecular assays are a relatively new type of influenza diagnostic test. These tests are similar to RT-PCR (which is also a molecular process and the gold standard for influenza virus detection), in that both tests use nucleic acid amplification, which detects influenza viruses in a respiratory specimen by amplifying (multiplying) certain nucleic acids (building blocks of genes) in the influenza virus genome.

Since 2014, other rapid influenza molecular assays have been approved by the FDA and are available for use in clinical settings. Of those, some are approved for point-of-care or bedside use, and do not require a clinical laboratory, including Cobas® Influenza A/B and Cobas® Influenza A/B RSV Assay by Roche Molecular Diagnostics; Xpert Xpress Flu and Xpert Xpress Flu/Respiratory syncytial virus (RSV) by Cepheid; Accula Flu A/ Flu B assay by Mesa Biotech Inc., and ID Now TM by Abbot.

Rapid influenza molecular assays have a strong ability to identify correctly patients with evidence of influenza virus infection (referred to as "high sensitivity," greater than 90%) and a strong ability to identify correctly patients without evidence of influenza virus infection, referred to as high specificity (90 to 100%). These assays produce results in 15 to 30 minutes, making them a convenient option for the clinical management of patients. Other rapid influenza molecular assays (such as the Cobas® Influenza A/B & RSV Assay by Roche Molecular Diagnostics) are approved that detect influenza A and B viruses and respiratory syncytial virus in respiratory specimens. These tests are particularly useful in the clinical management of young children with acute respiratory illness but can be used for persons of all ages.

Additionally, a number of other influenza molecular assays are FDA-approved for use in a moderately complex or complex hospital clinical laboratory. These assays may take more than one hour to produce results. Many of these molecular assays detect influenza A and B viruses as well as other respiratory viruses, such as adenovirus, coronavirus, human metapneumovirus (hMPV), human rhinovirus/enterovirus (HRV/ENT), parainfluenza virus (HPIVs), and RSV. Some also detect some respiratory bacterial infections.

Both rapid molecular and other molecular assays are more accurate than previously available influenza tests for use in clinical settings. These advances in molecular technology provide more-accurate influenza testing results and are likely to improve clinical management of patients with suspected influenza in ambulatory care clinics and emergency departments, and in hospitalized patients as well.

With regard to rapid influenza antigen detection tests, to address the issues identified during the pandemic, in 2011 the CDC, the Joint Commission, the Biomedical Advanced Research and Development Authority (BARDA), the Medical College of Wisconsin (MCW) and other public and private partners addressed key RIDT-related issues by:

- Creating the first method for systematically evaluating commercially available RIDTs, described in a 2012 Morbidity and Mortality Weekly Report (MMWR)
- Enhancing awareness among clinicians of appropriate RIDT protocols with new courses, videos, and decision-making tools
- Working with the FDA to reclassify RIDTs from Class I to Class II with Special Controls, thereby holding current and new RIDTs to higher performance standards

Reclassification means that RIDTs are now subject to the following requirements:

- Manufacturers must test their RIDTs annually to ensure they can detect currently circulating seasonal flu viruses. RIDTs with lower sensitivity to those flu viruses will need to indicate so on their labeling.
- RIDTs must meet minimum performance criteria, such as high sensitivity and high specificity to detect flu viruses in respiratory specimens compared to RT-PCR or viral culture. This means that currently, the FDA-approved RIDTs will now be more accurate in detecting flu viruses in respiratory specimens than previous RIDTs.
- In the event of a pandemic, manufacturers must test the reactivity of their RIDTs with the newly emergent flu virus as soon as virus samples become available.

- Since 2017 when reclassification of RIDTs occurred, manufacturers have made positive, steady changes to rapid influenza antigen detection tests, but more work still needs to be done.

Surveillance
Right-Sizing Initiative

The massive amount of laboratory testing that occurred during the 2009 H1N1 pandemic provided an opportunity for researchers to identify the optimal levels of influenza surveillance and laboratory testing needed in the United States, including ways to improve efficiency.

To answer those questions, in 2010, the CDC and the Association of Public Health Laboratories (APHL) began developing a "right-size" approach to influenza virologic surveillance which was based on extensive input from public-health laboratories and stakeholders. Since then, this right-size approach has helped public-health laboratories to:

- Standardize virologic surveillance practices, determine the optimal number of specimens to test to produce statistical confidence in resulting data, and define public-health surveillance priorities
- Adopt requirements, resources and statistical calculators that aid in planning and justifying budget and resource requests
- Increase the understanding and support from political leaders and the public
- Speak a common language between laboratories and epidemiologists
- Assist decision-makers in analyzing the impacts of budget decisions on national surveillance objectives, especially with regard to pandemic preparedness capacity

Prevention
Influenza Vaccines

The CDC and its partners have made significant progress in influenza surveillance; diagnostics; characterizing viruses for vaccine strain selection, and developing systems to evaluate the effectiveness of influenza vaccines over the last ten years. For example, with regard to vaccine development, by using newer production technologies, the CDC can now identify and provide candidate vaccine viruses for novel influenza threats to manufacturers within a matter of weeks.

This and other improvements have helped to better protect the public from seasonal and pandemic influenza threats through vaccination. However, to more fully protect Americans from seasonal and pandemic flu, more effective vaccines are needed and more people still need to receive annual flu vaccines.

In line with that public-health mission, more doses of seasonal vaccines and different vaccine products are available than ever before. In addition to trivalent inactivated vaccine and live attenuated influenza vaccine, the following vaccines have been approved by the FDA and are now available:

- A high dose vaccine that is designed specifically for people 65 and older to help create a stronger antibody response
- A trivalent flu vaccine made with adjuvant (an ingredient added to a vaccine that helps create a stronger immune response), which was approved for people 65 years of age and older
- The first United States-approved cell-based flu vaccine, which can potentially be made more quickly than traditional egg-based vaccines and does not require a large supply of eggs to produce
- Quadrivalent flu vaccines that protect against both lineages of influenza B viruses thus offering expanded protection against circulating influenza viruses
- Recombinant influenza vaccines, which do not require an egg-grown vaccine virus or eggs to produce, and which may be manufactured more quickly than egg-based vaccines.

The CDC is exploring new ways to further improve the influenza vaccine through the influenza vaccine improvement initiative (iVii). The initiative includes two primary goals.

- **Goal 1.** Build the evidence base for developing more-effective influenza vaccines, and increase the impact of vaccines that are currently available. This goal points to the need for deeper data, so during the 2018 to 19 season, the CDC increased the number and scope of Vaccine Effectiveness (VE) Network participants by over

1,500 children and adults, bringing the total number of participants enrolled to more than 10,500. The CDC also is increasing the diversity of people who can be enrolled in studies and has expanded VE monitoring through innovative use of healthcare and other data sources outside of the U.S. Flu VE Network. The laboratory process of evaluating vaccine response through the use of enhanced serologic and cellular testing has also been improved.

- **Goal 2.** Increase the capacity of the CDC laboratories to select, develop, evaluate and perform virus characterization to provide candidate vaccine viruses. To accomplish this, the CDC is employing state-of-the-art technologies to increase the volume of laboratory testing being done. The CDC also is working on developing new assays for manufacturers and regulatory laboratories and planning evaluation projects that support vaccine improvement.

The CDC also is focusing on expanding and improving global virus detection and improving vaccine effectiveness monitoring. This is being done through the expansion of next-generation sequencing (NGS) and fully transitioning to the Sequence-First initiative described earlier. In the process, the CDC has also worked with partners to automate the pipeline used to produce, store and share the enormous volume of NGS data.

The CDC also is piloting an advanced laboratory strategy to identify viruses, using antigenic data that are likely to predominate in the human population in future influenza seasons.

The CDC meets regularly with vaccine manufacturers and other World Health Organization Collaborating Centers (WHOCC) and Essential Regulatory Laboratories (ERL) including the FDA's Center for Biologics Evaluation and Research (CBER) to share information on a number of vaccine-related topics. Topics include the availability of candidate vaccine viruses for use in the development and production of seasonal influenza vaccines, the availability of protocols and reagents needed for the development, standardization, and regulation of influenza vaccines, and to discuss potential issues related to the timely production of seasonal influenza vaccines. The group meets from the time the vaccine composition is announced until vaccines are released for distribution to healthcare providers, for both the northern and southern hemisphere influenza seasons.

Separately, frequent Flu Risk Management Meetings (FRMM) serves as a venue to discuss issues relating to the U.S. Department of Health and Human Services (HHS) response to seasonal and pandemic influenza. Subjects for discussion include but are not limited to seasonal surveillance updates, the effectiveness of influenza vaccines, vaccine and antiviral stockpiles, emerging influenza virus surveillance, clinical trial response to influenza outbreaks of novel influenza viruses, and pandemic preparedness.

Treatment

The number of available approved and recommended treatment options have increased in the last ten years.

During the 2009 H1N1 pandemic, the influenza antiviral medication oseltamivir (oral oseltamivir, available under the trade name Tamiflu®) was used extensively for treatment, while zanamivir (inhaled, trade name Relenza®) was used less.

Oral oseltamivir's widespread use was due to it being approved, recommended and utilized for the treatment of patients hospitalized with severe influenza. It also was recommended for use in hospitalized patients with nonsevere influenza, although no antiviral medications were approved by the FDA for use in that group.

Outpatients could be prescribed either oral oseltamivir or inhaled zanamivir, which were both approved for early treatment of uncomplicated influenza by the FDA.

Of the two medications, the CDC was more concerned with the possibility of resistance emerging against oseltamivir, which did happen, but not often. The oseltamivir-resistant viruses that did emerge were not transmitted easily from person to person, and zanamivir was used effectively to treat them.

Beginning in April 2009 and continuing for a few years after the pandemic, the FDA's Emergency Investigational New Drug (EIND) program provided an application process that authorized investigational use of IV zanamivir for patients with severe and life-threatening influenza.

Later, on October 23rd, 2009, the FDA issued an Emergency Use Authorization (EUA) for IV Peramivir. At the time, IV Peramivir was an investigational intravenous antiviral drug used rarely to treat people who had been hospitalized with severe influenza. The drug was held in the Strategic National Stockpile (SNS) and distributed by the CDC under the EUA. Licensed clinicians were able to request this product through the CDC website electronic request system, and the product was delivered directly to hospital facilities until June 2010 when the EUA was terminated.

Following the pandemic, in December 2014, IV Peramivir was approved by the FDA for the early treatment of uncomplicated influenza in outpatients, which also opened up some off-label use in treating influenza in hospitalized patients. Previously, with the exception of the IV Peramivir EUA during the pandemic, oseltamivir and zanamivir were the only recommended antiviral medications for the treatment of influenza. (The other approved antiviral drugs—amantadine and rimantadine—were not and are still not recommended due to high levels of resistance detected in circulating influenza viruses). Roughly three years later, in September 2017, the FDA approved the first generic version of oseltamivir.

Oseltamivir, zanamivir, and IV peramivir are all neuraminidase-inhibitor (NI) influenza antiviral medications, so named because each works by targeting the neuraminidase surface protein of the influenza virus to stop the virus from being released from infected cells and spreading to healthy cells.

In December 2018, a new influenza antiviral medication called "oral baloxavir marboxil" (BXM) (trade name Xofluza®) was approved by the FDA and is recommended for the treatment of influenza. Baloxavir works differently, primarily by preventing an influenza virus from multiplying when it is inside a cell. Because baloxavir works differently, it is in a new class of antiviral medications called "cap-dependent endonuclease inhibitors" (CEN). Just as the neuraminidase-inhibitor medications, baloxavir has activity against both influenza A and B viruses. Baloxavir is approved for the early treatment of uncomplicated influenza in outpatients aged 12 years and older.

With more antiviral medications approved, recommended and available, treatment options have improved for both hospitalized patients with severe influenza and outpatients seeking treatment early for uncomplicated influenza. There remains a gap, however, in approved antiviral treatment options for hospitalized patients with nonsevere influenza, although the CDC and Infectious Diseases Society of America (IDSA) continues to recommend that those patients be treated with neuraminidase-inhibitor antiviral medications.

Decision-Making Tools
Risk Assessment (Influenza Risk Assessment Tool)
The 2009 H1N1 pandemic highlighted the public-health value of developing an objective, scientifically-based tool for assessing the potential pandemic risk posed to humans by influenza A viruses circulating in animals. To fill that need, the CDC developed an evaluation tool now called the "Influenza Risk Assessment Tool" (IRAT) with help from global animal and human health influenza experts. IRAT launched in 2011 and since then the CDC has used it to evaluate the potential risk posed by viruses that are not currently circulating in people. The IRAT relies on input from subject matter experts representing a variety of expertise in the study of influenza viruses. It uses 10 evaluation criteria grouped into major categories including properties of the virus, attributes of the human population, and epidemiology and ecology of the virus, to generate scores that indicate the potential risk of the virus to emerge as a pandemic virus, and the potential impact if it does.

The IRAT is not a prediction tool. Rather, the IRAT provides structure to prioritize and maximize investments in pandemic preparedness; identify key gaps in information; document transparently the data and scientific process used to inform management decisions associated with pandemic preparedness; provide a flexible means to easily and regularly update the risk assessment of novel flu viruses as new information becomes available; communicate effectively to the general public, policymakers, public-health laboratories, and other stakeholders; and provide a means to weigh the 10 evaluation criteria differently depending on whether the intent is to measure the ability of a virus to "emerge" as a pandemic-capable virus, or "impact" the human population after emerging.

Since its inception eight years ago, the IRAT has been used by the CDC to evaluate and inform pandemic preparedness decisions for 16 viruses, the results of which are listed at Summary of IRAT Results.

International Work

The CDC has strong global ties with other WHO Collaborating Centers for Influenza, National Influenza Centers (NICs) and ministries of health around the world. These collaborators provided critical data throughout the influenza pandemic on how, when and where the pandemic virus might be changing and if the monovalent pandemic vaccine would continue to be effective in preventing infection.

The CDC's Influenza Division formed an influenza international capacity-building initiative in 2004, which provided a five-year period of financial support for nine countries to improve laboratory diagnostics and sentinel surveillance for influenza-like illness and severe acute respiratory infection. In 2009, this number increased to 37 countries receiving support under 39 cooperative agreements.

Thus, the 2009 H1N1 pandemic occurred at a time when many of the 37 countries benefited from the newly established influenza surveillance and laboratory capacities. The pandemic provided the ultimate test to determine whether their laboratory diagnostics and surveillance systems were indeed strong enough to manage the massive surges in flu activity that would come their way.

Shortly after the pandemic, eight of the 37 countries transitioned to the program's second five-year period, called the "sustainability period." During this period, financial support was reduced as the programs focused on sustaining the gains made in laboratory diagnostics and surveillance. The countries focused on standardizing foundational aspects of influenza surveillance, including regular influenza activity reporting and sending viruses to the CDC and other WHO Collaborating Centers, all with an eye toward ensuring preparedness for the next pandemic.

Now, following 10 years of the pandemic's race around the globe, which caused hundreds of thousands of deaths worldwide, many countries have graduated from the sustainability period to maintenance and some are now developing in-country seasonal influenza vaccination programs based on their influenza surveillance data.

The 2009 H1N1 pandemic tested the U.S. laboratory and surveillance systems and highlighted many successes along the way, shining a light on one of the biggest takeaways of the 2009 H1N1 pandemic: develop seasonal influenza epidemiology and laboratory capacity that is flexible enough to handle the next pandemic.

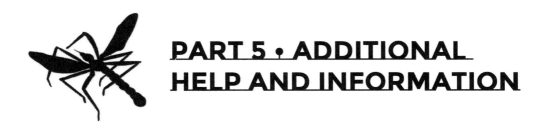

PART 5 • ADDITIONAL HELP AND INFORMATION

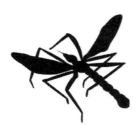

CHAPTER 41
Glossary of Terms Associated with Outbreaks, Epidemics, and Pandemics

accuracy: A measure of agreement between a test result and an accepted reference value. Example: if you have a standardized reference material at a known value (such as 180 mg/dl of cholesterol), accuracy measures how close the result of the test you are using will get to the known value. You may have a test that is very precise yet very inaccurate, which would be the case if your device measures 180 mg/dl of cholesterol reproducibly as 240 mg/dl.

adjuvant: A vaccine adjuvant is a substance that is added to a vaccine to increase and improve the body's immune response to the vaccine antigen(s). Antigens are the components of the flu vaccine that prompt your body to have an immune response. Vaccine adjuvants can allow flu vaccines to be produced using less antigen. Therefore, use of adjuvants can allow vaccine manufacturers to produce more doses of vaccine with less antigen.

airborne transmission: Occurs by dissemination of either airborne droplet nuclei (small-particle residue [5 μm or smaller] of evaporated droplets containing microorganisms that remain suspended in the air for long periods of time) or dust particles containing the infectious agent. Microorganisms carried in this manner can be dispersed widely by air currents and may become inhaled by a susceptible host in the same room or over a longer distance from the source patient, depending on environmental factors.

This glossary contains terms excerpted from documents produced by several sources deemed reliable.

anesthesia: A combination of medications administered to a patient to block pain and other sensations, at times rendering the patient unconscious, so that medical or surgical procedures can be performed; anesthesia can be general, regional or local

anesthetic: A drug that causes insensitivity to pain and is used for surgeries and other medical procedures.

anthrax: An acute infectious disease caused by the spore-forming bacterium *Bacillus anthracis*. Anthrax most commonly occurs in hoofed mammals and can also infect humans.

antibiotic: A drug that kills or stops the growth of bacteria. Antibiotics are a type of antimicrobial. Penicillin and ciprofloxacin are examples of antibiotics.

antibody: A protein made by plasma cells (a type of white blood cell (WBC)) in response to an antigen (a substance that causes the body to make a specific immune response). Each antibody can bind to only one specific antigen.

antigen: A substance or molecule that is recognized by the immune system. The molecule can come from foreign materials, such as bacteria or viruses.

antimicrobial: A substance, such as an antibiotic, that kills or stops the growth of microbes, including bacteria, fungi, or viruses. Antimicrobials are grouped according to the microbes they act against (antibiotics, antifungals, and antivirals). Also referred to as drugs.

antitoxin: Antibodies capable of destroying toxins generated by micro-organisms including viruses and bacteria.

assessment: The process of gathering evidence and documentation of a student's learning.

asthma: A chronic disease in which the bronchial airways in the lungs become narrowed and swollen, making it difficult to breathe.

attenuated vaccine: A vaccine in which live virus is weakened through chemical or physical processes in order to produce an immune response without causing the severe effects of the disease.

bacteria: Single-celled organisms that live in and around us with a distinct structure from other microbes. Bacteria can be helpful, but can also cause illnesses, such as strep throat, ear infections, and pneumonia.

blood transfusion: The administration of blood or blood products into a blood vessel.

blood: A tissue with red blood cells (RBCs), white blood cells, platelets, and other substances suspended in fluid called "plasma." Blood takes oxygen and nutrients to the tissues, and carries away wastes.

cancer: A term for diseases in which abnormal cells divide without control. Cancer cells can invade nearby tissues and can spread to other parts of the body through the blood and lymph systems.

cell: The individual unit that makes up the tissues of the body. All living things are made up of one or more cells.

central nervous system (CNS): Comprised of the nerves in the brain and spinal cord. These nerves are used to send electrical impulses throughout the body, resulting in voluntary and reflexive movement. Information about the environment is received by the senses and sent to the CNS, which causes the body to respond appropriately.

chemotherapy: Treatment with anticancer drugs.

chronic disease: A disease that has one or more of the following characteristics: is permanent; leaves residual disability; is caused by nonreversible pathological alteration; requires special training of the patient for rehabilitation; or may be expected to require a long period of supervision, observation, or care.

clinical trial: A research study in which one or more human subjects are prospectively assigned to one or more interventions (which may include placebo or other control) to evaluate the effects of those interventions on health-related biomedical or behavioral outcomes.

communicable disease: An infectious disease that is contagious and which can be transmitted from one source to another by infectious bacteria or viral organisms.

conjugate vaccine: A vaccine in which proteins that are easily recognizable to the immune system are linked to the molecules that form the outer coat of disease-causing bacteria to promote an immune response.

contagious disease: A very communicable disease capable of spreading rapidly from one person to another by contact or close proximity.

coronavirus: One of a group of viruses that have a halo or crown-like (corona) appearance when viewed under a microscope. These viruses are a common cause of usually mild to moderate upper-respiratory illness in humans and are associated with respiratory, gastrointestinal, liver, and neurologic disease in animals, but can be fatal.

culture: A test to see whether there are tuberculosis (TB) bacteria in your phlegm or other body fluids. This test can take two to four weeks in most laboratories.

diabetes: A disease in which blood glucose (blood sugar) levels are above or below normal.

diagnosis: The process of identifying a disease by the signs and symptoms.

diphtheria: A bacterial disease marked by the formation of a false membrane, especially in the throat, which can cause death.

disease: A state in which a function or part of the body is no longer in a healthy condition.

disinfection: The destruction of pathogenic and other kinds of microorganisms by physical or chemical means. Disinfection is less lethal than sterilization, because it destroys most recognized pathogenic microorganisms, but not necessarily all microbial forms, such as bacterial spores. Disinfection does not ensure the margin of safety associated with sterilization processes.

drug: Any substance, other than food, that is used to prevent, diagnose, treat, or relieve symptoms of a disease or abnormal condition.

encephalitis: Inflammation of the brain caused by a virus. Encephalitis can result in permanent brain damage or death.

endemic: The continual, low-level presence of disease in a community.

epidemic: A disease outbreak that affects many people in a region at the same time.

exercise: A type of physical activity that involves planned, structured, and repetitive bodily movement done to maintain or improve one or more components of physical fitness.

exposure: Contact with infectious agents (bacteria or viruses) in a manner that promotes transmission and increases the likelihood of disease.

fetus: A developing unborn offspring in the uterus (womb). This stage of pregnancy begins eight weeks after conception and lasts until birth.

genes: Genes, which are made up of DNA, are the basic units that define the characteristics of every organism. Genes carry information that determine traits, such as eye color in humans and resistance to antibiotics in bacteria.

genome: A genome is an organism's complete set of genes that carry the genetic instructions for building and maintaining that organism.

hand hygiene: A general term that applies to any one of the following: 1. handwashing with plan (nonantimicrobial) soap and water, 2. antiseptic handwash (soap containing antiseptic agents and water), 3. antiseptic hand rub (waterless antiseptic product, most often alcohol-based, rubbed on surfaces of hands), or 4. surgical hand antisepsis.

herd immunity: The resistance to a particular disease gained by a community when a critical number of people are vaccinated against that disease.

human immunodeficiency virus (HIV): HIV infects and destroys the body's immune cells and causes a disease called "acquired immunodeficiency syndrome (AIDS)."

immune system: A complex network of specialized cells, tissues, and organs that defends the body against attacks by disease-causing microbes.

immunity: Protection against a disease. Immunity is indicated by the presence of antibodies in the blood and can usually be determined with a laboratory test.

immunization: The process by which a person becomes immune, or protected, against a disease. This term is often used interchangeably with vaccination or inoculation. However, the term "vaccination" is defined as the injection of a killed or weakened infectious organism in order to prevent the disease. Thus, vaccination, by inoculation with a vaccine, does not always result in immunity.

inactivated vaccine: A vaccine made from a whole virus or bacteria inactivated with chemicals or heat.

incubation period: The time from contact with infectious agents (bacteria or viruses) to onset of disease.

infection: A state in which disease-causing microbes have invaded or multiplied in body tissues.

infectious agents: Organisms capable of spreading disease (e.g., bacteria or viruses).

inflammation: Redness, swelling, heat, and pain resulting from injury to tissue (parts of the body underneath the skin). Also known as "swelling."

influenza: A highly contagious viral infection characterized by sudden onset of fever, severe aches and pains, and inflammation of the mucous membrane.

lesion: An abnormal change in the structure of an organ, due to injury or disease.

lung: One of a pair of organs in the chest that supplies the body with oxygen and removes carbon dioxide from the body.

lymphocyte: A white blood cell central to the immune system's response to foreign microbes. B cells and T cells are lymphocytes.

macrophage: A large and versatile immune cell that devours and kills invading microbes and other intruders.

meningitis: Inflammation of the meninges, the membranes that envelop the brain and the spinal cord; may cause hearing loss or deafness.

microbes: Living organisms, such as bacteria, fungi, or viruses, which can cause infections or disease. Also referred to as germs.

mycobacterium tuberculosis (Mtb): Bacteria that cause latent TB infection and TB disease.

nursing: The profession concerned with the provision of care and services essential to the promotion, maintenance, and restoration of health by attending to a patient's needs.

organ: A part of the body that performs a specific function. For example, the heart is an organ.

organism: Any living thing, including humans, animals, plants, and microbes.

outbreak: Sudden appearance of a disease in a specific geographic area (e.g., neighborhood or community) or population (e.g., adolescents).

outpatient: A patient who visits a healthcare facility for diagnosis or treatment without spending the night, sometimes called a "day patient."

pandemic: An epidemic occurring over a very large geographic area.

parasites: Plants or animals that live, grow, and feed on or within another living organism.

pathogens: Organisms (e.g., bacteria, viruses, parasites and fungi) that cause disease in human beings.

personal protective equipment (PPE): It is specialized clothing or equipment worn by an employee for protection against a hazard (e.g., gloves, masks, protective eyewear, gowns). General work clothes (e.g., uniforms, pants, shirts or blouses) not intended to function as protection against a hazard are not considered to be personal protective equipment.

physical examination: An exam of the body to check for general signs of disease.

pneumonia: Inflammation of the lungs characterized by fever, chills, muscle stiffness, chest pain, cough, shortness of breath, rapid heartrate and difficulty breathing.

polysaccharide: A long, chain-like molecule made up of a linked sugar molecule. The outer coats of some bacteria are made of polysaccharides.

precaution: A condition in a recipient which may result in a life-threatening problem if the vaccine is given, or a condition which could compromise the ability of the vaccine to produce immunity.

pregnancy: The condition between conception (fertilization of an egg by a sperm) and birth, during which the fertilized egg develops in the uterus. In humans, pregnancy lasts about 288 days.

prevention: Actions that reduce exposure or other risks, keep people from getting sick, or keep disease from getting worse.

protein: A molecule made up of amino acids. Proteins are needed for the body to function properly. They are the basis of body structures, such as skin and hair, and of other substances, such as enzymes, cytokines, and antibodies.

pump: A device that is used to give a controlled amount of a liquid at a specific rate. For example, pumps are used to give drugs (such as chemotherapy or pain medicine) or nutrients.

quarantine: The isolation of a person or animal who has a disease (or is suspected of having a disease) in order to prevent further spread of the disease.

recombinant: Of or resulting from new combinations of genetic material or cells

seizure: The sudden onset of a jerking or staring spell. Many seizures following a vaccination are caused by fever. Seizures are also known as "convulsions."

side effect: A problem that occurs when treatment affects healthy tissues or organs. Some common side effects of cancer treatment are fatigue, pain, nausea, vomiting, decreased blood cell counts, hair loss, and mouth sores.

smallpox: An acute, highly infectious, often fatal disease caused by a poxvirus and characterized by high fever and aches with subsequent widespread eruption of pimples that blister, produce pus, and form pockmarks. Also called "variola."

specimen: A sample collected for laboratory testing. During outbreak investigations, samples may be collected from the blood, stool, or another location of a human or animal, and from food and the environment.

strain: A specific version of an organism. Many diseases, including HIV/AIDS and hepatitis, have multiple strains.

stroke: Also known as a "cerebrovascular accident" (CVA); caused by a lack of blood to the brain, resulting in the sudden loss of speech, language, or the ability to move a body part, and, if severe enough, death.

subunit vaccine: A vaccine that uses one or more components of a disease-causing organism, rather than the whole, to stimulate an immune response.

supportive care: Care given to improve the quality of life (QOL) of patients who have a serious or life-threatening disease.

surgery: A medical specialty concerned with manual or operative procedures used in the diagnosis and treatment of diseases, injuries, or deformities.

symptom: An indication that a person has a condition or disease. Some examples of symptoms are headache, fever, fatigue, nausea, vomiting, and pain.

T cell: A white blood cell that directs or participates in immune defenses.

tetanus: Toxin-producing bacterial disease marked by painful muscle spasms.

tissue: A group of similar cells joined to perform the same function.

toxin: Agent produced by plants and bacteria, normally very damaging to cells.

toxoid: A toxin, such as those produced by certain bacteria, that has been treated by chemical means, heat or irradiation and is no longer capable of causing disease.

typhoid fever: Typhoid fever is a life-threatening illness caused by the bacterium *Salmonella Typhi*. Persons with typhoid fever carry the bacteria in their bloodstream and intestinal tract.

vaccine: A product made from very small amounts of weak or dead germs that can cause diseases—for example, viruses, bacteria, or toxins. It prepares your body to fight the disease faster and more effectively so you won't get sick. Vaccines are administered through needle injections, by mouth, and by aerosol.

virulence: The relative capacity of a pathogen to overcome body defenses.

virus: A small organism that can infect a person and cause illness or disease.

x-ray: A type of high-energy radiation. In low doses, x-rays are used to diagnose diseases by making pictures of the inside of the body.

yoga: An ancient system of practices used to balance the mind and body through exercise, meditation (focusing thoughts), and control of breathing and emotions.

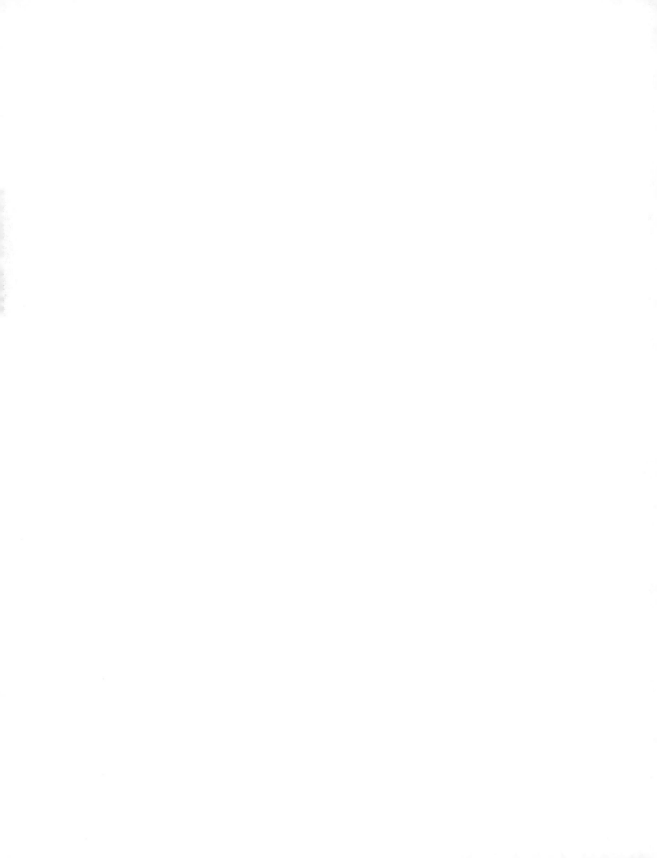

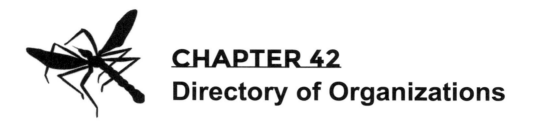

CHAPTER 42
Directory of Organizations

Government Organizations

Agency for Healthcare Research and Quality (AHRQ)
Office of Communications
5600 Fishers Ln.
Seventh Fl.
Rockville, MD 20847
Phone: 301-427-1104
Website: www.ahrq.gov

AIDS*info*
U.S. Department of Health and
Human Services (HHS)
P.O. Box 4780
Rockville, MD 20849-6303
Toll-Free: 800-HIV-0440
(800-448-0440)
Phone: 301-315-2816
Toll-Free TTY: 888-480-3739
Fax: 301-315-2818
Website: aidsinfo.nih.gov
E-mail: ContactUs@aidsinfo.nih.gov

Resources in this chapter were compiled from several sources deemed reliable; all contact information was verified and updated in January 2020.

Centers for Disease Control and Prevention (CDC)

1600 Clifton Rd.
Atlanta, GA 30329-4027
Toll-Free: 800-CDC-INFO
(800-232-4636)
Phone: 404-639-3311
Toll-Free TTY: 888-232-6348
Website: www.cdc.gov
E-mail: cdcinfo@cdc.gov

Centers for Medicare & Medicaid Services (CMS)

7500 Security Blvd.
Baltimore, MD 21244
Toll-Free: 877-267-2323
Phone: 410-786-3000
TTY: 410-786-0727
Toll-Free TTY: 866-226-1819
Website: www.cms.gov
E-mail: ContactUs@aidsinfo.nih.gov

Clinical Center (CC)

National Institutes of Health (NIH)
10 Center Dr.
Bethesda, MD 20892
Toll-Free: 800-411-1222
Phone: 301-496-2563
Toll-Free TTY: 866-411-1010
Website: clinicalstudies.info.nih.gov
E-mail: webmaster@cc.nih.gov

Health Resources and Services Administration (HRSA)

Information Center
P.O. Box 2910
Merrifield, VA 22116
Toll-Free: 888-275-4772
Toll-Free TTY: 877-489-4772
Fax: 703-821-2098
Website: www.hrsa.gov
E-mail: ask@hrsa.gov

HealthCare.gov

Centers for Medicare & Medicaid
Services (CMS)
Toll-Free: 800-318-2596
Toll-Free TTY: 855-889-4325
Website: www.healthcare.gov

healthfinder.gov

Office of Disease Prevention and
Health Promotion (ODPHP)
200 Independence Ave.
Washington, DC 20201
Website: www.healthfinder.gov
E-mail: healthfinder@hhs.gov

HIV.gov

Office of HIV/AIDS and Infectious
Disease Policy (OHAIDP)
330 C St., S.W.
Rm. L100
Washington, DC 20024
Website: www.hiv.gov

National Center for Health Statistics (NCHS)

3311 Toledo Rd.
Hyattsville, MD 20782-2064
Toll-Free: 800-CDC-INFO
(800-232-4636)
Phone: 301-458-4000
Toll-Free TTY: 888-232-6348
Website: www.cdc.gov
E-mail: www.cdc.gov/nchs/index.htm

National Health Information Center (NHIC)

U.S. Department of Health and
Human Services (HHS)
1101 Wootton Pkwy
Ste. LL100
Rockville, MD 20852
Fax: 240-453-8281
Website: www.health.gov/nhic
E-mail: nhic@hhs.gov

National Institute of Neurological Disorders and Stroke (NINDS)

NIH Neurological Institute
P.O. Box 5801
Bethesda, MD 20824
Toll-Free: 800-352-9424
Website: www.ninds.nih.gov
E-mail: DEA.Registration.Help@usdoj.gov

National Institutes of Health (NIH)

9000 Rockville Pike
Bethesda, MD 20892
Phone: 301-496-4000
TTY: 301-402-9612
Website: www.nih.gov

National Library of Medicine (NLM)

8600 Rockville Pike
Bethesda, MD 20894
Toll-Free: 888-FIND-NLM
(888-346-3656)
Phone: 301-594-5983
Website: www.nlm.nih.gov
E-mail: custserv@nlm.nih.gov

National Prevention Information Network (NPIN)

Centers for Disease Control and
Prevention (CDC)
P.O. Box 6003
Rockville, MD 20849-6003
Website: npin.cdc.gov
E-mail: NPIN-Info@cdc.gov

Office of Disease Prevention and Health Promotion (ODPHP)

Office of the Assistant Secretary for Health (OASH), Office of the Secretary
1101 Wootton Pkwy
Ste. LL100
Rockville, MD 20852
Fax: 240-453-8281
Website: health.gov
E-mail: odphpinfo@hhs.gov

U.S. Department of Agriculture (USDA)

1400 Independence Ave. S.W.
Washington, DC 20250
Phone: 202-720-2791
Website: www.usda.gov
E-mail: feedback@oc.usda.gov

U.S. Department of Health and Human Services (HHS)

200 Independence Ave., S.W.
Washington, DC 20201
Toll-Free: 877-696-6775
Website: www.hhs.gov

U.S. Drug Enforcement Administration (DEA)

Office of Diversion Control
8701 Morrissette Dr.
Springfield, VA 22152
Toll-Free: 800-882-9539
Phone: 202-307-1000
Website: www.dea.gov
E-mail: DEA.Registration.Help@usdoj.gov

U.S. Food and Drug Administration (FDA)

10903 New Hampshire Ave.
Silver Spring, MD 20993-0002
Toll-Free: 888-INFO-FDA
(888-463-6332)
Website: www.fda.gov

U.S. National Library of Medicine (NLM)

8600 Rockville Pike
Bethesda, MD 20894
Toll-Free: 888-FIND-NLM
(888-346-3656)
Phone: 301-594-5983
Website: www.nlm.nih.gov
E-mail: custserv@nlm.nih.gov

U.S. Social Security Administration (SSA)
Windsor Park Bldg.
6401 Security Blvd.
Baltimore, MD 21235
Toll-Free: 800-772-1213
Toll-Free TTY: 800-325-0778
Website: www.ssa.gov

USA.gov
Toll-Free: 844-USA-GOV1
(844-872-4681)
Website: www.usa.gov
E-mail: custserv@nlm.nih.gov

Private Organizations

American Academy of Family Physicians (AAFP)
11400 Tomahawk Creek Pkwy
Leawood, KS 66211-2680
Toll-Free: 800-274-2237
Phone: 913-906-6000
Fax: 913-906-6075
Website: www.aafp.org
E-mail: aafp@aafp.org

American Cancer Society (ACS)
250 Williams St., N.W.
Atlanta, GA 30303
Toll-Free: 800-ACS-2345
(800-227-2345)
Toll-Free TTY: 866-228-4327
Website: www.cancer.org

American Health Information Management Association (AHIMA)
233 N. Michigan Ave.
21st Fl.
Chicago, IL 60601-5809
Toll-Free: 800-335-5535
Phone: 312-233-1100
Fax: 312-233-1500
Website: www.ahima.org
E-mail: info@ahima.org

American Heart Association (AHA)
National Center
7272 Greenville Ave.
Dallas, TX 75231
Toll-Free: 800-AHA-USA-1
(800-242-8721)
Website: www.heart.org

American Lung Association® (ALA)

National Office
55 W. Wacker Dr.
Ste. 1150
Chicago, IL 60601
Toll-Free: 800-LUNGUSA
(800-586-4872)
Website: www.lung.org
E-mail: info@lung.org

American Medical Association (AMA)

AMA Plaza
330 N. Wabash Ave.
Ste. 39300
Chicago, IL 60611-5885
Phone: 312-464-4782
Website: www.ama-assn.org

Caregiver Action Network (CAN)

1150 Connecticut Ave., N.W.
Ste. 501
Washington, DC 20036-3904
Toll-Free: 855-CARE-640
(855-227-3640)
Phone: 202-454-3970
Website: caregiveraction.org
E-mail: info@caregiveraction.org

Cleveland Clinic

9500 Euclid Ave.
Cleveland, OH 44195
Toll-Free: 800-223-2273
Phone: 216-444-2200
Website: my.clevelandclinic.org

National Healthcare Anti-Fraud Association (NHCAA)

1220 L St., N.W.
Ste. 600
Washington, DC 20005
Phone: 202-659-5955
Fax: 202-785-6764
Website: www.nhcaa.org
E-mail: NHCAA@nhcaa.org

National Patient Advocate Foundation (NPAF)

Washington, DC
Phone: 202-347-8009
Website: www.npaf.org
E-mail: action@npaf.org

The Nemours Foundation/ KidsHealth®

10140 Centurion Pkwy N.
Jacksonville, FL 32256
Phone: 904-697-4100
Website: www.nemours.org

U.S. Preventive Services Task Force (USPSTF)

USPSTF Program Office
5600 Fishers Ln.
MS 06E53A
Rockville, MD 20857
Website: www.
uspreventiveservicestaskforce.org

World Health Organization (WHO)

20 Ave. Appia
1211 Geneva
Switzerland
Phone: +41-22-7912111
Fax: 41-22-791-4857
Website: www.who.int
E-mail: info@wilsonsdisease.org